The Psychopharmacology of Schizophrenia

The Psychopharmacology of Schizophrenia

A TITLE IN THE BRITISH ASSOCIATION FOR PSYCHOPHARMACOLOGY SERIES

Edited by

MICHAEL A REVELEY MD, PhD, FRCPsych

Professor of Psychiatry, Department of Psychiatry, University of Leicester, Leicester, UK

and

J F WILLIAM DEAKIN PhD, FRCPsych

Professor of Psychiatry and Director of the Neuroscience and Psychiatry Unit, School of Psychiatry and Behavioural Sciences, The University of Manchester, Manchester, UK

A member of the Hodder Headline Group
LONDON
Co-published in the United States of America by
Oxford University Press Inc., New York

First published in Great Britain in 2000 by
Arnold, a member of the Hodder Headline Group
338 Euston Road, London NW1 3BH

http://www.arnoldpublishers.com

Co-published in the United Stataes of America by
Oxford University Press Inc.,
198 Madison Avenue, New York 10016
Oxford is a registered trademark of Oxford University Press

Whilst the advice and information in this book are believed to be true and
accurate at the date of going to press, neither the authors nor the
publisher can accept any legal responsibility for any errors or omissions
that may be made. In particulàr (but without limiting the generality of the
preceding disclaimer) every effort has been made to check drug dosages;
however, it is still possible that errors have been missed. Furthermore,
dosage schedules are constantly being revised and new side-effects
recognized. For these reasons the reader is strongly urged to consult the
drug companies' printed instructions before admimistering any of the
drugs recommended in this book.

British Library Cataloguing in Publication Data
A catalogue record for this book is available from the British Library

Library of Congress Cataloging-in-Publication Data
A catalog record for this book is available from the Library of Congress

ISBN 0 340 75912 7

2 3 4 5 6 7 8 9 10

Commissioning Editor: Georgina Bentliff
Project Editor: Sarah de Souza
Production Editor: James Rabson
Production Controller: Priya Gohil

Typeset in 10/11pt Times by Phoenix Photosetting, Chatham, Kent
Printed and bound in Great Britain by
MPG Books Ltd, Bodmin, Cornwall

What do you think about this book? Or any other Arnold Title?
Please send your comments to feedback.arnold@hodder.co.uk

Contents

Colour plates appear between pages 150 and 151.

Contributors

Hassen A Al-Amin Clinical Brain Disorder Branch, Intramural Research Programs, National Institute of Mental Health, NIH Neuroscience Centre at St. Elizabeth's, Washington DC 20032, USA

Thomas R E Barnes MD, FRCPsych Professor of Clinical Psychiatry, Division of Neuroscience and Psychological Medicine, Imperial College School of Medicine, London, UK

Paul R Buckland BSc, PhD Reader, Division of Psychological Medicine, University of Wales College of Medicine, Heath Park, Cardiff, Wales, UK

David Cotter MRCPsych Department of Psychological Medicine, Department of Neuropathology, Institute of Psychiatry and King's College School of Medicine, De Crespigny Park, London, UK

Calum G Crosthwaite BSc (Hons) Research Assistant, Department of Psychiatry, University of Leicester School of Medicine, Clinical Sciences Building, Leicester Royal Infirmary, Leicester, UK

J F William Deakin BSc, PhD, FRCPsych Professor of Psychiatry, School of Psychiatry and Behavioural Sciences, The University of Manchester, Manchester, UK

Lars Farde MD, PhD Department of Clinical Neuroscience, Psychiatry Section, Karolinska Institute and Hospital, S-171 76, Stockholm, Sweden

Paul Fearon MRCPI, MRCPsych Department of Psychological Medicine, Institute of Psychiatry & King's College School of Medicine, De Crespigny Park, London, UK

Robert Kerwin MA, PhD, MB Bchir., DSc, FRCPsych Professor of Clinical Neuropharmacology, Institute of Psychiatry, De Crespigny Park, London, UK

Peter F Liddle Jack Bell Professor and Head, Schizophrenia Division, Department of Psychiatry, The University of British Columbia, Vancouver, BC, Canada

Stephen R Marder MD Psychiatry Service (116A), West Los Angeles Veterans Affairs Medical Center, Los Angeles, CA 90073, USA

Peter McGuffin MD, PhD, FRCP, FRCPsych Professor of Psychological Medicine, Institute of Psychiatry & King's College School of Medicine, De Crespigny Park, London, UK

Robin G McCreadie DSc, MD, FRCPsych Director of Clinical Research and Consultant Psychiatrist, Crichton Royal Hospital, Dumfries, Scotland, UK

Ann M Mortimer BSc, MB, ChB, MmedSc, FRCPsych Professor, Foundation Chair in Psychiatry, The School of Medicine, The University of Hull, Willerby, Hull, UK

Robin M Murray MD, DSc, FRCP, FRCPsych Institute of Psychiatry & King's College School of Medicine, De Crespigny Park, London SE5 8AF, UK

Stefan Pauli MD Department of Clinical Neuroscience, Psychiatry Section, Karolinska Institute and Hospital, S-171 76, Stockholm, Sweden

Michael A Reveley MD, PhD, FRCPsych Professor of Psychiatry, Department of Psychiatry, University of Leicester School of Medicine, Clinical Sciences Building, Leicester Royal Infirmary, Leicester, UK

Göran C Sedvall MD, PhD Department of Clinical Neuroscience, Psychiatry Section, Karolinska Institute and Hospital, S-171 76 Stockholm, Sweden

Sean A Spence Functional Neuroimaging Laboratory, The New York Hospital, Cornell Medical Center, New York NY 10021, USA

John L Waddington PhD, DSc Professor of Neuroscience, Department of Clinical Pharmacology, Royal College of Surgeons in Ireland, Dublin, Republic of Ireland

Daniel R Weinberger MD Clinical Brain Disorder Branch, Intramural Research Programs, National Institute of Mental Health, NIH Neuroscience Center at St. Elizabeths, Washington, DC 20032, USA

Donna Ames Wirshing Psychiatry Service (116A), West Los Angeles Veterans Affairs Medical Center, Los Angeles, CA 90073, USA

William C Wirshing MD Psychiatry Service (116A), West Los Angeles Veterans Affairs Medical Center, Los Angeles, CA 90073, USA

Preface

Schizophrenia is the most severe of the mental illnesses, often causing lifelong disability for its sufferers and a substantial financial burden to society, both in loss of productivity and in services to care for disabled people.

A great deal has been learnt over the latter part of this century about the treatment of schizophrenia. There was a time when the majority of patients with schizophrenia were in long stay institutions receiving, principally, custodial care, with only minimal hope for discharge from hospital. The discovery of chlorpromazine in the 1950s and widespread treatment with conventional antipsychotics has led to the discharge of many patients into the community and has prevented new long-term admissions. This development has brought its own problems, especially in the management of patients in the community, but there can be no doubt about the transformation of the quality of life of the majority of patients with schizophrenia because of the prevention of much of the disability of schizophrenia with effective pharmacological treatment combined with psychosocial support. With new understanding of how anti-psychotics work it is now possible to develop new psychopharmacological treatments which are targeted towards special symptoms and disabilities in schizophrenia, and which have fewer adverse effects.

Over the past decade, the decade of the brain, major advances have been made in understanding the brain mechanism underlying schizophrenia. It is now widely accepted that schizophrenia is a brain disorder. At last, the brainlessness of psychiatry is waning. Thus, the proper understanding of the psychopharmacology of schizophrenia requires not just the clinical understanding of the drugs and their use, but also an understanding of the basic and clinical sciences relevant to drug treatment. The aim of this book is to present the pharmacological treatment of schizophrenia in the context of the basic and clinical sciences underpinning clinical treatment.

The first chapter by Al-Amin and Weinberger reviews the dopamine hypothesis in the light of new evidence from molecular biology and points to new directions in understanding the pathophysiology of schizophrenia. Chapter 2 by Fearon, Cotter and Murray reviews the evidence for the neurodevelopmental theory of schizophrenia and presents a review of the mechanisms by which obstetric complications may interact with glutamate to contribute to the development of schizophrenia in early adult life. Chapter 3 by Kerwin provides an in-depth exploration of the molecular biology of dopamine and serotonin receptors and their relevance to the mechanisms of action of anti-psychotic medication. Chapter 4 by Deakin reviews the new neuropathology in which neurotransmitter circuits are visualized. Much evidence implicates glutamatergic abnormalities and this is leading to completely new treatment approaches. Chapter 5 by Buckland and McGuffin reviews the molecular genetics of schizophrenia particularly with regard to dopamine, serotonin and neurotensin receptors. Exciting prospects for identifying genes contributing to schizophrenic illness are discussed. The next three chapters describe the brain imaging of schizophrenia and provide a bridge from brain tissue to the living, functioning brain. Chapter 6 by Crosthwaite and Reveley reviews published CT and MRI studies relevant to the effects of brain structural deficits on prognosis, outcome and response to treatment. Chapter 7 by Liddle reviews functional imaging of schizophrenia as revealed by cerebral blood flow studies using PET, SPECT and fMRI. Cognitive and pharmacological activation studies have consistently revealed focal brain under and over activation as well as disturbances in relationships among brain areas mediating cognitive systems. In Chapter 8 Sedvall, Farde and Pauli examine the use of PET radioligands for the imaging of dopamine, serotonin and other receptors. The principles underlying the neuroimaging of receptors are thoroughly explained and their relevance to anti-psychotic drug treatment is presented. In subsequent chapters, Mortimer reviews the principal neurocognitive deficits in schizophrenia and the effects of anti-psychotic drug treatment in ameliorating these deficits. Barnes and Spence describe the principal types of movement disorders associated with schizophrenia and anti-psychotic drug treatments. They also explore their pathophysiology and approach to therapy. Marder, Wirshing and Wirshing discuss the management of acute and chronic schizophrenia with a particular focus on maximizing the efficacy of conventional anti-psychotic treatments. Waddington reviews the basic and clinical pharmacology of the new atypical anti-psychotics. McCreadie discusses the problems of delivering psychiatric care and support to patients in the community.

It has been clear for some time that schizophrenia is founded on genetic risk and early pathological changes that set the scene for later processes underlying psychotic breakdown and deterioration. None of these mechanisms has been precisely identified but the excellent contributions to this book capture the progress that is being made and show how drug treatments can interact at all stages in the evolution of this disease.

The editors are extremely grateful to all contributors for their manuscripts, and we hope the reader will find that this book clarifies further the relationship between the brain, schizophrenia and psychopharmacology.

November 1999
M.A.R.
J.F.W.D.

CHAPTER 1

Recent advances in schizophrenia research

HASSEN A. AL-AMIN AND DANIEL R. WEINBERGER

Introduction

Research in the last decade has confirmed that schizophrenia is a brain disorder that cannot be attributed solely to psychosocial factors. It is widely accepted from twin and adoption studies that schizophrenia has a significant genetic component (McGuffin *et al.*, 1995). However, the journey from genes to phenotype still seems to be a long and tortuous one, with new findings that add pieces to the puzzle without defining the framework, let alone solving it. The dopamine hypothesis, which is primarily based on the therapeutic effects of blocking dopaminergic D2 receptors, has failed to explain many aspects of schizophrenia, such as negative symptoms, cognitive deficits, and other neurochemical and pathological findings. Interest in dopamine interactions with the other neurotransmitter systems has contributed to the development of novel antipsychotics with better clinical efficacy and fewer side effects. However, the new psychopharmacology of the disorder is still short of explaining its pathophysiology.

As the search for clues to the pathophysiology of schizophrenia has turned in new directions, some surprising possibilities have emerged. For example, there has been increasing evidence from epidemiological (Green *et al.*, 1994; O'Reilly, 1994), post-mortem (Akbarian *et al.*, 1993a, 1993b, 1996), neuroimaging (Chua and Mckenna, 1995) and molecular biology (Nanko *et al.*, 1994; Barbeau *et al.*, 1995) studies that schizophrenia may result from a prenatal insult that affects the development of the brain and maturation of the cortex (Weinberger, 1995, 1996). In this regard, temporal and prefrontal cortices have been described as having abnormal cellular differentiation (Akbarian *et al.*, 1993a, 1993b, 1996), and functional studies have suggested that the connections between the prefrontal and temporolimbic cortices are dysfunctional (Frith, 1995; Weinberger, 1996).

The last decade has also provided new tools to study the effects of antipsychotics beyond their direct interaction with membrane receptors. It has become possible to demonstrate that neuroleptics can indirectly target the genome of the cell and alter the long-term expression of different proteins that may consequently remodel its functional identity (Hyman and Nestler, 1993). The gene modification by antipsychotics has shown specific regional patterns that may further the understanding of their therapeutic effects.

In this chapter we consider some of these new directions. We will first revisit the dopamine hypothesis, discuss recent research on various dopamine receptors and review their relation to the antipsychotic medications and the psychosis induced by dopamine agonists. Second, we will highlight the neurodevelopmental hypothesis of schizophrenia, discuss the proposed dysfunction of the temporolimbic–prefrontal connectivity, and finish this section with the findings of a potential developmental animal model. Last, we will look at the intracellular effects of antipsychotics and their relation to the circuitry implicated in schizophrenia.

Dopamine revisited

A major landmark in the history of the understanding and treatment of schizophrenia was the discovery that dopamine D2-blocking agents can control the hallucinations and delusions of schizophrenic patients (Delay and Deniker, 1952). The advent of many new antipsychotics, all of which showed a correlation between their clinical potency and their in-vitro affinity for binding to D2 receptors (Seeman *et al.*, 1976), encouraged the proposal that schizophrenia may result from increased dopamine. This was further supported by the finding that dopamine agonists can worsen psychotic symptoms in patients with schizophrenia (Lieberman *et al.*, 1987) and even induce paranoid ideation and hallucinations in normal individuals (for review *see* Antelman, 1991).

DOPAMINE RECEPTORS AND SCHIZOPHRENIA

Initial reports of increased dopamine levels in schizophrenic brains have not been replicated (Davis *et al.*, 1991; Hyde *et al.*, 1991). The hypothesis of dopamine over-activity was then extensively tested in the basal ganglia, because these nuclei are known to be rich in dopamine and are part of the limbic circuitry that controls the cognitive and emotional attributes of behaviour (Robbins and Everitt, 1982). Several post-mortem studies of schizophrenic brains showed increased dopamine D2 receptors in the striatum (Seeman, 1987, 1992a), but this increase has not been consistently replicated after controlling for the effects of antipsychotics (Knable *et al.*, 1994). One explanation for the increased D2 binding in schizophrenics is that chronic treatment with neuroleptics can increase the expression of D2 receptors and enhance the binding of the ligand. Chronic treatment with haloperidol, clozapine and remoxipride has resulted in upregulation of D2 receptors in primate brains (Lidow and Goldman-Rakic, 1994).

Neuroimaging studies using positron emission tomography (PET) and single photon emission computerized tomography (SPECT) allow in-vivo analysis of D2 receptors. In 1986, the first PET study with non-medicated schizophrenics showed elevated receptor D2 density (Wong *et al.*, 1986). However, later studies did not consistently demonstrate significant differences in dopamine D2 receptor density between normal controls and medication-free (Pilowsky *et al.*, 1994), or drug-naïve (Farde *et al.*, 1990) schizophrenics. In addition, PET and SPECT imaging were also used to assess the relationships between clinical response and D2 receptor occupancy. They showed that psychotic symptoms can persist even after full blockade of D2 receptors (Pilowsky *et al.*, 1993) and that some patients who had a good clinical response to clozapine showed low occupancy of D2 receptors (Farde *et al.*, 1992). Furthermore, association studies of the D2 receptor gene and its alleles did not show any abnormalities in schizophrenic patients (Comings *et al.*, 1991). Thus, although the D2 receptors may have a role in the therapeutic effects of typical neuroleptics, evidence for D2 receptor alteration as a cause of schizophrenia is lacking.

The dopamine hypothesis was re-invigorated after two major recent findings: (i) gene cloning techniques allowed the identification of five distinct types of dopamine receptors, and (ii) clozapine was found to have high affinity to dopamine D4 receptors. Interest in D4 receptors was further enhanced by evidence that these receptors are expressed in regions that are anatomically and functionally implicated in schizophrenia, such as the frontal cortex, medial temporal cortex, and other limbic regions (Seeman, 1992b). As there is no specific ligand for D4 receptors, researchers assessed their abundance by subtracting the binding of ligands with affinities to receptors D2, D3, and D4 from those that bind to receptors D2 and D3 only. Postmortem studies of schizophrenic brains have reported higher levels of D4 receptor binding in the putamen (Seeman *et al.*, 1993, 1995) and nucleus accumbens (Murray *et al.*, 1995), using this subtractive binding approach. Again, other studies using the same and/or different ligands did not replicate this upregulation of D4 receptors in schizophrenia, and some question whether D4 receptors are found in the putamen (Reynolds and Mason, 1994, 1995). Flamez *et al.* (1994) used [³H]clozapine as a ligand and did not find D4 receptors in post-mortem human brains. No neuroimaging studies have been published on D4 receptors in schizophrenia.

The cloning and sequencing of the D4 receptor gene has revealed multiple allelic variations based on the number of repeats of a 48 base-pair segment in exon III corresponding to the third cytoplasmic loop of the receptor protein. These allelic variants have different affinities for clozapine (Van Tol *et al.*, 1992). In view of the genetic component in schizophrenia, several studies have attempted to find if there is an association between the different alleles of the D4 receptor gene and schizophrenia. No association between schizophrenia and the variants of the D4 receptor gene have been found (Campion *et al.*, 1994; Maier *et al.*, 1994; Daniels *et al.*, 1994; Macciardi *et al.*, 1994a, 1994b; Petronis *et al.*, 1995). A rare deletion variant, two single base-pair substitutions (Seeman *et al.*, 1994; Cichon *et al.*, 1995), and a null mutation of the first exon (Nothen *et al.*, 1994) have also been discovered in the D4 receptor gene, but none of these have been found to be associated with schizophrenia. Other studies have checked if the polymorphic variations could determine the variability in the clinical response to clozapine but none of the receptor D4 allelic variants have consistently predicted the response to clozapine (Shaikh *et al.*, 1993; Rao *et al.*, 1994; Kennedy *et al.*, 1994). In conclusion, more studies with specific ligands are needed to confirm possible elevation of D4 receptors in schizophrenia, but it is clear that the D4 receptor gene is not genetically linked to schizophrenia.

The other dopamine receptor that has been considered to be related to schizophrenia or its treatment is the D3 receptor, whose expression was found to be mainly in limbic regions, including the shell of the nucleus accumbens and islands of Calleja (Camacho-Ochoa *et al.*, 1995). Post-mortem studies have demonstrated that the expression of dopamine D3 receptor mRNA is absent in the parietal and motor cortices in patients with schizophrenia (Schamuss *et al.*, 1993) but the same regions showed higher expression of a modified D3 receptor (D3nf) that results from cleavage of an atypical intron of dopamine D3 receptor pre-mRNA (Schamuss, 1996). Another study of a small post-mortem sample claimed upregulation of D3 receptors in schizophrenic striatum (Gurevich *et al.*, 1997). Earlier association studies have suggested that individuals homozygous for both alleles of the BalI polymorphism at the D3 receptor gene, showed a twofold higher risk of schizophrenia (Schwartz *et al.*, 1993). However, in another study that used the reliable 'haplotype relative risk' strategy with parental chromosomes as controls, the dopamine D3 receptor gene was not found to be associated with schizophrenia (Macciardi *et al.*, 1994a). Hence, more research is needed to clarify the role of dopamine D3 receptors in the pathophysiology of schizophrenia.

DOPAMINE HYPOTHESIS AND EFFECTS OF ANTIPSYCHOTICS

Another often-cited weakness of the dopamine hypothesis involves the time course of the clinical effects of antipsychotics. While neuroleptics block D2 receptors shortly after crossing the blood–brain barrier, their antipsychotic effects do not reach a clinically significant level until, on average, one to two weeks later (Kane and Lieberman, 1987). In addition, antipsychotics neither cure the illness, nor stop the relapse of symptoms completely, and about 30% of patients are refractory to treatment with dopamine blockers (Kane and Lieberman, 1987). In this regard, the atypical neuroleptics (e.g. clozapine, risperidone, sertindole, and olanzapine), which are generally less specific blockers of dopamine, may be superior to haloperidol and result in less extrapyramidal symptoms (EPS) (for review *see* Borison, 1995). Meltzer (1995) suggested that the unique effects of clozapine are secondary to its differential effects on the serotonin and dopamine receptors, e.g. high affinity to 5HT-2 with relatively weak affinity for D2 receptors. This receptor profile has prompted the use of the term serotonin–dopamine antagonists (SDAs) and some authors have rediscovered the hypothesis, from the LSD era of the 1950s, that serotonin may have a role in the aetiology of schizophrenia.

Kapur and Remington (1996) suggested that the blockade of serotonin by antipsychotics disinhibits dopamine and thus decreases the negative symptoms at the level of prefrontal cortex. However, Carpenter (1995) questioned the effects of atypical neuroleptics on negative symptoms, arguing that the enhanced effects on negative symptoms could be related to alleviation of secondary negative symptoms, e.g. EPS, increased activation or amelioration of depression. Other studies have also reported that the cognitive functions that are subserved in large part by the prefrontal cortex (Goldberg and Weinberger, 1994) do not improve with clozapine.

DRUG-INDUCED PSYCHOSIS

One of the corner-stones in the dopamine hypothesis is the observation that dopamimetic drugs can elicit psychotic symptoms in normal individuals. These symptoms, however, are primarily paranoid ideation and hallucinations (Antelman, 1991), which represent only a small part of the constellation of symptoms seen in schizophrenia. Hyperdopaminergia, even if it exists, would not explain the deficit symptoms and the abnormalities in memory and executive functions, which are more enduring than are paranoid ideation and hallucinations. In contrast, there is evidence that deficit symptoms may be related to decreased dopamine in the mesocortical system (Weinberger *et al.*, 1988). In rats, clozapine increases dopamine release in the prefrontal cortex (Moghaddam, 1994a). In primates prefrontal dopamine is important for the performance on working memory tests that depends on normal frontal lobe function (Arnsten *et al.*, 1995). Furthermore, in schizophrenics, dopamine agonists enhance the performance on Wisconsin Card Sorting Test (WCST), a cognitive test that relies also on working memory and prefrontal activity (Daniel *et al.*, 1991). These observations suggest that, at least in terms of certain cognitive functions that are related to prefrontal cortex, if dopamine is a factor, it may be because its activity is too low, not too high.

Alteration of other neurotransmitters has also been associated with psychosis, including the serotonin, glutamate, acetylcholine, and adrenergic systems. These systems interact with each other and with dopamine, and any alteration in one can have significant impact on the others, depending on the region studied and the subtypes of receptors involved (for reviews *see* Joyce, 1993; Moghaddam, 1994b). The psychosis induced by phencyclidine (PCP), a non-competitive antagonist of the NMDA glutamate receptor, is of particular interest. PCP-induced psychosis has been proposed as a better model of schizophrenia because it can result in both positive and negative symptoms (Javitt and Zukin, 1991). Several other studies have repeatedly implicated the glutamatergic system in schizophrenia (Olney and Farber, 1995; for review *see* Halberstadt, 1995). However, the role of this system in the therapeutic effects of antipsychotics is not clear and the benefits of using glycine or cycloserine (both of which augment glutamate effects at NMDA receptors) as an adjuvant treatment in schizophrenia have not been confirmed (Deutsch *et al.*, 1989; Cascella *et al.*, 1994; Waziri, 1996). Perhaps, the most compelling reason to suspect a role for glutamate is its importance as a neurotransmitter in intracortical and corticofugal projections. To the extent that such projections may be dysfunctional in schizophrenia (Weinberger and Lipska, 1995), glutamatergic function would be implicated.

To summarize, the data on dopamine receptors are inconclusive and do not support its direct genetic linkage to schizophrenia. Dopamine blockade may have a therapeutic effect on positive symptoms, but the results may be different depending on the regions of brain involved. Dopamine hyperactivity does not explain the negative symptoms and cognitive deficits in schizophrenia. Finally, dopamine (and other neurotransmitter) abnormalities could be secondary to a more generalized alteration of cortical development and function (Jaskiw and Weinberger, 1992), where antipsychotics may differentially modify these abnormalities depending on the characteristics of the targeted regions.

Schizophrenia: neurodevelopmental perspective

Several lines of evidence continue to accumulate and converge suggesting that schizophrenia, at least in many cases, may result from an abnormality in brain development (for reviews *see* Weinberger, 1995, 1996; Weinberger and Lipska, 1995). This hypothesis is based on the notion that early prenatal insults can alter the maturation of the brain and result in dysfunctional cortical development that manifest as schizophrenia in early adulthood. The pathophysiologic events from the lesion to the dysfunction are still obscure, probably because multiple neuronal factors and pathways are entangled with variable genetic and environmental constructs. This may also help explain the heterogeneity in schizophrenia and the high variability seen in almost all the neurobiological aspects of the disorder.

NEURODEVELOPMENTAL MIENS OF SCHIZOPHRENIA

The following is a brief summary of the lines of evidence that support the neurodevelopmental hypothesis of schizophrenia. While the evidence is indirect and circumstantial, it is considerable.

(*a*) Retrospective (Walker and Lewine, 1990) and prospective studies (Jones *et al.*, 1994) have shown that children, even infants, who subsequently develop schizophrenia as adults have more abnormalities in neuromotor, affective, and psychosocial functions than controls.

(*b*) Schizophrenic patients have a slightly but significantly higher frequency of minor physical anomalies (like low-set ears and facial muscle irregularities) and abnormal dermatoglyphics, which are both indicators of fetal maldevelopment during the early second trimester (Green *et al.*, 1994).

(*c*) Potential fetal exposure to influenza during the second trimester has been associated with increased risk of schizophrenia, suggesting that viral disturbance of brain maturation occurs in some cases of schizophrenia (for review *see* O'Reilly, 1994).

(*d*) Obstetric complications and low birth weight are more frequent in patients with schizophrenia than in controls, including siblings (McNeil, 1988, Rifkin *et al.*, 1994).

(*e*) Neuroimaging studies with computerized tomography (CT) and magnetic resonance imaging (MRI) have repeatedly shown enlarged ventricles (*see* Chua and Mckenna, 1995, for a review), reduced cerebral volume (Nasrallah *et al.*, 1990), and decreased volumes of mesial temporolimbic structures (Marsh *et al.*, 1994). Post-mortem studies of brains from schizophrenic patients have demonstrated almost similar findings, including 4–6% reduction of brain volume (Pakkenberg, 1987), larger lateral ventricles, and smaller limbic temporal lobe structures (Bogerts *et al.*, 1986; Brown *et al.*, 1986). Most of these findings have been seen at the onset of the illness (Weinberger *et al.*, 1982) and remain static with minimal progression over time (Illowsky *et al.*, 1988; Marsh *et al.*, 1994) and no change with treatment (Weinberger *et al.*, 1980).

(*f*) Most histopathologic studies of schizophrenia have reported an absence of gliosis (Roberts and Crow, 1987). This suggests that after maturation of the brain there are no progressive degenerative or inflammatory processes involved. Lesions prior to the third trimester generally do not result in gliosis.

(*g*) Genetic studies have shown that two alleles of the neurotrophin-3 gene (a trophic factor essential for the growth of embryonic cells) are associated with schizophrenia (Nanko *et al.*, 1994; Hattori and Nanko, 1995). The embryonic isoform of the neural cell adhesion molecule (NCAM) is highly polysialylated (PSA-NCAM) and is necessary for the axonal growth and connectivity between neurons. PSA-NCAM showed less expression in the hippocampus of schizophrenic patients (Barbeau *et al.*, 1995). The possibility that such factors regulate neurodevelopment may contribute to the understanding of the neurobiology of schizophrenia.

(*h*) In vivo ¹H magnetic resonance spectroscopy showed reduced *N*-acetyl-aspartate (NAA) concentrations in the dorsal prefrontal cortex and hippocampal region of patients with schizophrenia, including neuroleptic-naïve patients. No changes were found in the mapping of choline-containing compounds (CHO) signal intensity (Bertolino *et al.*, 1996). The latter suggests the absence of gliosis or a neurodegenerative process while reduction of NAA is compatible with neuronal pathology in the aforementioned areas.

INTRACORTICAL 'DYSCONNECTION': POTENTIAL TEMPLATE FOR THE PUZZLE

Further support for the neurodevelopmental hypothesis comes from studies of putative cytoarchitectural abnormalities found in the post-mortem brains of schizophrenic patients. The most provocative findings are: (i) the superficial layers in the parahippocampal gyrus are underdeveloped (Jakob and Beckmann, 1986), (ii) reduced number of neurons in the granular layer of dentate gyrus (Bogerts *et al.*, 1986) and in entorhinal cortex (Falkai and Bogerts, 1991), especially in superficial laminae (Arnold *et al.*, 1991), and (iii) decreased number of interneurons in layers II of the lateral temporal, prefrontal (Akbarian *et al.*, 1993a, 1993b) and cingulate cortices (Benes, 1991) with higher density of pyramidal cells in the layer V of the same regions (Benes, 1991; Akbarian *et al.*, 1993a, 1993b). These abnormalities are all suggestive of disturbed neuronal differentiation or arrested migration of cells at a premature position (Akbarian *et al.*, 1996). Such a failure of migration suggests an abnormal brain developmental process during the second trimester of pregnancy (Rakic, 1988; Rakic *et al.*, 1994). These developmental changes could conceivably alter communication between different cortical regions resulting in faulty processing of information (Weinberger and Lipska, 1995).

Thus, the pathological findings in the prefrontal and temporolimbic regions are suggestive of abnormal neurodevelopment, and they may underlie some of the cognitive deficits in schizophrenia. Patients with schizophrenia usually show a wide range of impaired performance on neuropsychological tests that assess working memory and so-called executive functions (Goldberg and Weinberger, 1994). Although variable in degree, the deficits in memory and executive functions are very common and consistent in patients with schizophrenia, as demonstrated by studies of monozygotic twins that are discordant for schizophrenia (Goldberg *et al.*, 1990). The relationships between memory and executive functions and the temporal and prefrontal cortices, respectively, are well known (Goldman-Rakic and Friedman, 1991). However, the deficits in these functions as seen in patients with schizophrenia do not merely reflect absence of these regions *per se*, as the localized lesions in these cortices do not result in the similar deficits seen in schizophrenia (Randolph *et al.*, 1992). This supports the speculative notion that there is an alteration in their functional connectivity that manifests as cognitive deficits in schizophrenia (Weinberger and Lipska, 1995). However, further research is needed to clarify the relation between dysfunctional intracortical connections and the signs and symptoms of schizophrenia.

A failure of temporolimbic–prefrontal connectivity has also been inferred from PET studies of regional cerebral blood flow (rCBF) in patients with schizophrenia. The most impressive result of these studies is the failure to activate the dorsolateral prefrontal cortex during the performance of working memory tasks like the WCST (Weinberger and Berman, 1996) and verbal recall tasks (Liddle, 1995), but not during simple cognitive and motor tasks (Weinberger and Berman, 1988; Berman and Weinberger, 1991; Frith, 1995). Hypoactivation of the prefrontal cortex appears to be dependent upon the demands of the task performed at the time of the study. Studies of monozygotic twins that are discordant for schizophrenia have replicated this cognition-dependent 'hypofrontality' (Berman *et al.*, 1992) and in addition have shown hyperactivation of the hippocampus during these tasks which is not present in normal controls or unaffected twins (Weinberger *et al.*, 1993). As the performance on these tasks relies on circuitry between prefrontal, parietal and temporolimbic cortices (Goldman-Rakic and Friedman, 1991), this abnormal hypoactivation of prefrontal cortex and hyperactivation of hippocampus reflects a dysfunction in this circuit. In view of the abnormal pathology in the temporal and prefrontal lobes, this temporolimbic prefrontal 'dysconnectivity' has been viewed as a pathophysiologic substrate of the core cognitive deficit in schizophrenia, and may also underlie the classic psychotic behaviour in schizophrenia (Weinberger and Lipska, 1995).

DEVELOPMENTAL ANIMAL MODEL OF SCHIZOPHRENIA

Several animal models have attempted to simulate the cortical maldevelopment in schizophrenia by using generalized insults like hypoxia, nutritional deprivation, and irradiation. However, the first model to cover the developmental aspect of a cortical lesion in neonatal rats and the relation of the emergent behaviour to the known phenomenologic and neurobiologic aspects of schizophrenia, came from studies by Lipska, Jaskiw and Weinberger (1993). The cortical lesion was induced by injecting the neurotoxin, ibotenic acid, into the ventral hippocampus (VH) at postnatal day seven. The neurotoxin selectively damages the VH neurons without affecting the majority of extrinsic synaptic connectivities or the local axonal fibres projecting to other areas. The major finding from this model is that the rats do not show any grossly abnormal behaviour until challenged or stressed. Then they show abnormal behaviours only after puberty but not before (Lipska *et al.*, 1993). The findings from this animal model will be discussed in the context of different categories of validity as an animal model of schizophrenia, namely face, predictive, and construct validity.

Face validity   This refers to the features in this model which mimics certain aspects in schizophrenia. These features are as follows.

(*a*) Postpubertal onset of abnormal hyperresponsive behaviours that were not evident before adulthood. These behaviours include increased locomotion after exposure to a novel environment, saline injection, or amphetamine, and increased stereotypy after apomorphine (Lipska *et al.*, 1993). The neonatal lesioned rats showed also abnormal prepulse inhibition of startle which is also evident in patients with schizophrenia (Lipska *et al.*, 1995a). The abnormal behaviours are suggestive of increased dopaminergic function in the striato-limbic system, another feature that has been associated with schizophrenia.
(*b*) Cognitive and social abnormalities were also seen in this model, as lesioned rats showed impaired performance on a delayed alternation cognitive task and social interaction assessment (Lipska *et al.*, 1996). These deficits may model some of the negative symptoms in schizophrenia.
(*c*) The lesioned rats showed an exaggerated behavioural response to MK-801, a non-competitive NMDA antagonist, where they manifested increased hyper-locomotion and enhanced stereotypy when compared to sham controls (Al-Amin *et al.*, 1996). This is suggestive of an altered NMDA glutamate system, which has also been implicated in patients with schizophrenia who are also hyperresponsive to NMDA antagonists (Itil *et al.*, 1967; Lahti *et al.*, 1995)).

Predictive validity   This involves testing the effectiveness of various neuroleptics in blocking the hyperactivity and enhanced stereotypy seen in this model. Except for the alternation task and impaired social interaction, all the aforementioned abnormal behaviours were blocked with both typical and atypical antipsychotics (Lipska and Weinberger, 1994; Al-Amin *et al.*, 1996). In view of the specific effects of clozapine being more effective in treating psychotic symptoms of schizophrenia and in having no propensity to produce EPS or tardive dyskinesia, it is interesting to note that in this rat model clozapine was more effective than haloperidol in reversing stress-induced hyperlocomotion (Lipska *et al.*, 1993; Lipska and Weinberger, 1994); and increased apomorphine-induced stereotypies were not seen after withdrawal of clozapine, as occurred after withdrawal of haloperidol (Lipska and Weinberger, 1994; Lipska *et al.*, 1995b). This normalization by the antipsychotics suggests the possibility that the neuropharmacological alterations induced by these drugs can somehow compensate for the developmental dysfunction/'dysconnection' induced by the neonatal lesions of the temporolimbic region.

The dopamine-dependent abnormal behaviours do not seem to be related to the loss of VH *per se*, as the same lesion in adults produces a different pattern of abnormal behaviours both in terms of severity and type of responses (Lipska *et al.*, 1992; 1994) . Similarly, the possibly altered NMDA system in the neonatal lesioned rats is not apparent before puberty, and the same cortical lesion in adults does not produce exaggerated responses to MK-801 (Al-Amin *et al.*, 1997). This further supports the impact of the developmental stage on the functional activity of the intra-cortical connections, where a primary disruption of the temporolimbic projections appears to lead to impairment in the maturation of other cortical and subcortical systems.

Construct validity   This model is limited in terms of this category. Although abnormal cellularity of the hippocampal region has been demonstrated in several post-mortem studies of schizophrenic brains (Bogerts *et al.*, 1986; Arnold *et al.*, 1991; Akbarian *et al.*, 1993b), the induced pathology in these rats exceeds any demonstrable pathology in schizophrenia. Furthermore, the rat model mimics certain aspects of schizophrenia but it is far from being representative of the whole syndrome of schizophrenia, as the behavioural and cognitive aspects in patients with schizophrenia are more complex than can be assessed in rats. However, this model provides a convincing mechanism that supports the possibility of an early neonatal lesion leading to onset of abnormal dopamine-dependent behaviours and abnormal NMDA system function in adults. Furthermore, similar lesions in monkeys have reproduced some of the findings discussed above (Kolachana *et al.*, 1996; Beauregard and Bachevalier, 1996). Novel antipsychotics can also be tested in this model by studying their ability to block the behavioural abnormalities. Finally, the understanding of the relationships between early temporolimbic pathology and its impact on the development of widespread neural systems may help to further elucidate altered mechanisms in schizophrenia.

The neurodevelopmental perspective in schizophrenia is ascertained in this model by timing the lesion during a critical period of neurodevelopment. In rats, the brain undergoes significant development in the first two weeks postnatally, corresponding in many respects to the second trimester of gestation in the neurodevelopment of a primate brain (Stanfield and Cowan, 1988). This period corresponds also to the proposed time when neurodevelopment in schizophrenia is affected. In schizophrenia we do not know the nature of the defect that is disrupting neurodevelopment, but conceptually this model provides the opportunity of timing a neonatal insult and of studying its effect on the structure and function of the brain at a later stage. It seems that the early loss of VH output connections is compensated by unknown mechanisms and only after puberty does this loss lead to abnormal responses to stress and other pharmacological stimuli. The driving force behind this loss of compensation seems to be dependent on the exact timing of two related factors: the loss of VH projections, and its impact on the development of the brain. In rats the VH projects strongly to the medial prefrontal cortex and nucleus accumbens.

Effects of neuroleptics on gene activation

Antipsychotics have been used for over 40 years, but we still do not know how they exert their therapeutic effects and why a good clinical response evolves over a period of time. The interaction between antipsychotics and receptors is transduced almost immediately into modulation of enzymes that affect different second messengers like cAMP (Krebs, 1989). However, repeated exposure to drugs or other stimuli may also result in more dramatic morphological and functional changes such as upregulation of receptors, changes in the permeability of ion channels, and other variations in synaptic plasticity that ultimately can modify cognitive functions like memory and learning. Such long-term changes involve protein synthesis which requires waves of gene activation over relatively long periods. These transcriptional gene activation events are regulated by a sequential course of intermediary processes where, after the initial receptor-mediated transduction event, a set of genes is transcribed and the proteins formed will modulate the transcription of another set of genes, and so on. The transcription of the first wave of genes is not dependent on protein synthesis as many environmental (e.g. stress) and pharmacological (e.g. dopamine agonists) stimuli can induce their expression within minutes. These genes, known as immediate early genes (IEGs), are the initiators of a cascade of events that alter the expression of other genes and ultimately the physiologic mechanisms of the cell (Hyman and Nestler, 1993).

In the last few years animal studies have shown that antipsychotics can trigger the expression of immediate early genes such as *c-fos*, *c-jun*, *fos B*, and many others (Robertson and Fibiger, 1992; Merchant and Dorsa, 1993). These genes, known also as proto-oncogenes, are involved in the regulation of the transcription of downstream genes. For example, the dimer formed by binding c-fos and c-jun proteins is activated by phosphokinase C to bind to DNA at a transcriptional complex site called AP-1, which modulates a new wave of gene activation, e.g. the transcription of the neurotensin/neuromedin (*NT/N*) gene. The blockade of *c-fos* mRNA by using antisense *c-fos* oligodeoxynucleotide results in attenuation of *NT/N* mRNA expression induced by haloperidol (Merchant, 1994). Although the role of gene activation in the therapeutic effects of antipsychotics effects involves complex regulatory mechanisms that need further exploration, the genetic process illuminates some aspects of the time course of their effects. In the following section, we will focus on the effects of antipsychotics on *c-fos* induction in rats as clinical doses of the typical and atypical neuroleptics have shown differential anatomical patterns of *c-fos* expression that may relate to some of their specific clinical characteristics.

PARALLELS BETWEEN C-FOS INDUCTION AND CLINICAL PROFILES

Both typical and atypical neuroleptics share the property of inducing *c-fos* in nucleus accumbens neurons (Deutch *et al.*, 1992; Robertson and Fibiger, 1992; Fink-Jensen and Kristensen, 1994; Robertson *et al.*, 1994). More specifically, the shell compartment of nucleus accumbens is the region that shows increased *c-fos* after administration of each and every neuroleptic (Deutch *et al.*, 1992; Robertson and Fibiger 1992; MacGibbon *et al.*, 1994). Clinically these drugs share the property of ameliorating the positive symptoms of schizophrenia. On the other hand the atypical neuroleptics differ from the typical ones in that (i) they have a reduced EPS liability (Borison, 1995) and (ii) they may be clinically superior, e.g. clozapine can help 35% of the patients who have been refractory to treatment with typical neuroleptics (Kane *et al.*,

1988). The first difference has its parallel in the regional pattern of c-fos expression. The typical neuroleptics (e.g. haloperidol, chlorpromazine, fluphenazine, and thio-ridazine), which often produce EPS, induce higher c-fos expression in the dorsolateral striatum than do the atypical ones (Deutch et al., 1992; Roberston and Fibigier, 1992; Merchant and Dorsa, 1993; Fink-Jensen and Kristensen, 1994; Roberston et al., 1994). Further support for this distinction comes from metoclopramide, a dopamine antagonist that produces EPS but has no antipsychotic activity. It also induces c-fos in the dorsolateral striatum (Deutch et al., 1992; Roberston et al., 1994). The atypical neuroleptics (e.g. clozapine, remoxipride, sertindole, and fluper-lapine) produce much less EPS and they do not induce c-fos expression in the dorso-lateral striatum (Deutch et al., 1992; Robertson and Fibigier, 1992; Merchant and Dorsa, 1993; Fink-Jenson and Kristensen 1994; MacGibbon et al., 1994; Roberston et al., 1994). The second difference, which is related to the enhanced clinical efficacy of clozapine, may also have a parallel in the pattern of clozapine-induced c-fos. Clozapine and other novel atypical agents like fluperlapine, RMI-81852, remox-ipride, melprone, tiospirone, and quetiapine induce IEGs in the medial prefrontal cortex while the typical drugs like haloperidol, fluphenazine, and chlorpromazine do not (Robertson et al., 1994; Deutch and Duman, 1996). Two exceptions have been noted: first molindone activates c-fos in the prefrontal cortex, and second, risperi-done does not show such activation (Robertson et al., 1994). However, other researchers have demonstrated activation of c-fos in prefrontal cortex by higher doses of risperidone (Fink-Jensen and Kristensen, 1994). To some degree these results are still preliminary in that varying methods and doses have been utilized.

C-fos EXPRESSION: REGIONAL SPECIFICITY VS. RECEPTOR PROFILE

Although each neuroleptic has a somewhat different receptor affinity profile, all neuroleptics alter gene expression in the nucleus accumbens. Preliminary data have suggested that the effects of neuroleptics on c-fos induction in the nucleus accum-bens are mediated by a mechanism that involves dopamine receptors, as their effects on c-fos induction are not seen in dopamine-depleted animals (Robertson and Fibiger, 1992). However, it is difficult to explain why clozapine and some other atyp-icals do not induce c-fos in the dorsolateral striatum even at relatively high doses where they would be occupying a majority of dopamine receptors (Deutch et al., 1992; Robertson and Fibiger 1992). Thus, either clozapine-induced c-fos expression reflects modulation at different isoforms of D2 receptors or is mediated via an unknown dopamine receptor that is active in the nucleus accumbens but not in the dorsolateral striatum (Weinberger and Lipska, 1995; Deutch and Duman, 1996).

In this regard, it is worth noting that the nucleus accumbens, mainly the shell com-partment, receives – at least in the rat – convergent inputs from both the prefrontal and temporolimbic cortices, suggesting that the nucleus accumbens acts as a relay station that can modulate information processed in these cortical regions. Indeed, glutamatergic terminals from the hippocampus and from the prefrontal cortex synapse in close proximity to the dopaminergic terminals from the ventral tegmental area on intrinsic GABA neurons of the nucleus accumbens (Sesack and Pickel, 1990, 1992). One can speculate that the long-term effects of neuroleptics may involve indirect compensation of abnormal temporolimbic prefrontal connectivity at the level of this convergence on intrinsic nucleus accumbens neurons. Again, the fact that the dorsolateral striatum receives major projections from the sensorimotor cortex and not from the prefrontal or temporolimbic cortices may help to explain the relation between the unique effects of typical neuroleptics in the dorsolateral striatum and their high frequency of motor side effects.

In contrast to *c-fos* expression in the nucleus accumbens, induction of this IEG in prefrontal cortex by clozapine is not dependent on dopamine, as clozapine-induced Fos expression is not altered by dopamine depletion (Robertson and Fibiger, 1992) or by pretreatment with sulpiride (D2/3/4 antagonist) and SCH23390 (D1/5 antagonist) (Deutch and Duman, 1996). Blockade of 5-HT-2 and alpha-1 adrenergic receptors by ritanserin and prazosin, respectively, also did not induce Fos protein in prefrontal cortex, thus likely excluding these receptors as possible mediators of this specific regional expression (Fink-Jensen *et al.*, 1995; Deutch and Duman 1996). Deutch and Duman excluded also the role of 5HT-2c and muscarinic receptors, but found that dopamine agonists can also enhance Fos expression in the prefrontal cortex (Deutch and Duman 1996). This is reminiscent of the possibility that clozapine's effect on negative symptoms is mediated through increasing dopamine release in the prefrontal cortex (Kapur and Remington, 1996). However, further research is needed to understand better the events leading to prefrontal IEG expression, and to clinical response. The quite unique effects of clozapine on *c-fos* expression in the prefrontal cortex may highlight its better clinical position in view of the major role of prefrontal cortex in the proposed defect in intracortical connections (Weinberger and Lipska, 1995). In other words, by targeting the prefrontal cortex, the gene activation events that are initiated by clozapine may affect the error in information processing at its primary site and thus may give better control of the symptoms.

To summarize, neuroleptics can activate IEGs that play a role in regulating long-term events in the cell and ultimately basic changes in its function. The variation in the anatomical distribution of c-fos protein expression after different neuroleptics may shed some light on the anatomical regions that mediate their clinical effects. It also supports the possibility that neuroleptics may act by compensating for the proposed intracortical 'dysconnection'.

Conclusions

The data reviewed in this chapter highlight several recent new directions in schizophrenia research that merit further investigation and confirmation. The pathophysiology of schizophrenia cannot be attributed to dopamine hyperactivity or any single neurotransmitter abnormality. The understanding of the interactions between different neurotransmitter systems and their impact on behaviour may help in designing novel antipsychotics with a better clinical profile. However, the modification of these systems in schizophrenia appears to be better understood in relation to the cortical maldevelopment that is implicated in the disorder. Post-mortem, neuroimaging, and neurocognition studies support dysfunctional temporolimbic prefrontal connectivity.

The intracortical 'dysconnectivity' and the compelling evidence that schizophrenia is a neurodevelopmental disorder may provide a better framework to study the neurobiology of schizophrenia and put the pieces of the puzzle together. Neonatal cortical lesions in rats and primates appear to represent a model to investigate the impact of disturbed neurodevelopment on the neural substrates of schizophrenic behaviour. This model also imitates many features of schizophrenia and may be useful in testing new therapies. The genetic effects of neuroleptics show distinct regional patterns of gene expression that may better explain their clinical profile, and further support the importance of targeting intracortical and subcortical coupling to compensate for the disordered behaviour in schizophrenia.

References

Akbarian, S., Bunney Jr., W.E., Potkin, S.G. *et al*. (1993a) Altered distribution of nicotinamide-adenine dinucleotide phosphate-diaphorase cells in frontal lobe of schizophrenics implies disturbances of cortical development. *Arch Gen Psychiatry*, **50**(3), 169–77.

Akbarian, S., Kim, J.J., Potkin, S.G. *et al*. (1996) Maldistribution of interstitial neurons in prefrontal white matter of the brains of schizophrenic patients. *Arch Gen Psychiatry*, **53** (5), 425–36.

Akbarian, S., Vinuela, A., Kim, J.J. *et al*. (1993b) Distorted distribution of nicotinamide-adenine dinuclcotide phosphate-diaphorase neurons in temporal lobe of schizophrenics implies anomalous cortical development. *Arch Gen Psychiatry*, **50**(3), 178–87.

Al-Amin, H.A., Lipska, B.K. and Weinberger, D.R. (1996) Differential effects of haloperidol and clozapine on the MK-801-induced behaviors in rats with neonatal hippocampal lesions. *Abstr Am Coll Neuropsychopharmacol*, **35**, 196.

Al-Amin, H.A., Lipska, B.K., Lillrank, S.M. *et al*. (1997) Postpubertal modulation of NMDA system after neonatal ventral hippocampus (VH) lesions in rats. *Abstr Soc Neurosci*, **23**, 1363.

Antelman, S.M. (1991) Possible animal model of some of the schizophrenia and their response to drug treatment. In S.R. Steinhaur, J.H. Gruzlier and J. Zubin (eds), *Handbook of schizophrenia, vol 5: Neuropsychology, psychophysiology and information processing*. Amsterdam: Elsevier Science Publishers, 161–80.

Arnold, S.E., Hyman, B.T., Van Hoesen, G.W. and Damasio, A.R. (1991) Some cytoarchitectural abnormalities of the entorhinal cortex in schizophrenia. *Arch Gen Psychiatry*, **48** (7), 625–32.

Arnsten, A.F., Cai, J.X., Steere, J.C. and Goldman-Rakic, P.S. (1995) Dopamine receptor mechanisms contribute to age-related cognitive decline: the effects of quinpirole on memory performance in monkeys. *J Neurosci*, **15** (5 Pt 1), 3429–39.

Barbeau, D., Liang, J.J., Robitalille, Y. *et al*. (1995) Decreased expression of the embryonic form of the neural cell adhesion molecule in schizophrenic brains. *Proc Natl Acad Sci USA*, **92** (7), 2785–89.

Beauregard, M. and Bachevalier, J. (1996) Neonatal insult to the hippocampal region and schizophrenia: a review and a putative animal model. *Can J Psychiatry*, **41**, 446–56.

Benes, F.M. (1991) Evidence for neurodevelopment disturbances in anterior cingulate cortex of post-mortem schizophrenic brain. *Schizophr Res*, **5** (3), 187–8.

Berman, K.F. and Weinberger, D.R. (1991) Functional localization in the brain in schizophrenia. In A. Tasman (ed.), *American Psychiatric Press review of Psychiatry, Vol 10*. Washington, DC: APPA Press, 24–59.

Berman, K.F., Torrey, E.F., Daniel, D.G. and Weinberger, D.R. (1992) Regional cerebral blood flow in monozygotic twins discordant and concordant for schizophrenia. *Arch Gen Psychiatry*, **49**, 927–34.

Bertolino, A., Nawroz, S., Mattay, S.M. *et al.* (1996) Regionally specific pattern of neurochemical pathology in schizophrenia as assessed by multislice proton magnetic resonance spectroscopic imaging. *Am J Psychiatry*, **153**, 1554–63.

Bogerts, B., Falkai, P. and Tutsch, J. (1986) Cell numbers in the pallidum and hippocampus of schizophrenics. In C. Shagass *et al.* (eds), *Biologic psychiatry*. Amsterdam: Elsevier, 1178–80.

Borison, R. L. (1995) Clinical efficacy of serotonin–dopamine antagonists relative to classic neuroleptics. *J Clin Psychopharmacol*, **15** (1 Suppl 1), 24S-29S.

Brown, R., Colter, N. and Corsellis, J.A.N. (1986) Postmortem evidence of structural brain changes in schizophrenia. Differences in brain weight, temporal horn area and parahippocampal gyrus compared with affective disorder. *Arch Gen Psychiatry*, **43**, 36–42.

Camacho-Ochoa, M., Walker, E.L., Evans, D.L. and Piercey, M.F. (1995) Rat brain binding sites for pramipexole, a clinically useful D3-preferring dopamine agonist. *Neurosci Lett*, **196** (1–2), 97–100.

Campion, D., d'Amato, T., Bastard, C. *et al.* (1994) Genetic study of dopamine D1, D2, and D4 receptors in schizophrenia. *Psychiatry Res*, **51** (3), 215–30.

Carpenter Jr., W.T. (1995) Serotonin-dopamine antagonists and treatment of negative symptoms. *J Clin Psychopharmacol*, **15** (1 Suppl 1), 30S-35S.

Cascella, N.G., Macciardi, F., Cavallini, C. and Smeraldi, E. (1994) d-cycloserine adjuvant therapy to conventional neuroleptic treatment in schizophrenia: an open-label study. *J Neural Transm Gen Sect*, **95** (2), 105–11.

Chua, S.E. and McKenna, P.J. (1995) Schizophrenia: a brain disease? A critical review of structural and functional cerebral abnormality in the disorder. *Br J Psychiatry*, **166**, 563–82.

Cichon, S., Nothen, M.M., Catalano, M. *et al.* (1995) Identification of two novel polymorphisms and a rare deletion variant in the human dopamine D4 receptor gene. *Psychiatr Genet*, **5** (3), 97–103.

Comings, D.E., Comings, B.G., Muhleman, D. *et al.* (1991) The dopamine D2 receptor locus as a modifying gene in neuropsychiatric disorders. *J Am Med Assoc*, **266**, 1793–1800.

Daniel, D.G., Weinberger, D.R., Jones, D.W. *et al.* (1991) The effect of amphetamine on regional cerebral blood flow during cognitive activation in schizophrenia. *J Neurosci*, **11**, 1907–17.

Daniels, J., Williams, J., Mant, R. *et al.* (1994) Repeat length variation in the dopamine D4 receptor gene shows no evidence of association with schizophrenia. *Am J Med Genet*, **54** (3), 256–8.

Davis, K.L., Kahn, R.S., Ko, G. and Davidson, M. (1991) Dopamine in schizophrenia: a review and reconceptualization. *Am J Psychiatry*, **148**, 1474–86.

Delay, J. and Deniker, P. (1952) Le traitement des psychoses par une methode neurolyptique derivée de l'hibernotherapi. In *Congrès des medicins aliensites et neurologistes de France*, vol 50, Luxemberg, 497.

Deutch, A.Y. (1994) Identification of the neural systems subserving the actions of clozapine: clues from immediate-early gene expression. *J Clin Psychiatry*, **55**, 37–42.

Deutch, A.Y. and Duman, R.S. (1996) The effects of antipsychotic drugs on Fos protein expression in the prefrontal cortex: cellular localization and pharmacological characterization. *Neuroscience*, **70** (2), 377–89.

Deutch, A.Y., Lee, M.C. and Iadarola, M.J. (1992) Regionally specific effects of atypical antipsychotic drugs on striatal Fos expression: the nucleus accumbens shell as a locus of antipsychotic action. *Mol Cell Neurosci*, **3**, 332–41.

Deutsch, S.I., Mastropaolo, J., Schwartz, B.L. *et al.* (1989) A 'glutamatergic hypothesis' of schizophrenia: rationale for pharmacotherapy with glycine. *Clin Neuropharmacol*, **12**, 1–13.

Falkai, P. and Bogerts, B. (1991) Qualitative and quantitative assessment of pre-alpha cell clusters in the entorhinal cortex of schizophrenics. A neurodevelopmental model of schizophrenia? *Schizophr Res*, **4**, 357–8.

Farde, L., Nordstrom, A.L., Weisel, F.A. *et al.* (1992) Positron emission tomographic analysis of central D1 and D2 receptor occupancy in patients treated with classical neuroleptics and clozapine. *Arch Gen Psychiatry*, **49**, 538–44.

Farde, L., Weisel, F.A., Stone-Elander, S. *et al.* (1990) D2 dopamine receptors in neuroleptic naive schizophrenic patients: a positron emission tomography study with [¹¹C]raclopride. *Arch Gen Psychiatry*, **47**, 213–19.

Fink-Jensen, A. and Kristensen, P. (1994) Effects of typical and atypical neuroleptics on Fos protein expression in the rat forebrain. *Neurosci Lett*, **182** (1), 115–18.

Fink-Jensen, A., Ludvigsen, T.S. and Korsgaard, N. (1995) The effect of clozapine on Fos protein immunoreactivity in the rat forebrain is not mimicked by the addition of alpha 1–adrenergic or 5HT-2 receptor blockade to haloperidol. *Neurosci Lett*, **194** (1–2), 77–80.

Flamez, A., De Backer, J.P., Wilezak, N. *et al.* (1994) ³H-clozapine is not a suitable radioligand for the labeling of D4 dopamine receptors in post-mortem human brain. *Neurosci Letters*, **175**, 17–20.

Frith, C. (1995) Functional imaging and cognitive abnormalities. *Lancet*, **346**, 615–20.

Goldberg, T.E., Ragland, D.R., Gold, J.M. *et al.* (1990) Neuropsychological assessment of monozygotic twins discordant for schizophrenia. *Arch Gen Psychiatry*, **47**, 1066–72.

Goldberg, T.E. and Weinberger, D.R. (1994) The effects of clozapine on neurocognition: an overview. *J Clin Psychiatry*, **55** (Suppl B), 88–90.

Goldman-Rakic, P.S. and Friedman, H.R. (1991) The circuitry of working memory revealed by anatomy and metabolic imaging. In H.S. Levin, H.M. Eisenberg and A.L. Benton (eds), *Frontal Lobe Function and Dysfunction*, New York: Oxford University Press, 72–91.

Green, M.F., Bracha, H.S., Satz P. and Christenson, C.D. (1994) Preliminary evidence for an association between minor physical anomalies and second trimester neurodevelopment in schizophrenia. *Psychiatry Res*, **53** (2), 119–27.

Gurevich, E.V., Bordelon, Y., Shapiro, R.M. *et al.* (1997) Mesolimbic dopamine D3 receptors and use of antipsychotics in patients with schizophrenia. A postmortem study. *Arch Gen Psychiatry*, **54**, 225–32.

Halberstadt, A.L. (1995) The phencyclidine-glutamate model of schizophrenia. *Clin Neuropharmacol*, **18** (3), 237–49.

Hattori, M. and Nanko, S. (1995) Association of neurotrophin-3 gene variant with severe forms of schizophrenia. *Biochem Biophys Res Commun*, **209** (2), 513–18.

Hyde, T., Casanova, M., Kleinman, J.E. and Weinberger, D.R. (1991) Neuroanatomical and neurochemical pathology in schizophrenia. In A. Tasman (ed.), *American psychiatric press review of psychiatry*, vol 10, Washington, DC: APPA Press, 275–81.

Hyman, S.E. and Nestler, E.J. (eds) (1993) The molecular foundation of psychiatry. Washington, DC: American Psychiatric Press.

Illowsky, B., Juliano, D.M., Bigelow, L.B. *et al.* (1988) Stability of CT scan findings in schizophrenia: results of an 8 year follow-up study. *J Neurol Neurosurg Psychiatry*, **51**, 209–13.

Itil, T., Keskiner, A., Kiremitci, N. and Holden, J.M.C. (1967) Effect of phencyclidine in chronic schizophrenia. *Can J Psychiatry*, **12**, 209–12.

Jakob, H. and Beckmann, H. (1986) Prenatal developmental disturbances in the limbic allocortex in schizophrenics. *J Neural Transm*, **65**, 303–26.

Jaskiw, G.E. and Weinberger, D.R. (1992) Dopamine and schizophrenia—a cortically corrective perspective. *Semin Neurosci*, **4**, 179–88.

Javitt, D.C. and Zukin, S.R. (1991) Recent advances in the phencyclidine model of schizophrenia. *Am J Psychiatry*, **148**, 1301–8.

Jones, P., Rodgers, B., Murray, R. and Marmot, M. (1994) Child developmental risk factors for adult schizophrenia in the British 1946 birth cohort. *Lancet*, **344**, 1398–402.

Joyce, J.N. (1993) The dopamine hypothesis of schizophrenia: limbic interactions with serotonin and norepinephrine. *Psychopharmacology (Berl)*, **112** (1 Suppl), S16–34.

Kane, J.M. and Lieberman, J. (1987) Maintenance pharmacotherapy in schizophrenia. In H.Y. Meltzer (ed.), *Psychopharmacology, the third generation of progress: the emergence of molecular biology and biological psychiatry*, New York, Raven Press, 1103–9.

Kane, J.M., Honigfeld, G., Singer, J. *et al.* (1988) Clozapine for the treatment-resistant schizophrenic: a double-blind comparison with chlorpromazine. *Arch Gen Psychiatry*, **45**, 789–96.

Kapur, S. and Remington, G. (1996) Serotonin-dopamine interaction and its relevance to schizophrenia. *Am J Psychiatry*, **153** (4), 466–76.

Kennedy, J.L., Petronis, A., Gao, J. *et al.* (1994) Genetic studies of DRD4 and clinical response to neuroleptic medications. *Am J Hum Genet*, **55**, 3.

Knable, M.B., Hyde, T.M., Herman, M.M., *et al.* (1994) Quantitative autoradiography of dopamine -D1 receptors, D2 receptors, and dopamine uptake sites in postmortem striatal specimens from schizophrenic patients. *Biol Psychiatry*, **36**, 827–35.

Kolachana, B.S., Saunders, R.C., Bachevalier, J. and Weinberger, D.R. (1996) Abnormal prefrontal cortical regulation of striatal dopamine release after neonatal medial temporal-limbic lesions in rhesus monkey. *Abstr Soc Neurosci*, **22**, 1974.

Krebs, E.G. (1989) Role of cyclic AMP-dependent protein kinase in signal transduction. *J Am Med Assoc*, **262**, 1815–18.

Lahti, A.C, Koffel, B., LaPorte, D. and Tamminga, C.A. (1995) Subanesthetic doses of ketamine stimulate psychosis in schizophrenia. *Neuropsychopharmacology*, **13**, 9–19.

Liddle, P.F. (1995) Brain imaging. In S.R. Hirsch and D.R. Weinberger (eds), *Schizophrenia*. London: Blackwood, 425–39.

Lidow, M.S. and Goldman-Rakic, P.S. (1994) A common action of clozapine, haloperidol, and remoxipride on D1– and D2–dopaminergic receptors in the primate cerebral cortex. *Proc Natl Acad Sci USA*, **91** (10), 4353–6.

Lieberman, J.A., Kane, J.M. and Alvir, D.J. (1987) Provocative tests with psychostimulant drugs in schizophrenia. *Psychopharmacology*, **91**, 415–33.

Lipska, B.K., Jaskiw, G.E., Chrapusta, S., *et al.* (1992) Ibotenic acid lesion of the ventral hippocampus differentially affects dopamine and its metabolites in the nucleus accumbens and prefrontal cortex in the rat. *Brain Res*, **585** (1–2), 1–6.

Lipska, B.K., Jaskiw, G.E. and Weinberger, D.R. (1993) Postpubertal emergence of hyper-responsiveness to stress and to amphetamine after neonatal excitotoxic hippocampal damage: a potential animal model of schizophrenia. *Neuropsychopharmacology*, **9** (1), 67–75.

Lipska, B.K., Jaskiw, G.E. and Weinberger, D.R. (1994) The effects of combined prefrontal cortical and hippocampal damage on dopamine-related behaviors in rats. *Pharmacol Biochem Behav*, **48** (4), 1053–7.

Lipska, B.K. and Weinberger, D.R. (1994) Subchronic treatment with haloperidol and clozapine in rats with neonatal excitotoxic hippocampal damage. *Neuropsychopharmacology*, **10** (3), 199–205.

Lipska, B.K., Swerdlow, N.R., Geyer, M.A. *et al.* (1995a) Neonatal excitotoxic hippocampal damage in rats causes post-pubertal changes in prepulse inhibition of startle and its disruption by apomorphine. *Psychopharmacology (Berl)*, **122** (1), 35–43.

Lipska, B.K., Chrapusta, S.J., Egan, M.F. and Weinberger, D.R. (1995b) Neonatal excitotoxic ventral hippocampal damage alters dopamine response to mild repeated stress and to chronic haloperidol. *Synapse*, **20** (2), 125–30.

Lipska, B.K., Moghaddam, B., Sams-Dodd, F. *et al.* (1996) Neonatal hippocampal damage in the rat models negative symptoms of schizophrenia. *Abstr Am Coll Neuropsychopharmacol*, **35**, 127.

Macciardi, F., Verga, M., Kennedy, J.L. *et al.* (1994a) An association study between schizophrenia and the dopamine receptor genes DRD3 and DRD4 using haplotype relative risk. *Hum Hered*, **44** (6), 328–36.

Macciardi, F., Petronis, A., Van Tol, H.H. *et al.* (1994b) Analysis of the D4 dopamine receptor gene variant in an Italian schizophrenia kindred. *Arch Gen Psychiatry*, **51** (4), 288–93.

MacGibbon, G.A., Lawlor, P.A., Bravo, R. and Dragunow, M. (1994) Clozapine and haloperidol produce a differential pattern of immediate early gene expression in rat caudate-putamen, nucleus accumbens, lateral septum and islands of Calleja. *Brain Res Mol Brain Res*, **23** (1–2), 21–32.

Maier, W., Schwab, S., Hallmayer, J. *et al.* (1994) Absence of linkage between schizophrenia and the dopamine D4 receptor gene. *Psychiatry Res*, **53** (1), 77–86.

Marsh, L., Suddath, R.L., Higgins, N. and Weinberger, D.R. (1994) Medial temporal lobe structures in schizophrenia: relationship of size to duration of illness. *Schizophr Res*, **11**, (3), 225–38.

McGuffin, P., Owen, M.J., and Farmer, A.E. (1995) Genetic basis of schizophrenia. *Lancet*, **346**, 678–82.

McNeil, T.F. (1988) Obstetric factors and perinatal injuries. In M.T. Tsuang and J.C. Simpson (eds), *Handbook of schizophrenia, vol 3: nosology, epidemiology, and genetics*, New York: Elsevier, 319–44.

Meltzer, H.Y. (1995) Role of serotonin in the action of atypical antipsychotic drugs. *Clin Neurosci*, **3** (2), 64–75.

Merchant, K.M. (1994) c-fos antisense oligonucleotide specifically attenuates haloperidol-induced increases in neurotensin/neuromedin N mRNA expression in rat dorsal striatum. *Mol Cell Neurosci*, **5** (4), 336–44.

Merchant, K.M. and Dorsa, D.M. (1993) Differential induction of neurotensin and c-fos gene expression by typical versus atypical antipsychotics. *Proc Natl Acad Sci USA*, **90** (8), 3447–51.

Moghaddam, B. (1994a) Preferential activation of cortical dopamine neurotransmission by clozapine: functional significance. *J Clin Psychiatry*, **55** (Suppl B), 27–9.

Moghaddam, B. (1994b) Recent basic findings in support of excitatory amino acid hypothesis of schizophrenia. *Prog Neuropsychopharmacol Biol Psychiatry*, **18** (5), 859–70.

Murray, A.M., Hyde, T.M., Knable, M.B. *et al.* (1995) Distribution of putative D4 dopamine receptors in postmortem striatum from patients with schizophrenia. *J Neurosci*, **15** (3 Pt 2), 2186–91.

Nanko, S., Hattori, M., Kuwata, S. *et al.* (1994) Neurotrophin-3 gene polymorphism associated with schizophrenia. *Acta Psychiatr Scand*, **89** (6), 390–2.

Nasrallah, H.A., Coffman, J.A., Schwarzkopf, S.B. *et al.* (1990) Reduced cerebral volume in schizophrenia. *Schizophr Res*, **3**, 17.

Nothen, M.M., Cichon, S., Hemmer, S. *et al.* (1994) Human dopamine D4 receptor gene: frequent occurrence of a null allele and observation of homozygosity. *Hum Mol Genet*, **3** (12), 2207–12.

Olney, J.W. and Farber, N. B. (1995) Glutamate receptor dysfunction and schizophrenia. *Arch Gen Psychiatry*, **52** (12), 998–1007.

O'Reilly, R.L. (1994) Viruses and schizophrenia. *Aust N Z J Psychiatry,* **28** (2), 222–8.

Pakkenberg, B. (1987) Post-mortem study of chronic schizophrenic brains. *Br J Psychiatry*, **151**, 744–52.

Petronis, A., Macciardi, F., Athanassiades, A. *et al.* (1995) Association study between the dopamine D4 receptor gene and schizophrenia. *Am J Med Genet*, **60** (5), 452–5.

Pilowsky, L.S., Costa, D.C., Ell, P.J. et al (1993) Antipsychotic medication D2 dopamine receptor blockade and clinical response: an ^{123}I-IBZM SPET (single photon emission tomography) study. *Psychol Med*, **23**, 791–7.

Pilowsky, L.S., Costa, D.C., Ell, P.J. et al (1994) D2 dopamine receptor binding in the basal ganglia of antipsychotic-free schizophrenic patients: an ^{123}I-IBZM single photon emission computerized tomography study. *Br J Psychiatry*, **164**, 16–26.

Rakic, P. (1988) Specification of cerebral cortical areas. *Science*, **241**, 170–6.

Rakic, P., Cameron, R.S. and Komuro, H. (1994) Recognition, adhesion, transmembrane signaling and cell motility in guided neuronal migration. *Curr Opin Neurobiol*, **4** (1), 63–9.

Randolph, C., Gold, J.M., Carpenter, C. *et al.* (1992) Release from proactive interference: determination of performance and neuropsychological correlates. *J Clin Exp Neuropsychol*, **14**, 785–800.

Rao, P.A., Pickar, D., Gejman, P.V. *et al.* (1994) Allelic variation in the D4 dopamine receptor (DRD4) gene does not predict response to clozapine. *Arch Gen Psychiatry*, **51** (11), 912–17.

Reynolds, G.P. and Mason, S.L. (1994) Are striatal dopamine D4 receptors increased in schizophrenia? *J Neurochem*, **63** (4), 1576–7.

Reynolds, G.P. and Mason, S.L. (1995) Absence of detectable striatal dopamine D4 receptors in drug-treated schizophrenia. *Eur J Pharmacol*, **281** (2), R5–6.

Rifkin, L., Lewis, S., Jones, P. *et al.* (1994) Low birth weight and schizophrenia. *Br J Psychiatry*, **165** (3), 357–62.

Robbins, T.W. and Everitt, B.J. (1982) Functional studies of the central catecholamines. *Int Rev Neurobiol*, **23**, 303–65.

Roberts, G.W. and Crow, T.J. (1987) The neuropathology of schizophrenia – a progress report. *Br Med Bull*, **43**, 599–615.

Robertson, G.S. and Fibiger, H.C. (1992) Neuroleptics increase c-fos expression in the forebrain: contrasting effects of haloperidol and clozapine. *Neuroscience*, **46** (2), 315–28.

Robertson, G.S., Matsumura, H. and Fibiger, H.C. (1994) Induction patterns of Fos-like immunoreactivity in the forebrain as predictors of atypical antipsychotic activity. *J Pharmacol Exp Ther*, **271** (2), 1058–66.

Schamuss, C., Haroutunian, V., Davis, K.L. and Davidson, M. (1993) Selective loss of dopamine D3 receptor mRNA expression in the parietal and motor cortex in patients with chronic schizophrenia. *Proc Natl Acad Sci USA*, **90**, 8942–6.

Schamuss, C. (1996) Enhanced cleavage of an atypical intron of dopamine D3–receptor premRNA in chronic schizophrenia. *J Neurosci*, **16**, 7902–9.

Schwartz, J.C., Levesque, D., Martres, M.P. and Sokoloff, P. (1993) Dopamine D3 receptor: basic and clinical aspects. *Clin Neuropharmacol*, **16** (4), 295–314.

Seeman, P. (1987) Dopamine receptors and the dopamine hypothesis of schizophrenia. *Synapse*, **1**, 133–52.

Seeman, P. (1992a) Elevated D2 in schizophrenia. *Neuropsychopharmacology*, **1**, 55–7.

Seeman, P. (1992b) Dopamine receptor sequences. Therapeutic levels of neuroleptics occupy D2 receptors, clozapine occupies D4. *Neuropsychopharmacology*, **7**, 261–84.

Seeman, P., Guan, H.C., Van Tol, H.H. and Niznick, H.B. (1993) Dopamine D4 receptors elevated in schizophrenia. *Nature*, **365**, 441–4.

Seeman, P., Ulpian, C., Chouinard, G. *et al.* (1994) Dopamine D4 receptor variant, D4GLYCINE194, in Africans, but not in Caucasians: no association with schizophrenia. *Am J Med Genet*, **54** (4), 384–90.

Seeman, P., Guan, H.C., and Van Tol, H.H. (1995) Schizophrenia: elevation of dopamine D4–like sites, using [^{3}H]nemonapride and [^{125}I]epidepride. *Eur J Pharmacol*, **286** (2), R3–5.

Seeman, P., Lee, T., Chou-Wong, M. *et al.* (1976) Antipsychotic drug dose and neuroleptic/dopamine receptors. *Nature*, **261**, 717–18.

Sesack, S.R. and Pickel, V.M. (1990) In the rat medial accumbens, hippocampal and catecholaminergic terminals converge on spiny neurons and are in opposition to each other. *Brain Res*, **527**, 266–79.

Sesack, S.R. and Pickel, V.M. (1992) Prefrontal cortical efferents in the rat synapse on unlabeled neuronal targets of catecholamine terminals in the nucleus accumbens septi and on dopamine neurons in the ventral tegmental area. *J Comp Neurol* **320**, 145–60.

Shaikh, S., Collier, D.H., Kerwin, R.W. *et al.* (1993) Dopamine D4 receptor subtypes and response to clozapine. *Lancet*, **341**, 116.

Stanfield, B.B and Cowan, W.M. (1988) The development of the hippocampal region. In A. Peters and E.G. Jones (eds), *Cerebral cortex, development and maturation of cerebral cortex*, vol 7. New York: Plenum Press, 91–131.

Van Tol, H.H., Wu, C.M., Guan, H.C. *et al.* (1992) Multiple dopamine D4 receptor variants in the human population. *Nature*, **358**, 149–92.

Walker, E. and Lewine, R. (1990) Prediction of adult-onset schizophrenia from childhood home movies of the patients. *Am J Psychiatry*, **147**, 1052–6.

Waziri, R. (1996) Glycine therapy of schizophrenia: some caveats. *Biol Psychiatry*, **39** (3), 155–6.

Weinberger, D.R. (1995) From neuropathology to neurodevelopment. *Lancet*, **346**, 552–7.

Weinberger, D.R. (1996) On the plausibility of 'the neurodevelopmental hypothesis' of schizophrenia. *Neuropsychopharmacology*, **14** (3S), 1S–11S.

Weinberger, D.R., Berman, K.F. and Illowsky, B. (1988) Physiological dysfunction of dorsolateral prefrontal cortex in schizophrenia. III. A new cohort and evidence for monoaminergic mechanism. *Arch Gen Psychiatry*, **45**, 609–15.

Weinberger, D.R. and Berman, K.F. (1988) Speculation on the meaning of cerebral metabolic 'hypofrontality' in schizophrenia. *Schizophr Bull*, **14**, 157–68.

Weinberger, D.R. and Berman, K.F. (1996) Prefrontal function in schizophrenia: confounds and controversies. *Phil Trans R Soc Lond B*, **351**, 1495–503.

Weinberger, D.R., Berman, K.F., Ostrem, J.L. *et al.* (1993) Disorganization of prefrontal-hippocampal connectivity in schizophrenia: A PET studies of discordant MZ twins. *Abstr Soc Neurosci*, **19**, 7.

Weinberger, D.R., Bigelow, L.B., Kleinman, J.E. *et al.* (1980) Cerebral ventricular enlargement in chronic schizophrenia: association with poor response to treatment. *Arch Gen Psychiatry*, **37**, 11–14.

Weinberger, D.R. and Lipska, B.K. (1995) Cortical maldevelopment, antipsychotic drugs, and schizophrenia: a search for common ground. *Schizophr Res*, **16**, 87–110.

Weinberger, D.R., DeLisi, L.E., Perman, G. *et al.* (1982) Computed tomography scans in schizophreniform disorder and other acute psychiatric patients. *Arch Gen Psychiatry*, **39**, 778–83.

Wong, D.F., Wagner Jr., H.N., Tune, L.E. *et al.* (1986) Positron emission tomography reveals elevated D2 dopamine receptors in drug-naïve schizophrenics. *Science*, **234**, 1558–63.

CHAPTER 2

Is the association between obstetric complications and schizophrenia mediated by glutamatergic excitotoxic damage in the fetal/neonatal brain?

PAUL FEARON, DAVID COTTER AND ROBIN M. MURRAY

Introduction

The idea that some early onset psychotic conditions have a neurodevelopmental origin was popular a century ago (Clouston; 1891: Southard, 1915), and re-emerged in the mid-1980s (Murray *et al.*, 1985; Weinberger, 1987; Murray and Lewis, 1987). In this chapter we will briefly review the evidence that an early brain lesion can predispose an individual to the later development of schizophrenia before considering the possibility that glutamate neurotoxicity in the developing brain may be the crucial pathogenic mechanism.

Evidence of abnormal development

CHILDHOOD DYSFUNCTION

Clinical and epidemiological studies have reported a range of cognitive, personality and social functioning deficits in preschizophrenic children (Jones *et al.*, 1994; Done *et al.*, 1994; Cannon *et al.*, 1995, 1997). These studies have been extensively reviewed elsewhere (Chua and Murray, 1996; Jones and Done, 1997; Davies *et al.*, 1997) and will not be discussed further here, except to say that the findings are obviously compatible with the idea that the childhood dysfunction is secondary to an underlying brain abnormality.

NEUROLOGICAL SIGNS

An increased prevalence of 'soft' neurological signs is seen in adult schizophrenic patients; these have been associated with poor academic achievement and premorbid asociality (Quitkin *et al.*, 1976); similar neurological signs are seen in preschizophrenic children (Fish *et al.*, 1992). Walker and Lewine (1990), who examined home movies of preschizophrenic children, noted more postural and upper limb movement abnormalities than in their well siblings; these abnormalities were most noticeable in the first two years of life, and ameliorated thereafter (Walker *et al.*, 1996), raising the possibility of ongoing recovery from an early lesion.

MINOR PHYSICAL ANOMALIES

Indirect evidence implicating prenatal developmental disruption in schizophrenia comes from the reported increase in minor physical anomalies (MPAs) (Clouston, 1891; O'Callaghan *et al.*, 1991a; Green *et al.*, 1994; McGrath *et al.*, 1995) and dermatoglyphic abnormalities (Davis and Bracha, 1996; Fananas *et al.*, 1996). MPAs are trivial alterations in ectodermal development such as malformed ears or high arched palate and are thought to develop during the second trimester. Dermatoglyphic patterns are formed in the late first and second trimesters and remain unchanged thereafter. Thus, such abnormalities can be regarded as 'fossilized' evidence of developmental disruption during the period when they were formed. This corresponds to the time during which the brain, another ectodermally derived structure, is undergoing its most extensive period of development.

MPAs could be secondary to either genetic or environmental effects, but Griffiths *et al.* (1998) have shown that familial schizophrenics do not show an excess of MPAs while non-familial patients, especially males, do. This implies that they are secondary to some environmentally induced disruption of fetal development.

Obstetric complications

The overwhelming majority of studies examining the histories of schizophrenic patients have reported an excess of obstetric complications (OCs) compared to controls (McNeil and Kaij, 1978; Parnas *et al.*, 1982; Lewis and Murray, 1987; O'Callaghan *et al.*, 1992a; McNeil, 1995; McGrath and Murray, 1995; Geddes and Lawrie, 1995).

Three recent studies have been particularly convincing. First, Kendell *et al.* (1996) compared the obstetric records of 115 Scottish schizophrenics with 115 matched controls; the former were more likely to have had both pregnancy (odds ratio 6.2) and perinatal (odds ratio 18.0) complications; the highest odds ratio for any individual complication was pre-eclampsia (odds ratio 9.0). Second, in a similar study from Sweden, Hultman *et al.* (1997) showed that 82 schizophrenics were more likely to have severe obstetric complications than 214 matched controls (odds ratio 3.7). Third, Jones *et al.* (1998), who carried out a cohort study of 11 017 individuals born in north Finland in 1966, found that the 76 who developed schizophrenia were seven times more likely to have had perinatal complications and six times more likely to be premature than the remainder of the cohort. These authors calculated that the population attributable risk was 6.8% for detectable perinatal complications and 4.6% for low birth weight. The highest risk for any individual complication was for placental infarction.

HYPOXIC/ISCHAEMIC DAMAGE

McNeil (1994) has long maintained that those OCs that are associated with hypoxia (e.g. pre-eclampsia, placental infarction, preterm birth, prolonged labour, prolapsed cord) are especially common in schizophrenics. However, small sample size has limited the power of most studies to examine the effects of individual complications. Therefore, Geddes *et al.* (1999) carried out a collaborative meta-analysis of 11 studies which had used the scale of Lewis *et al.* (1989) to interview mothers retrospectively about their offsprings' gestation; data were available for 700 schizophrenics and 835 controls. The OCs particularly implicated included: low birthweight; prematurity, requiring resuscitation or being placed in an incubator; and premature rupture of membranes.

As part of the same meta-analysis, Verdoux *et al.* (1997) noted that the earlier the onset of psychosis, the more likely patients were to have suffered an OC. Thus, this study confirms previous reports that the excess of OCs is largely confined to schizophrenics with an onset before 25 years of age.

Several groups have found an association between OCs and childhood dysfunction (Walker and Neumann, 1995), especially in male preschizophrenics (Rifkin *et al.*, 1994). Neurological signs have also been reported, especially in those schizophrenics who had suffered OCs (Cantor-Graee *et al.*, 1994; Walker and Neumann, 1995).

PRENATAL VIRAL INFECTION

Schizophrenia is associated with smaller head circumference at birth (McNeil *et al.*, 1993; Rifkin *et al.*, 1994; Kunugi *et al.*, 1995; Hultman *et al.*,1997), a finding suggestive of some impairment of fetal brain growth. One possible explanation is prenatal exposure to a viral infection causing subtle damage to the fetal brain. This explanation is supported by the finding from the Finnish cohort study described above (Jones *et al.*, 1998) that maternal fever in mid–late gestation carried almost a fourfold excess risk of later schizophrenia.

The excess of late winter/early spring births among schizophrenics is well replicated (Torrey *et al.*, 1997), particularly among those schizophrenics born in urban rather than rural settings (Machon *et al.*, 1983; Takei *et al.*, 1995; O'Callaghan *et al.*, 1995; Verdoux *et al.*, 1997). Thus, any candidate viral infection should show a pattern of transmission that is facilitated by winter and by urban crowding. The epidemiology of influenza conforms to such a pattern, and some, but not all, studies have reported an increase in births of schizophrenics in the four to five months following influenza epidemics (e.g. Mednick *et al.*, 1988; O'Callaghan *et al.*, 1991b; Sham *et al.*, 1992; McGrath and Murray, 1995).

Neuroimaging

Numerous CT and MRI studies of schizophrenics have shown enlarged cerebral ventricles (Woodruff and Murray, 1994); other commonly reported findings include decrements in the volume of temporal lobe structures such as the hippocampus. Four MRI studies have reported a significant reduction in overall cortical grey matter volume of the order of 5–10% (Zipursky *et al.*, 1992; Harvey *et al.*, 1993; Pieri *et al.*, 1995; Lim *et al.*, 1995) compared to control subjects. Wright *et al.* (1999) have used pixel-based analytical methods to establish where these cortical volume decrements are most pronounced; the maximal differences between schizophrenics and controls lay in the insula and temporal poles.

Most follow-up imaging studies have suggested that these changes do not progress over time (Nasrallah *et al.*, 1986; Illowski *et al.*, 1988) though some (e.g. DeLisi *et al.*, 1992; Rapoport *et al.*, 1997) dispute this. Evidence that such findings have their origins early in life comes from occasional case reports of abnormal scans obtained prior to the onset of psychosis (O'Callaghan *et al.*, 1988). Furthermore, developmental brain lesions, such as aqueduct stenosis, arachnoid and septal cysts, and agenesis of the corpus callosum (Owens *et al.*, 1980; O'Callaghan *et al.*, 1992b) occur with excess frequency in schizophrenia.

Several studies have found an association between changes on CT and MRI and premorbid psychopathology (Weinberger *et al.*, 1980; Harvey *et al.*, 1993). Walker *et al.* (1996) have related observations made of childhood video recordings to MRI scans in schizophrenics and their healthy siblings; early childhood neuromotor defects and negative affect were associated with greater ventricular size in the adult patients.

Evidence that the changes are developmental also comes from the work of Bullmore *et al.* (1997) who reasoned that damage in the latter part of gestation would lead to loss of normal cerebral asymmetry, a decrease in the volume of white matter connecting tracts, and loss of the normal correlations in volume between different regions of the brain.

Certainly, considerable evidence shows first that schizophrenic subjects have more symmetrical brains than normals (Crow *et al.*, 1989; Bilder *et al.*, 1994: Bullmore *et al.*, 1995; Sharma *et al.*, 1995). Second, some, but not all, studies show a decrease in the volume of the corpus callosum, the largest white matter tract (Woodruff *et al.*, 1993, 1995). Third, in normal subjects, the volumes of frontal and temporal structures are highly correlated. However, such correlations are much lower in male schizophrenics, suggesting developmental dysplasia (Woodruff *et al.*, 1997; Bullmore *et al.*, 1997).

Van Os *et al.* (1997) postulated that if MRI changes are secondary to abnormalities of development during gestation, then they should be found particularly in those schizophrenics who show dermatoglyphic abnormalities. They found such a relationship in 28 male schizophrenics, between reduced total a-b ridge count and both frontal CSF and third ventricular volume, and between total finger ridge count and both total cerebral and temporal lobe volume.

Neuropathology

Macroscopic investigations of schizophrenic brains demonstrate reduced brain weight, length (Bruton *et al.*, 1990; Johnstone *et al.*, 1994) and ventricular enlargement (Pakkenberg, 1987; Bruton *et al.*, 1990). Other findings include decreased volume of the hippocampus (Bogerts *et al.*, 1985; Falkai and Bogerts, 1986; Jeste and Lohr, 1989), parahippocampal gyrus (Bogerts *et al.*, 1985; Falkai *et al.*, 1988) and parahippocampal gyrus thickness (Brown *et al.*, 1986; Altshuler *et al.*, 1990). Not all of these findings have been replicated; notably four studies have failed to find reduced hippocampal volume (Heckers *et al.*, 1990; Altshuler *et al.*, 1990; Benes *et al.*, 1991a; Bruton *et al.*, 1990). Other structures which may show volume loss include the thalamus, basal ganglia, cerebellum and brain stem (*see* review by Arnold and Trojanowski, 1996).

To date, microscopic studies have focused largely on the medial temporal and frontal cortical regions. Reductions in hippocampal pyramidal neuron number (Falkai and Bogerts, 1986; Jeste and Lohr, 1989) and size (Benes *et al.*, 1991a; Arnold *et al.*, 1995; Zaidel *et al.*, 1997) have been described, but reports of altered pyramidal neuron density have been less consistent (for review *see* Arnold and Trojanowski, 1996). The absence of fibrillary gliosis (Falkai and Bogerts, 1986; Roberts *et al.*, 1987), implies that these alterations have not arisen from an adult onset degenerative process.

Within the frontal cortex, laminar-specific reductions in neuronal and interneuronal densities (Benes *et al.*, 1986, 1991) and neuronal size (Benes *et al.*, 1991a) have been described. However, Akbarian *et al.* (1995) were unable to replicate the finding of reduced frontal neuronal density, while Selemon *et al.* (1995) reported a generalized increase in neuronal density.

Alterations in neuronal size and density are important, but they could be secondary to neuroleptic medication and fixation artefact rather than schizophrenia itself. Since alterations in lamination or orientation could not be explained thus, such findings are particularly important. Furthermore, because of the unique, orderly sequence of neuronal migration during fetal life, alterations in lamination can provide clues to the timing of any developmental deviation found.

Jakob and Beckmann (1986) reported displacement of some layer II cells of the limbic cortex into layer III and concluded that these findings represented abnormal lamination due to altered neuronal migration during the second trimester. Akbarian *et al.* (1993a, 1993b, 1996) have demonstrated more convincing abnormalities in the distribution of nicotinamide–adenine dinucleotide phosphate diaphorase (NADPH-d) in the frontal and temporal cortex of schizophrenics; this is consistent with a disturbance of either the normal pattern of programmed cell death or the orderly migration of neurons towards the cortical plate during the second or third trimesters. Other studies have demonstrated altered arrangement of neurons in the entorhinal cortex (Arnold *et al.*, 1991a), anterior cingulate (Benes *et al.*, 1986; Benes and Bird, 1987) and the prefrontal cortex (Benes *et al.*, 1991b; Anderson *et al.*, 1996).

Pyramidal cell disorientation in the CA1–prosubiculum, CA1–CA2 and CA2–CA3 interface zones (Kovelman and Scheibel, 1984; Conrad *et al.*, 1991; Zaidel *et al.*, 1997) has also been described. Scheibel and Conrad, (1993) suggested that since these interface zones represent embryologically distinct boundaries, they may be especially susceptible to developmental insult. However, these findings have not been consistently replicated (Christison *et al.*, 1989; Benes *et al.*, 1991a; Arnold *et al.*, 1995; Cotter *et al.*, 1997).

The investigation of dendrites, synapses and the adhesion characteristics of neurons in schizophrenic subjects has added a new dimension to post-mortem studies. Golgi studies have demonstrated decreased dendritic spines (Glantz and Lewis, 1995). These alterations have been confirmed in ultrastructural studies, which have shown abnormal dendritic spine clustering (Ong and Garey, 1993). Likewise, the synaptic markers GAP 43 (Perrone-Bizzozero *et al.*, 1996), synaptophysin and SNAP-35 (Glantz and Lewis, 1994; Eastwood *et al.*, 1995a), synapsin (Browning *et al.*, 1993), and the encoding mRNA for synaptophysin (Eastwood *et al.*, 1995b) are reduced in schizophrenia. The embryonic form of the neural cell adhesion molecule (NCAM) family, which is an essential trophic factor during neurodevelopment, has been found to be reduced in the hippocampus in schizophrenia (Barbeau *et al.*, 1995).

Causes of the brain abnormalities

Both genetic and early environmental factors appear to contribute to the structural brain changes found in schizophrenia. Thus, the first-degree relatives of schizophrenics are more likely to have larger lateral ventricles than controls (Weinberger *et al.*, 1981; Delisi *et al.*, 1986). Sharma *et al.* (1998) have shown that in families that are multiply affected with schizophrenia, those unaffected relatives who appear to be transmitting the disorder have similarly enlarged lateral ventricles to their affected kin. This implies that increased ventricular volume represents, in these multiply affected families at least, a marker of the genetic vulnerability to the illness.

However, imaging studies of monozygotic twins discordant for schizophrenia indicate that the ill twins show greater ventricular enlargement and smaller brains than their well co-twins (Reveley *et al.*, 1982, 1984; Suddath *et al.*, 1990). Reveley *et al.* (1982, 1984) also found that the well monozygotic co-twins displayed a degree of ventricular enlargement intermediate between that of their ill co-twins and control twins. A plausible explanation is that both members of the twin pair share a genetic predisposition to ventricular enlargement, but this is compounded by the additional effect of an early cerebral insult in the twin who becomes ill.

Obstetric complications have emerged as possible causes of this early insult. Studies of preterm infants have shown that they are at risk of hypoxia/ischaemia and resultant intra- and periventricular haemorrhage (Paneth *et al.*, 1994; Kempley *et al.*, 1996; Penrice *et al.*, 1996). The consequences of periventricular haemorrhage include ventricular enlargement and cortical and corpus callosal abnormalities (Stewart and Kirkbride, 1996; Leviton and Gilles, 1996). Recent evidence suggests that such brain abnormalities persist as the preterm individuals grow up into adolescence (Stewert and Kirkbride, 1996). Some studies of schizophrenics have found a relationship between OCs and lateral ventricular enlargement (reviewed by McGrath and Murray, 1995; Woerner *et al.*, 1997).

The question that obviously arises is how hypoxic–ischaemic damage at or before birth increases the later risk of schizophrenia. We will now review data suggesting that hypoxic/ischaemic neurotoxicity may be mediated through glutamatergic overactivity.

Glutamate in brain development

Glutamate, the major excitatory neurotransmitter within the brain (Fonnum, 1984), has two main classes of receptor. The first, the ionotropic receptor, comprises three families, namely N-methyl-D-aspartate (NMDA), amino-3-hydroxy-5-methyliso-azole-4-propionic acid (AMPA) and kainate. The second form of glutamate receptor, the metabotropic receptor, is a G-protein coupled receptor that acts through cyclic AMP or phosphoinositide.

In addition to its role as a neurotransmitter, the glutamatergic system plays central roles in synaptic remodelling, learning and neuronal maintenance, and in brain development (Mattson, 1988). Glutamate stimulates protein synthesis in developing neurons and provokes synaptic maturation (Aruffo *et al.*, 1987). NMDA receptor stimulation promotes granule cell survival (Balazs *et al.*, 1988) and neurite outgrowth (Pearce *et al.*, 1987), while non-NMDA receptor activation promotes synaptogenesis (Mattson, 1988). Furthermore, neurotrophins such as NGF, BDNF, and NT3, which play a critical role in the outgrowth of dendrites in developing neurons, require glutamate receptors in order to function normally. In short, since glutamate is involved in the regulation of neuronal development, it follows that alterations in its expression may disturb this process.

GLUTAMATE AND NEUROTOXICITY

Cerebral hypoxia and ischaemia can lead to over-stimulation of glutamate receptors in the brain and result in dysregulation of intracellular calcium homeostasis which induces neuronal injury and death (Olney, 1978). The primary cause of pre/perinatal hypoxia in the developing brain is reduced placental or pulmonary gas exchange, with superimposed chronic hypoxia worsening the outcome.

Those areas of the brain which are particularly vulnerable to excitotoxic damage in the postnatal rat, namely the hippocampus, corpus striatum and the cerebral cortex, are also the most vulnerable to hypoxic–ischaemic damage and contain large numbers of glutamate receptors (McDonald and Johnston, 1990; Trescher *et al.*, 1994). This neurotoxic effect has been well described for the three classes of ionotropic receptor, but recent evidence suggests that class I metabotropic receptors may also contribute (Bruno *et al.*, 1995). Glutamate receptor antagonists such as phenylcyclidine and dizocilpine (MK801) are known to protect against some of this damage (Lyeth *et al.*, 1989).

CRITICAL DEVELOPMENTAL PERIODS

The impact of any toxic influence on the brain depends not only on the severity and duration of the insult but also on its timing. The developing brain differs from the adult brain in having less white matter, and in having temporary structures such as the germinal matrix, and a 'subplate' zone between the immature cerebral cortex and white matter containing fetal neurons and synapses; this disappears after the sixth postnatal month. In addition, the fetal brain produces more neurons than are later necessary and about twice as many synapses are present in certain regions of the fetal cerebral cortex than in adulthood (Huttenlocher and Courten, 1987).

These extensive organizational changes within the developing brain create 'critical periods' of selective vulnerability to damage (Johnston, 1995). Consequently, hypoxia–ischaemia can lead to different neurodevelopmental outcomes depending on the exact timing of the insult. This may explain some of the variation in outcomes from cerebral palsy, epilepsy and other overt neurological deficits in cases of more severe hypoxic/ischaemic encephalopathy (Nyakas *et al.*, 1996), to the subtle neuromotor, neuropsychological, and social deficits exhibited by some preschizophrenic children.

NEURONAL VULNERABILITY

Neurons are at increased risk of neurotoxic damage during the later periods of fetal development when both they and the glutamatergic system exhibit greater functional maturity. Immature neurons require less energy because of their low level of differentiation (Bickler *et al.*, 1993). However, during the second trimester and perinatal period, neurons require increasing amounts of energy for proliferation, migration and differentiation. The increased sensitivity of the glutamatergic system also makes the perinatal period a time of particular vulnerability to hypoxic/ischaemic injury (Slotkin *et al.*, 1986). While immature neurons survive prolonged hypoxia in the absence of glutamatergic synapses, the development of such synapses heralds neuronal death under hypoxic conditions (Rothman, 1983). The density and functional reactivity of postsynaptic cortical NMDA receptors in the rat is enhanced in the early postnatal period (McDonald *et al.*, 1990; Kumar *et al.*, 1994).

These immature NMDA receptors conduct greater amounts of calcium, are more easily stimulated by glycine (a co-agonist with glutamate at these receptors), and are less easily blocked by magnesium than the adult receptor (Barnashev *et al.*, 1992; Burgard and Habitz, 1993; Kato and Yoshimura, 1993; Sheng *et al.*, 1994). Therefore, their presence makes the immature brain vulnerable to pathological enhancement of glutamate release during hypoxia/ischaemia. Fortunately, presynaptic glutamatergic release in response to hypoxia /ischaemia is reduced in the immature brain (Cherici *et al.*, 1991) and this may provide some protection from the increased postsynaptic sensitivity to glutamatergic activity.

Glutamate in schizophrenia

Dysfunction of the glutamatergic system was first proposed as a causal factor in schizophrenia by Kim and colleagues (1980) following their report of reduced amounts of glutamate in the cerebrospinal fluid in schizophrenic subjects. Although this finding was not replicated (Perry, 1982), research into the role of glutamate was given impetus by the discovery that the NMDA receptor antagonist phenylcyclidine (PCP) (Lodge *et al.*, 1987), and indeed a range of other NMDA receptor antagonists (Kristensen *et al.*, 1992; Grotta, 1994), can produce schizophrenia-like symptoms in normal subjects.

Post-mortem investigations provided further evidence of glutamatergic abnormalities in schizophrenia. Kerwin *et al.*, (1988) found a loss of non-NMDA glutamatergic kainate receptors in the hippocampus and later localized this finding to the CA4 and CA3 subregions (Kerwin *et al.*, 1990). Brain regions other than the hippocampus have also been examined with increased kainate and aspartate (a marker for glutamatergic neurons) binding described in the frontal cortex (Deakin *et al.*, 1989).

With the cloning of several mRNAs encoding the non-NMDA glutamatergic receptors in rat brain, these mRNAs were investigated in schizophrenia. There is a loss of the non-NMDA mRNA in the hippocampus (Harrison *et al.*, 1991), which specifically involves mRNA for both the GluR1 and GluR2 AMPA-preferring non-NMDA receptor genes (Eastwood *et al.*, 1995a). Akbarian and colleagues (1996) investigated the expression pattern of five mRNAs for NMDA receptor subunits by in-situ hybridization (NR1/NR2A-D) in prefrontal, parietotemporal and cerebellar cortex. They found elevated expression solely of the NR2D subunit family in the prefrontal area, and interpreted the findings as evidence against a generalized deficit in NMDA mediated neurotransmission. Because the NR2D subunit is required for the formation of neuronal and synaptic connections in situations of reduced presynaptic activity (as in immature synapses), Akbarian and colleagues suggested that their findings might be related to diminished frontal activation in schizophrenia.

There is thus a substantial body of evidence demonstrating changes in glutamatergic transmission in schizophrenia. The best replicated are those alterations in the hippocampus, wherein diminished NMDA modulatory site binding and non-NMDA receptor and gene expression have been described.

How do glutamatergic changes relate to schizophrenic symptoms?

Olney and Farber (1995) have proposed a theory of NMDA receptor hypofunction that they claim can account for many of the features of schizophrenia. They hypothesize that a reduction of NMDA receptors, particularly in the corticolimbic regions, results in a reduction of inhibitory modulation (via reduced glutamate-dependent GABA activity), producing an effective overstimulation of certain pathways in the brain which leads to schizophrenic symptoms. In support of their theory, they point out that those NMDA antagonists that produce psychotic symptoms also cause degenerative changes in the corticolimbic regions of the brain in rats.

As mentioned above, the NMDA receptor is critical for the normal development of systems of neurons. At about the eighth month of gestation, the maximum number of axonal–dendritic spines is glutamatergic. If the NMDA receptor is then blocked, the migration of neurons along the radial glia is inhibited. Thus, an excitotoxic event such as hypoxia could lead to a loss of NMDA receptor-bearing GABAergic neurons, thus causing faulty or arrested migration of such neurons.

In Olney and Faber's model, the early defect remains quiescent until corticolimbic circuits form their adult connections in adolescence. At this point, the receptor hypofunction on GABA neurons manifests itself as a reduction of the usual inhibitory tone to parts of the corticolimbic system, thus producing overstimulation. Intriguingly, Farber *et al.* (1992, 1995) have demonstrated that prepubertal rats are insensitive to the neurotoxic effects of NMDA antagonists, a finding mirrored by the relative rarity of psychosis induced by ketamine (a short-acting dissociative anaesthetic agent with phenylcyclidine-receptor binding properties) in prepubertal children. Perhaps some key maturational event during adolescence renders the brain vulnerable to the effects of NMDA receptor hypofunction.

Hippocampal damage

Lipska and colleagues, using a model in which rats have undergone a hippocampal excitotoxic lesion in the early neonatal period, have shown that this relatively circumscribed lesion can produce more widespread cortical effects involving deafferentation of other cortical and subcortical sites from their usual hippocampal connections (Lipska *et al.*, 1993; Lipska and Weinberger, 1993; Weinberger and Lipska, 1995). They suggest that the animal suffers a deficit in glutamatergic neurons emanating from the hippocampal formation and grows into a condition of dopamine stress hyper-responsivity. Prior to puberty, these developmentally disconnected rats show no signs of limbic or striatal dopaminergic malfunction. However, shortly after the onset of puberty, they show exaggerated exploratory behaviour after exposure to environmental stress and to amphetamine, suggestive of hyper-responsiveness of limbic dopamine systems. This appears to be independent of gonadal hormonal changes (Lipska and Weinberger, 1994). They speculate that this delayed onset of abnormal activity until adolescence may be due to a critical developmental milestone that occurs during or after puberty, perhaps involving greater cortical control of dopamine as the intracortical circuitry matures.

The attractions of this model are that it mimics the hippocampal damage postulated to result from pre- or perinatal hypoxia in some cases of schizophrenia. As early as 1970, Mednick suggested that hippocampal damage, secondary to perinatal hypoxic–ischaemic damage, could predispose individuals to later schizophrenia. However, it is only recently that researchers have tested this hypothesis. Stefanis *et al.* (1999) carried out MRI scans on 21 schizophrenics without a history of OCs who came from multiply affected families (in whom genetic factors can be presumed to play an overwhelming role) and 26 schizophrenics without any family history of psychosis but with a history of severe OCs. The former group showed no decrement in hippocampal volume compared to 26 control subjects, but the latter had significantly smaller hippocampi, especially on the left. Thus, hippocampal volume reduction in schizophrenia appears to be determined by hypoxic–ischaemic damage rather than abnormal genes; the fact that only a minority of schizophrenics have suffered such damage provides one explanation why reduction in hippocampal volume has only been found in some series of schizophrenics (*vide supra*).

Conclusions

Thus, an initial glutamatergic excitotoxic event in early development could account for some of the neurobiological features of schizophrenia. These could come about through direct cell damage/death at the time of the initial insult, or as a consequence of altered glutamatergic activation which may occur thereafter, since the latter is known to be central to the normal development, migration and connectivity of neurons.

Furthermore, microtubule assembly, which dictates neuronal cytoarchitecture (Nunez, 1986) is activated by glutamate-dependent phosphorylation (Bigot *et al.*, 1991). It is therefore possible that the reduced MAP2 and MAP5 expression in the subiculum and entorrhinal cortex (Arnold *et al.*, 1991b), and elevated expression of non-phosphorylated MAP2 in the left subiculum (Cotter *et al.*, 1997), could be the manifestation of altered glutamatergic function.

Given the crucial role of glutamate, GABA and dopamine as neurotransmitters in the adult, any disruption of the balance between them is likely to have profound consequences not only for the development, but also ultimately for the functioning of the adult brain.

It is unlikely that any single mechanism will account for all cases of schizophrenia. However, the concept of a fetal or perinatal glutamatergic excitotoxic event causing altered neuronal circuitry is consistent with the known neurochemical and neuropathological findings in the adult schizophrenic brain, and it allows for a latency period between the initial insult and subsequent first psychotic episode.

References

Akbarian, S., Bunney, W.E., Potkin, S.G. *et al.* (1993a) Altered distribution of nicotinamide-adenosine dinucleotide phosphate-diaphorase cells in frontal lobe of schizophrenics implies disturbances of cortical development. *Arch Gen Psychiatry*, **50**, 169–77.

Akbarian, S., Vinuela, A., Kim, J.J. *et al.* (1993b) Distorted distribution of nicotinamide-adenosine dinucleotide phosphate-diaphorase cells in temporal lobe of schizophrenics implies anomalous cortical development. *Arch Gen Psychiatry* **50**, 178–87.

Akbarian, S., Kim, J.J., Potkin, S.G. *et al.* (1995) Gene expression for glutamic acid decarboxylase is reduced without loss of neurons in prefrontal cortex of schizophrenics. *Arch Gen Psychiatry*, **52**(4); 258–66.

Akbarian, S., Kim, J.J., Potkin, S.G., Hetrick, W.P., Bunney, W.E. and Jones, E.G. (1996) Maldistribution of interstitial neurons in prefrontal white matter of the brains of schizophrenic patients. *Arch Gen Psychiatry*, **53**(5), 425–36.

Altshuler, L., Conrad, A., Kovelman, J.A. and Scheibel, A.B. (1987) Hippocampal pyramidal cell orientation in schizophrenia. *Arch Gen Psychiatry*, **44**, 994–8.

Altshuler, L.L., Casanova, M.F., Goldberg, T.E. and Kleinman, J.E. (1990) The hippocampus and parahippocampus in schizophrenia, suicide, and control brains. *Arch Gen Psychiatry*, **47**(11), 1029–34.

Anderson, S., Volk, D. and Lewis, D.A. (1996) Increased density of microtubule associated protein immunoreactive neurons in the prefrontal white matter of schizophrenic subjects. *Schizophr Res*, **19**, 1211–19.

Arnold, S.E., Hyman, B.T., Hoesen, G.W.V. and Damasio, A.R. (1991a) Some cytoarchitectural abnormalities of the entorhinal cortex in schizophrenia. *Arch Gen Psychiatry*, **48**, 625–32.

Arnold, S.E., Lee, V.M.Y., Gur, R.E. and Trojanowski, J.Q. (1991b) Abnormal expression of two microtubule associated proteins (MAP2 and MAP5) in specific subfields of the hippocampal formation in schizophrenia. *Proc Natl Acad Sci USA*, **88**, 10850–4.

Arnold, S.E., Franz, B.R., Gur, R.C. *et al.* (1995) Smaller interneuron size in schizophrenia in hippocampal subfields that mediate cortical-hippocampal interactions. *Am J Psychiatry* **152**, 738–48.

Arnold, S.E. and Trojanowski, J.Q. (1996) Recent advances in defining the neuropathology of schizophrenia. *Acta Neuropath*, **92**, 217–31.

Aruffo, C., Ferszt, R., Hildebraudt, A.G. and Cervos Navarro, J. (1987) Low doses of L-monosodium glutamate promote neuronal growth and differentiation *in vitro. Dev Neurosci*, **9**, 228–39.

Balazs, R., Jorgensen, O.S. and Hack, N. (1988) *N*-methyl-D-aspartate promotes the survival of cerebellar granule cells in culture. *Neuroscience*, **27**, 437–51.

Barbeau, D., Liang, J.J., Robitaille, Y., Quirion, R. and Srivastava, L.K. (1995) Decreased expression of the embryonic form of the neural cell adhesion molecule in schizophrenic brains. *Proc Natl Acad Sci USA*, **92**, 2785–9.

Barnashev, N., Schoepfer, R., Monyer, H. *et al.* (1992) Control by asparagine residues of calcium permeability and magnesium blockade in the NMDA receptor. *Science*, **257**, 1415–19.

Benes, F.M., Davidson, J. and Bird, E.D. (1986) Quantitative cytoarchitectural studies of the cerebral cortex of schizophrenics. *Arch Gen Psychiatry*, **43**, 31–5.

Benes, F.M. and Bird, E.D. (1987) An analysis of the arrangement of neurons in the cingulate cortex of schizophrenic patients. *Arch Gen Psychiatry*, **44**, 608–16.

Benes, F.M., Sorensen, I. and Bird, E.D. (1991a) Reduced neuronal size in posterior hippocampus of schizophrenic patients. *Schizophr Bull*, **17**(4), 597–608.

Benes, F.M., McSparren, J., Bird, E.D., San Giovanni, J.P. and Vincent, S. L. (1991b) Deficits in small interneurons in prefrontal and cingulate cortices of schizophrenic and schizoaffective patients. *Arch Gen Psychiatry*, **48**, 996–1001.

Bickler, P.E., Gallego, S.M. and Hansen, B.M. (1993) Developmental changes in intracellular calcium regulation in rat cerebral cortex during hypoxia. *J Cereb Blood Flow Metab*, **13**(5), 811–9.

Bigot, D., Matus, A. and Hunt, S.P. (1991) Reorganisation of the cytoskeleton in rat neurons following stimulation with excitatory amino acids in vitro. *Eur J Neurosci*, **3**, 551–8.

Bilder, R.M., Wu, H., Bogerts, B. *et al.* (1994) Abnormal cortical asymmetry and sulcal prominence are independent predictors of schizophrenia. *Schizophr Res*, **11**, 131.

Bogerts, B., Meertz, E. and Schonfeldt-Bausch, R. (1985) Basal ganglia and limbic system pathology in schizophrenia: a morphometric study of brain volume and shrinkage. *Arch Gen Psychiatry*, **42**, 784–91.

Brown, R., Colter, N., Corsellis, J.A.N. *et al.* (1986) Postmortem evidence of structural brain changes in schizophrenia: differences in brain weight, temporal horn area, and parahippocampal gyrus compared with affective disorder. *Arch Gen Psychiatry*, **43**, 36–42.

Browning, M.D., Dudeck, E.M., Rapier, J.L., Leonard, S. and Freedman, R. (1993) Significant reductions in synapsin but not synaptophysin specific activity in the brains of some schizophrenics. *Biol Psychiatry*, **34**, 528–35.

Bruno, V., Copani, A., Knopfel, T. *et al.* (1995) Activation of metabotropic glutamate receptors coupled to inositol phospholipid hydrolysis amplifies NMDA-induced neuronal degeneration in cultured cortical cells. *Neuropharmacology*, **34**(8), 1089–98.

Bruton, C.J., Crow, T.J., Frith, C.D., Johnstone, E.C., Owens, D.G.C. and Roberts, G.W.(1990) Schizophrenia and the brain: A prospective clinico-neuropathological study. *Psychol Med* **20**, 285–304.

Bullmore, E., Brammer, M., Harvey, I., Murray, R.M. and Ron, M. (1995) Cerebral hemispheric asymmetry revisited: effects of handedness, gender and schizophrenia measured by radius of gyration in magnetic resonance images. *Psychol Med*, **25**, 349–63.

Bullmore, E.T., O'Connell, P., Frangou, S. and Murray, R.M. (1997) Schizophrenia as a developmental disorder of neural network integrity: the dysplastic net hypothesis. In M.S. Keshavan and R.H. Murray (eds), *Neurodevelopment and adult psychopathology*. Cambridge: Cambridge University Press, 253–66.

Burgard, E.C. and Habitz, J.J. (1993) Developmental changes in NMDA and non-NMDA receptor-mediated synaptic potentials in rat neocortex. *Dev Brain Res*, **56**, 257–62.

Cannon, M., Kargin, M., Jones, P.B., Hollis, C. and Murray, R.M. (1995) Predictors of adult psychosis in children who present to a child psychiatry clinic. *Schizophr Res*, **15**, 191.

Cannon, M., Jones, P.B., Gilvarry, C. *et al.* (1997) Premorbid social functioning in schizophrenia and bipolar disorder: similarities and differences. *Am J Psychiatry*, **154**(11), 1544–50.

Cantor-Graee,E., McNeil, T.F., Nordstrom, L. G. and Rosenlund, T. (1994) Obstetric complications and their relationship to other etiological risk factors in schizophrenia: a case control study. *J Nerv Ment Dis*, **182**, 645–50.

Cherici G., Alesiani, M., Pellegrini-Giampietro, E. and Moroni, F. (1991) Ischaemia does not induce the release of excitotoxic amino acids from the hippocampus of newborn rats. *Dev Brain Res*, **60**, 235–40.

Christison, G.W., Casanova, M.F., Weinberger, D.F., Rawlings, R. and Kleinman, J.E. (1989) A quantitative investigation of hippocampal pyramidal cell size, shape and variation of orientation in schizophrenia. *Arch Gen Psychiatry*, **46**, 1027–32

Chua, S.E. and Murray, R.M. (1996) The neurodevelopmental theory of schizophrenia: evidence concerning structure and neuropsychology. *Acta Neuropsychiatrica*, **8**(2), 25–34.

Clouston, T.S. (1891) *The neuroses of development*. Edinburgh: Oliver & Boyd.

Conrad, A.J., Abebe, T., Ron, A., Forsythe, S. and Scheibel, B. (1991) Hippocampal pyramidal cell disarray in schizophrenia as a bilateral phenomenon. *Arch Gen Psychiatry*, **48**, 413–17.

Cotter, D., Doshi, B., Kerwin, R. and Everall. I. (1997) Alterations in hippocampal non-phosphorylated MAP2 protein expression in schizophrenia. *Brain Res.* **765**(2), 238–46.

Crow, T.J., Ball, J., Bloom, S.R. *et al.* (1989) Schizophrenia as an anomaly of development of cerebral asymmetry. A postmortem study and a proposal concerning the genetic basis of the disease. *Arch Gen Psychiatry*, **46**(12), 1145–50.

Davies, N., Russell, A., Jones, P.B. and Murray, R.M. (1997) What characteristics of schizophrenia predate psychosis? *J Psychiat Res*, 32(3–4), 121–31.

Davis, J.O. and Bracha, H.S. (1996) Prenatal growth markers in schizophrenia: A monozygotic co-twin control study. *Am J Psychiatry*, 153(9), 1166–72.

Deakin, J.F.W., Simpson, M.D.C., Gilchrist, A.C. *et al.* (1989) Frontal cortical and left temporal glutamatergic dysfunction in schizophrenia. *J Neurochem*, 52, 1781–6.

DeLisi, L.E., Goldin, L.R., Hamovit, J.R., Maxwell, M.E., Kurtz, D. and Gershon, E.S. (1986) A family study of the association of increased ventricular size with schizophrenia. *Arch Gen Psychiatry*, 43(2): 148–53.

DeLisi, L.E., Stritzke, P., Riordan, H. *et al.* (1992) The timing of brain morphological changes in schizophrenia and their relationship to clinical outcome. *Biol Psychiatry* 31(3), 241–54.

Done, D.J., Crow, T.J., Johnstone, E.C. and Sacker, A. (1994) Childhood antecedents of schizophrenia and affective illness. *Br Med J*, 309, 699–703.

Eastwood, S.L., McDonald, B., Burnet, P.W.J., Beckwith, J.P., Kerwin, R.W. and Harrison, P.J. (1995a) Decreased expression of mRNAs encoding non-NMDA glutamate receptors GluR1 and GluR2 in medial temporal lobe neurons in schizophrenia. *Mol Brain Res*, 29, 211–23.

Eastwood, S.L., Burnet, P.J. and Harrison, P.J. (1995b) Altered synaptophysin expression as a marker of synaptic pathology in schizophrenia. *Neuroscience*, 66, 201–6.

Falkai, P. and Bogerts, B. (1986) Cell loss in the hippocampus of schizophrenics. *Eur Arch Psychiat Neurol Sci*, 236, 154–61.

Falkai, P., Bogerts, B. and Rozumek, M. (1988) Limbic pathology in schizophrenia: the internal region-a morphometric study. *Biol. Psychiatry*, 24, 515–21.

Fananas, L., Van Os, J. and Murray, R.M. (1996) Dermatoglyphic a-b ridge count as a possible marker for developmental insult in schizophrenia: replication in two samples. *Schizophr Res*, 20, 307–14.

Farber, N.B., Price, M.T., Labruyere, J., Fuller, T.A. and Olney, J.W. (1992) Age dependency of NMDA antagonistic neurotoxicity. *Soc Neurosci Abstr* 18, 1148.

Farber, N.B., Wozniak, D.F., Price, M.T. *et al.* (1995) Age specific neurotoxicity in the rat associated with NMDA receptor blockade: potential relevance to schizophrenia? *Biol Psychiatry*, 38(12), 788–96.

Fish, B., Marcus, J., Hans, S.L., Auerbach, J.G. and Perdue, S. (1992) Infants at risk for schizophrenia: sequelae of genetic neurointegrative defect. *Arch Gen Psychiatry* 49, 221–35.

Fonnum, F. (1984) Glutamate: a neurotransmitter in mammalian brain. *J Neurochem*, 42(1), 1–11.

Geddes, J.R. and Lawrie, S.M. (1995) Obstetric complications and schizophrenia: a meta-analysis. *Br J Psychiatry*, 167(6), 786–93.

Geddes, J.R., Verdoux, H., Takei, N., Lawrie, S.M. and Murray, R.M. (1999) Individual patient data meta-analysis of the association between schizophrenia and abnormalities of pregnancy and labour. *Schizophr Bull*, (in press).

Glantz, L.A. and Lewis, D.A. (1994) Synaptophysin and not RAB3A is specifically reduced in the prefrontal cortex of schizophrenic subjects. *Soc Neurosci Abstr*, 20, 622.

Glantz, L.A. and Lewis, D.A. (1995) Assessment of spine density on layer III pyramidal cells in the prefrontal cortex of schizophrenic subjects. *Soc Neurosci Abstr*, 21, 239.

Green, M.F., Bracha, H.S., Satz,P. and Christenson, C.D. (1994) Preliminary evidence for an association between minor physical anomalies and second trimester neurodevelopment in schizophrenia. *Psychiat Res*, 53(2): 119–27.

Griffiths, T.D., Sigmunsson, T., Takei, N., Rowe, D. and Murray, R.M. (1998) Neurological abnormalities in familial and sporadic schizophrenia. *Brain*, 121(2), 191–203.

Grotta, J. (1994) Safety and tolerability of the glutamate receptor antagonist CGS 19755 in acute stroke patients. *Stroke*, 25, 255.

Harrison, P., McLaughlin, D. and Kerwin, R.W. (1991) Decreased hippocampal expression of a glutamate receptor gene in schizophrenia. *Lancet*, **337**, 450–2.

Harvey, I., Ron, M.A., Du Boulay, G., Wicks, D., Lewis, S.W. and Murray, R.M. (1993) Reduction of cortical volume in schizophrenia on magnetic resonance imaging. *Psychol Med*, **23**(3), 591–604.

Heckers, S., Heinsen Y.C. and Beckmann, H. (1990) Limbic structures and lateral ventricles in schizophrenia: a quantitative postmortem study. *Arch Gen Psychiatry*, **47**, 1016–22.

Hultman, C.M., Ohman, A., Cnattingius, S., Wieselgren, I.M. and Lindstrom, L.H. (1997) Prenatal and neonatal risk factors for schizophrenia. *Br J Psychiatry*, **170**, 128–33.

Huttenlocher, P.R. and Courten, C. (1987) The development of synapses in striate cortex of man. *Hum Neurobiol*, **6**, 1–9.

Illowsky, B., Juliano, D.M., Bigelow, L.B. and Weinberger, D.R. (1988) Stability of CT scan findings in schizophrenia. *J Neurol Neurosurg Psychiatry*, **51**, 209–13.

Ishimaru, M., Kurumagi, A. and Toru, M. (1994) Increases in strychnine-insensitive glycine binding sites in cerebral cortex of chronic schizophrenics: evidence for glutamate hypothesis. *Biol Psychiatry*, **35**, 84–95.

Jacob, H. and Beckmann, H. (1986) Prenatal development disturbances in the limbic allocortex in schizophrenics. *J Neural Trans*, **65**, 303–26.

Jeste, D.V. and Lohr, J.B. (1989) Hippocampal pathologic findings in schizophrenia: a morphometric study. *Arch Gen Psychiatry*, **46**, 1019–24.

Johnstone, E.C., Bruton, C.J., Crow, T.J., Frith, C.D. and Owens, D.G. (1994) Clinical correlates of postmortem brain changes in schizophrenia: decreased brain weight and length correlate with indices of early impairment. *J Neurol Neurosurg Psychiatry*, **57**(4), 474–9.

Johnston, M. (1995) Neurotransmitters and vulnerability of the developing brain. *Brain Dev*, **17**, 301–6.

Jones, P.B., Rodgers, B., Murray, R.M. and Marmot, M.(1994) Child developmental risk factors for schizophrenia. *Lancet* **344**, 1398–402.

Jones, P. and Done, J. (1997) From birth to onset: a developmental perspective of schizophrenia in two national birth cohorts. In M.S. Keshavan and R.M. Murray (eds), *Neurodevelopmental origins of psychopathology*, Cambridge: Cambridge University Press, 119–53.

Jones, P., Rantakallio, P., Hartikainen, A.L., Isohanni, M. and Sipila, P. (1998) Schizophrenia as a long-term outcome of pregnancy, delivery, and perinatal complications: a 28-year follow-up of the 1966 north Finland general population birth cohort. *Am J Psychiatry*, **155**(3), 355–64.

Kato, N. and Yoshimura, H. (1993) Reduced Mg^{2+} block of NMDA receptor-mediated synaptic potentials in developing visual cortex. *Proc Natl Acad Sci USA*, **90**, 7114–18.

Kempley, S.T., Vyas, S., Bower, S., Nicolaides, K.H. and Gamsu, H. (1996) Cerebral and renal artery blood flow velocity before and after birth. *Early Hum Dev*, **46**(1–2), 165–74.

Kendell, R.E., Juszczak,E. and Cole, S.K. (1996) Obstetric complications and schizophrenia: a case control study based on standardised obstetric records. *Br J Psychiatry*, **168**(5), 556–61.

Kerwin, R.W., Patel, S., Meldrum, B.S., Czudek, C. and Reynolds, G.P. (1988) Asymmetrical loss of glutamate receptor subtype in left hippocampus in schizophrenia. *Lancet* **i**, 583–4.

Kerwin, R.W., Patel, S. and Meldrum, B.S. (1990) Autoradiographic localisation of the glutamate receptor system in control and schizophrenic post-mortem hipppocampal formation. *Neuroscience*, **39**, 25–32.

Kim, J.S., Kornhuber, H.H., Schmid-Burgk, W. and Holzmuller, B. (1980) Low cerebrospinal fluid glutamate in schizophrenia patients and a new hypothesis in schizophrenia. *Neurosci Lett*, **20**, 379–82.

Kovelman, J.A. and Scheibel, A.B. (1984) A neurohistological correlate of schizophrenia. *Biol Psychiatry*, **19**, 1601–21.

Kristensen, J.D., Svennson, B. and Gordh, T. (1992) The NMDA-receptor antagonist CPP abolishes neurogenic 'wind-up' pain after intrathecal administration in humans. *Pain*, **51**, 249–53.

Kornhuber, J., Mack-Burkhardt, F., Riederer, P. *et al.* (1989) [³H]MK-801 binding sites in postmortem brain regions of schizophrenic patients. *J Neural Transm*, **77**, 231–6.

Kumar, A., Schliebs, R. and Bigl, V. (1994) Postnatal development of NMDA, AMPA and kainate receptors in individual layers of rat visual cortex and the effect of monocular deprivation. *Int J Dev Neurosci*, **12**, 31–41.

Kunugi, H., Takei, N., Murray, R.M., Saito, K. and Nanko, S. (1995) Small head circumference at birth in schizophrenia. *Schizophr Res*, **20**, 165–70.

Leviton, A. and Gilles, F. (1996) Ventriculomegaly, delayed myelination, white matter hypoplasia, and 'periventricular' leukomalacia: how are they related? *Pediatr Neurol*, **15**(2), 127–36.

Lewis, S.W. and Murray, R.M. (1987) Obstetric complications, neurodevelopmemtal deviance and risk of schizophrenia. *J Psychiatr Res*, **21**, 413–21.

Lewis, S.W., Owen, M.J. and Murray, R.M. (1989) Obstetric complications and schizophrenia; methodology and mechanisms. In: S.C. Schulz and C.A. Tamminga (eds), *Schizophrenia: a scientific focus*, New York: Oxford University Press, 56–68.

Lim, K., Tew, W., Koshner, M. *et al.* (1995) Cortical grey matter volume deficit is present in first episode schizophrenia. *Schizophr Res*, **15**, 95–6.

Lipska, B.K. and Weinberger, D.R. (1993) Delayed effects of neonatal hippocampal damage on haloperidol-induced catalepsy and apomorphine-induced stereotypic behaviors in the rat. *Dev Brain Res*, **75**, 213–22.

Lipska, B.K., Jaskiw,G.E. and Weinberger, D.R. (1993) Postpubertal emergence of hyper-responsiveness to stress and amphetamine after neonatal excitotoxic damage. *Neuropsychopharmacology*, **9**, 67–75.

Lipska, B.K. and Weinberger, D.R. (1994) Gonadectomy does not prevent novelty or drug-induced motor hyperresponsiveness in rats with neonatal hippocampal damage. *Dev Brain Res*, **78**, 253–8.

Lodge, D., Aram, J.A., Church J. *et al.* (1987) Excitatory amino acids and phenylcyclidine-like drugs. In T.P. Hicks, D. Lodge, and H. McLennan (eds), *Excitatory amino acid transmission*. New York: Alan R. Liss, 83–90.

Lyeth, B.G., Jenkins, L.W., Ham, R.J. *et al.* (1989) Pretreatment with MK-801 reduces behavioural deficits following traumatic brain injury. *Abst Soc Neurosci*, **15**, 113.

Machon, R.A., Mednick, S.A. and Schulsinger, F. (1983) The interaction of seasonality, place of birth, genetic risk and subsequent schizophrenia in a high risk sample [published erratum appears in *Br J Psychiatry* 1987 Jul;**151**,124] *Br J Psychiatry*, **143**, 383–8.

Mattson, M.P. (1988) Neurotransmitters in the regulation of neuronal cytoarchitecture. *Brain Res Rev*, **13**, 179–212.

McDonald, J.W. and Johnston, M.V. (1990) Physiological and pathophysiological roles of excitatory amino acids during central nervous system development. *Brain Res Rev*, **15**, 41–70.

McDonald, J.W., Johnston M.V. and Young, A.B. (1990) Differential ontogenic development of three receptors comprising the NMDA receptor/channel complex in the rat hippocampus. *Exp Neurol*, **110**, 237–47.

McGrath, J.J., van Os, J., Hoyos, C., Jones, P.B., Harvey, I. and Murray, R.M. (1995) Minor physical anomalies in the functional psychoses: associations with clinical and putative aetiological variables. *Schizophr Res*, **18**, 9–20.

McGrath, J. and Murray, R.M. (1995) Risk factors for schizophrenia; from conception to birth. In S. Hirsch and D. Weinberger (eds), *Schizophrenia*. Oxford: Blackwell Science, 187–205.

McNeil, T.F. and Kaij, L. (1978) Obstetric factors in the development of schizophrenia: complications in the births of preschizophrenics and in reproductions by schizophrenic parents. In L.C. Wynne, R.L. Cromwell and S. Matthysse (eds), *The nature of schizophrenia: new approaches to research and treatment.* New York: John Wiley, 401–29.

McNeil, T.F., Cantor-Graae, E., Norstrom, L.G. and Rosenlund, T. (1993) Head circumference in 'preschizophrenic' and normal controls. *Br J Psychiatry*, **153**, 191–7.

McNeil, T.F. (1994) Presentation at the seventh congress of the Association of European Psychiatrists.

McNeil, T.F. (1995) Perinatal risk factors and schizophrenia. Selective review and methodological concerns. *Epidemiol Rev*, **17**, 107–12.

Mednick, S., Machon, R.A. and Huttunen, M.O. (1988) Adult schizophrenia following prenatal exposure to an influenza epidemic. *Arch Gen Psychiatry*, **45**, 189–92.

Murray, R.M., Lewis, S.W. and Reveley, A.M. (1985) Towards an aetiological classification of schizophrenia. *Lancet*, **i**, 1023–6.

Murray, R.M. and Lewis, S.W. (1987) Is schizophrenia a neurodevelopmental disorder? *Br Med J*, **295**, 681-2.

Nasrallah, H.A., Olson,S.C., McCalley, W.M., Chapman, S. and Jacoby, C.G. (1986) Cerebral ventricular enlargement in schizophrenia. A preliminary follow-up study. *Arch Gen Psychiatry*, **43**(2), 157–9.

Nunez, J. (1986) Differential expression of microtubule components during brain development. *Dev Neurosci*, **8**, 125–41.

Nyakas, C., Buwalda, B. and Luiten, P.G. (1996) Hypoxia and brain development. *Prog Neurobiol*, **49**(1), 1–51.

O'Callaghan E., Larkin, C., Redmond, O., Stack, J., Ennis, J.T. and Waddington, J.L. (1988) 'Early onset schizophrenia' after teenage head injury. A case report with magnetic resonance imaging. *Br J Psychiatry*, **153**, 394–6.

O'Callaghan, E., Larkin, C., Kinsella, A. and Waddington, J.L. (1991a) Familial, obstetric, and other clinical correlates of minor physical anomalies in schizophrenia. *Am J Psychiatry,* **148**, 479–83.

O'Callaghan, E., Sham, P., Takei, N., Glover, G. and Murray, R.M. (1991b) Schizophrenia after prenatal exposure to 1957 A2 influenza epidemic. *Lancet*, **i**, 1248–50.

O'Callaghan, E., Gibson, T., Colohan, H.A. *et al.* (1992a) Risk of schizophrenia in adults born after obstetric complications and their association of early onset of illness. *Br Med J*, **305**, 1256–9.

O'Callaghan, E., Buckley, P., Redmond, O., Stack, J., Ennis, J.T., Larkin, C. and Waddington, J.L. (1992b) Abnormalities of cerebral structure in schizophrenia on magnetic resonance imaging: interpretation in relation to the neurodevelopmental hypothesis. *J Royal Soc Med*, **85**, 227–31.

O'Callaghan, E., Cotter, D., Colgan, K., Larkin, C., Walsh, D. and Waddington, J.L. Confinement of winter birth excess in schizophrenia to the urban-born and its gender specificity. (1995) *Br J Psychiatry*, **166**(1), 51–4.

Olney, J.W. (1978) Neurotoxicity of excitatory amino acids. In E.G. McGeer, J.W. Olney, and P.L. McGeer (eds), *Kainic acid as a tool in neurobiology.* New York: Raven Press, 95–121.

Olney, J.W. and Farber, N.B. (1995) Glutamate receptor dysfunction and schizophrenia. *Arch Gen Psychiatry* **52**, 998–1007.

Ong, W.Y. and Garey, L.J. (1993) Ultrastructural features of biopsied temporopolar cortex (area 38) in a case of schizophrenia. *Schizophr Res*, **10**, 15–27.

Owens, D.G.C., Johnstone E.C., Bydder, G.M. *et al.* (1980) Unsuspected organic disease in chronic schizophrenia demonstrated by computed tomography. *J Neurol Neurosurg Psychiat*, **43**, 1065–70.

Pakkenberg, B. (1987) Post-mortem study of chronic schizophrenic brains. *Br J Psychiatry*, **151**, 744–52.

Paneth, N., Pinto-Martin, J., Gardiner, J. *et al.* (1993) Incidence and timing of germinal matrix/intraventricular hemorrhage in low birth weight infants. *Am J Epidemiol*, **137**(11), 1167–76.

Parnas, J., Schulsinger, F., Teasdale, T.W., Schulzinger, H., Feldman, P.M. and Mednick, S.A. (1982) Perinatal complications and clinical outcome within the schizophrenia spectrum. *Br J Psychiatry*, **140**, 416–20.

Pearce, I.A., Cambray-Deakin, M.A. and Burgoyne, R.D. (1987) Glutamate acting on NMDA receptors stimulates neurite outgrowth from cerebellar granule cells. *FEBS Lett*, **223**, 143–7.

Penrice, J., Cady, E.B., Lorek A. *et al.* (1996) Proton magnetic resonance spectroscopy of the brain in normal preterm and term infants, and early changes after perinatal hypoxia-ischemia. *Pediatr Res*, **40**(1), 6–14.

Perrone-Bizzozero, N.A., Sower A.C., Bird, E.D., Benowitz, L.I. and Ivins, K.J. (1996) Levels of the growth associated protein GAP-43 are selectively increased in association cortices in schizophrenia. *Proc Natl Acad Sci USA*, **93**, 14182–7.

Perry, T.L. (1982) Normal cerebrospinal fluid and brain glutamate levels in schizophrenia do not support the hypothesis of glutamatergic neuronal dysfunction. *Neurosci Lett*, **28**, 81–5.

Pieri, J., Gupta, B.K., Bagwell, W. *et al.* (1995) MRI abnormalities in first episode schizophrenia: association in neurological impairment. *Schizophr Res*, **15**, 90.

Quitkin, F., Rifkin, A. and Klein, D.F. (1976) Neurological soft signs in schizophrenia and character disorders. *Arch Gen Psychiatry*, **33**, 845–53.

Rapaport, J., Giedd, J., Rad, J., Jacobsen, L., Kumra, S. and Lenane, M. (1997) Accelerated increase in brain ventricular volume at 2 year rescan for childhood onset schizophrenics. *Schizophr Res*, **24**, 154.

Reveley, A.M., Reveley, M.A., Clifford, C.A. and Murray, R.M. (1982) Cerebral ventricular size in twins discordant for schizophrenia. *Lancet*, **i**, 540–1.

Reveley, A.M., Reveley, M.A. and Murray, R.M. (1984) Cerebral ventricular enlargement in non-genetic schizophrenia: a controlled twin study. *Br J Psychiat*, **144**, 89–93.

Rifkin, L., Lewis, S., Jones, P. B., Toone, B.K. and Murray, R.M. (1994) Low birth weight and schizophrenia. *Br J Psychiatry*, **165**, 357–62.

Roberts, G.W., Colter, N., Lofthouse, R., Johnstone, E.C. and Crow, T.J. (1987) Is there gliosis in schizophrenia? Investigation of the temporal lobe. *Biol Psychiatry*, **22**, 1459–68.

Rothman, S.M. (1983) Synaptic activity mediates death of hypoxic neurons. *Science*, **220**, 536–7.

Scheibel, A.B. and Conrad, A.S. (1993) Hippocampal dysgenesis in mutant mouse and schizophrenic man: is there a relationship? *Schizophr Bull*, **19**(1), 21–33.

Selemon, L.D., Rajkowska,G. and Goldman-Rakic, P.S. (1995) Abnormally high neuronal density in the schizophrenic cortex. A morphometric analysis of prefrontal area 9 and occipital area 17. *Arch Gen Psychiatry*, **52**(10), 805–18.

Sham, P., O'Callaghan, E., Takei, N., Murray, G., Hare, E. and Murray, R. (1992) Schizophrenic births following influenza epidemics: 1939–1960. *Br J Psychiatry*, **160**, 461–6.

Sharma, T., Lewis, S., Barta, P. *et al.* (1995) Loss of cortical asymmetry in familial schizophrenia. *Schizophr Res*, **18**, 184.

Sharma, T., Lancaster, E., Lee, D. *et al.* (1998) Brain changes in schizophrenia. Volumetric MRI study of families multiply affected with schizophrenia – the Maudsley Family Study 5. *Br J Psychiatry*, **173**, 132–8.

Sheng, M., Cummings, J., Rolau, L.A., Jan, Y.N. and Jan, L.Y. (1994) Changing subunit composition of heteromeric NMDA receptors during development of rat cortex. *Nature*, **368**, 144–7.

Slotkin, T.A., Cowdery, T.S., Orband, L., Pachman, S. and Whitmore W.L. (1986) Effects of neonatal hypoxia on brain development in the rat: immediate and long-term biochemical alterations in discrete regions. *Brain Res*, **374**, 63–74.

Southard, E.E. (1915) On the topographical distribution of cortex lesions and anomalies in dementia praecox. *Am J Insanity*, **71**, 603–71.

Stefanis, N., Frangou, S., Yakeley, J., Sharma,T., O'Connell, P., Morgan, K., Sigmunsson, T., Taylor, M. and Murray, R.M. (1999) Hippocampal volume reduction in schizophrenia is secondary to pregnancy and birth complications. *Biol Psychiatry*, (in press).

Stewart, A. and Kirkbride, V. (1996) Very preterm infants at fourteen years: relationship with neonatal ultrasound brain scans and neurodevelopmental status at one year. *Acta Paediatr* (Suppl), **416**, 44–7.

Suddath, R.L., Christison, G.W., Torrey, E.F., Casanova, M. and Weinberger, D.R. (1990) Anatomical abnormalities in the brains of mojnozygotic twins discordant for schizophrenia. *N Engl J Med*, **322**, 789–94.

Takei, N., Sham, P.C., O'Callaghan, E., Glover, G. and Murray, R.M. (1995) Schizophrenia: increased risk associated with winter and city birth – a case-control study in 12 regions within England and Wales. *J Epidemiol Community Health*, **49**(1), 106–7.

Torrey, E.F., Miller, J., Rawlings, R. and Yolken, R.H. (1997) Seasonality of births in schizophrenia and bipolar disorder: a review of the literature. *Schizophr Res*, **24**, 260.

Trescher, W.H., McDonald, J.W. and Johnston, M.V. (1994) Quinolinate-induced injury is enhanced in developing rat brain. *Brain Res Dev*, **83**(2), 224–32.

Van Os, J., Woodruff, P., Fananas, L., Shuriquie, N., Howard, R. and Murray, R.M. (1997) Temporal origin of cerebral structural abnormalities in schizophrenia: Associations with second trimester dermatoglyphic ridge counts. *Schizophr Res*, **24**, 158.

Verdoux, H., Geddes, J.R., Takei, N. *et al.* (1997) Obstetric complications and age at onset in schizophrenia: an international collaborative meta-analysis of individual patient data. *Am J Psychiatry*, **154**(9), 1220–7.

Walker, E. and Lewine, R.J. (1990) Prediction of adult-onset schizophrenia from childhood home movies of the patients. *Am J Psychiatry*, **147**(8), 1052–6.

Walker, E.F. and Neumann, C.S. (1995) Neurodevelopmental models of schizophrenia: the role of central nervous system maturation in the expression of neuropathology. In J.L. Waddington and P.F. Buckley (eds), *The neurodevelopmental basis of schizophrenia*. New York: R.G. Landes, 1–16.

Walker, E.F., Lewine, R.R.J., Neumann, C. (1996) Childhood behavioral characteristics and adult brain morphology in schizophrenia. *Schizophr Res*, **22**, 93–101.

Weinberger, D.R., Cannon-Spoor, E., Potkin, S.G. and Wyatt, R.J. (1980) Poor premorbid adjustment and CT scan abnormalities in chronic schizophrenia. *Am J Psychiatry*, **137**, 1410–13.

Weinberger, D.R., DeLisi, L.E., Neophytides, A.N. and Wyatt, R.J. (1981) Familial aspects of CT scan abnormalities in chronic schizophrenic patients. *Psychiat Res*, **4**, 65–71.

Weinberger, D.R. (1987) Implications of normal brain development for the pathogenesis of schizophrenia. *Arch Gen Psychiatry*, **44**(7), 660–9.

Weinberger, D.R., Lipska, B.K. (1995) Cortical maldevelopment, antipsychotic drugs and schizophrenia: a search for common ground. *Schizophr Res*, **16**, 87–110.

Woerner, M., Gunduz, H., Ma, J., Alvir, J., Bilder, J. and Lieberman, J. (1997) Obstetric complications and brain MRI findings in schizophrenia. *Schizophr Res*, **24**, 160.

Woodruff, P.W.R., Perlson, G.D., Geer, M.J., Bartta, P.E. and Chilcoat, H.G. (1993) A computerised magnetic resonance image study of corpus callosum morphology in schizophrenia. *Psychol Med*, **23**, 45–56.

Woodruff, P.W.R. and Murray, R.M. (1994) The aetiology of brain abnormalities in schizophrenia. In: R. Ancill (ed.), *Schizophrenia: exploring the spectrum of psychosis*. Chichester: John Wiley, 95–144.

Woodruff, P.W.R., McManus, I.C. and David, A.S. (1995) Meta-analysis of corpus callosum size in schizophrenia. *J Neurol Psychiatry*, **58**, 457–61.

Woodruff, P.W.R., Wright, I.C., Shuriquie, N. *et al.* (1997) Structural brain abnormalities in male schizophrenics reflect fronto-temporal dissociation. *Psychol Med*, **27**(6), 1257–66.

Wright, I., Ellison, Z., Sharma, T., Friston, K., Murray, R.M. and McGuire, P. (1999) Mapping of grey matter changes in schizophrenia. *Schizophr Res*, **35**, 1–14.

Zaidel, D.W., Esiri, M.M. and Harrison, P.J. (1997) Size, shape and orientation of neurons in the left and right hippocampus: investigation of normal asymmetries and alterations in schizophrenia. *Am J Psychiatry*, **154**, 812–18.

Zipursky, R.B., Lim, K.O., Sullivan, E.V., Brown, B.W. and Pfefferbaum, A. (1992) Widespread cerebral gray matter volume deficits in schizophrenia. *Arch Gen Psychiatry*, **49**(3), 195–205.

CHAPTER 3

The neuropharmacology of schizophrenia: past, present and future

ROBERT KERWIN

Introduction

In the past 40 years the neurochemical theories underlying the mechanism of action of antipsychotics have nearly come full circle. Although the role of the dopamine D2 receptor seemed dominant, patients were trapped by a group of inevitable neurological and endocrine side-effects. Similarly, because there were few plausible alternative theories, drug discovery in this area was stagnant for want of alternative therapeutic targets. However, recent discoveries have turned attention away from the D2 receptor and towards both novel members of the dopamine receptor family and serotonin receptors, giving rise to the present generation of antipsychotics. For the future, neurochemical systems such as the inhibitory GABA and excitatory glutamate systems are being considered as possible therapeutic targets. Nevertheless, further discoveries in molecular biology and regional anatomy continue to suggest that D2 receptors may ultimately be the ideal therapeutic target, if regional selectivity can be achieved. The aim of this review will be to consider this progress from a historical perspective.

The past

THE DOPAMINE HYPOTHESIS OF SCHIZOPHRENIA

At its simplest, the dopamine hypothesis states that functional overactivity at some point in mesolimbic systems, if not the primary defect, is at least responsible for the generation of positive psychotic symptoms (Crow, 1980). Prior to the discovery of dopamine receptors, Carlsson and Lindqvist (1963) showed that chronic treatment of rats with chlorpromazine increased the production of dopamine metabolites, indicating overall functional blockade of the dopamine system. Soon afterwards it was shown that chlorpromazine and similar major tranquilizers could block the specific behavioural consequences of dopamine releasing drugs (Randrup and Munkvad, 1967).

An adenylate cyclase linked to a dopamine receptor was discovered and antipsychotic drugs shown to inhibit the generation of cyclic AMP through this system (Snyder *et al.*, 1974). The presence of another dopamine receptor, the D2 receptor, was inferred by the ability of neuroleptics to displace [^{3}H]spiperone bound to brain membranes. The clinical efficacy of neuroleptics was found to parallel their affinity for the D2 receptor and not the D1 receptor (Lee *et al.*, 1978). Finally, Johnstone *et al.* (1978) showed that with flupenthixol, only the α-isomer containing D2 receptor blockade was an effective antipsychotic. However, the drive to find alternative targets for antipsychotics came from a variety of clinical and experimental findings. Clinically the severe extrapyramidal and endocrine side-effects associated with the typical antipsychotic drugs were a major impediment, as was the 20% non-response rate and relative intractability of negative symptoms (Kerwin, 1992). Experimentally, the D2 receptor hypothesis has not completely withstood the test of time in its ability to stimulate drug discovery. It has proven difficult to demonstrate in direct assays the hypothesized hyperactivity in the dopamine systems. Early work on levels of dopamine or its metabolites were confused by the effect of the dopamine receptor blockade in life (for a review of this field *see* Reynolds, 1988). A replicable increase in dopamine in the left amygdala remains the most enduring abnormality found in the transmitter system itself (Reynolds, 1983). Attempts to demonstrate elevated levels of D2 receptors in post-mortem brains were similarly confounded by the effect of prior treatment, but on the whole a weak consensus for a drug-independent elevation of levels of D2 receptors remains (Lee and Seeman, 1978; Owen *et al.*, 1978). The most recent cracks in the dopamine hypothesis have come with the advent of functional imaging with Positron Emission Tomography (PET) or Single Photon Emission Tomography (SPET) of dopamine receptors. There is now a large literature on dopamine receptor concentrations in patients with schizophrenia compared to controls. Only one study (Wong *et al.*, 1986) showed increased D2 receptors while a majority of studies found normal levels (e.g. Martinot *et al.*, 1991; Farde *et al.*, 1993, Pilowsky *et al.*, 1994).

Another area of functional imaging that has weakened the all-embracing form of the D2 receptor hypothesis for drug effect comes from occupancy studies of D2 receptors. Wolkin *et al.* (1989) and Pilowsky *et al.* (1992) demonstrated that complete D2 receptor blockade was not always associated with clinical response. The most important studies in this area, however, came with the work of Farde *et al.*

(1994) and Pilowsky *et al.* (1993) who showed that the atypical antipsychotic clozapine produced a superior clinical response, despite low occupancy. This work therefore suggests that there are alternative therapeutic targets in the brain which can
effectively treat schizophrenia without the inevitable side-effects of D2 blockade.
More recently, the same effect has been reported with the novel antipsychotic olanzapine (Pilowsky *et al.*, 1996). Thus, clozapine and olanzapine form a group of drugs
which probably treat schizophrenia via non-D2 receptor sites.

The present

NOVEL DOPAMINE RECEPTORS, 5HT RECEPTORS AND THE PRESENT GENERATION OF NEW ANTIPSYCHOTICS

The dopamine receptor system

Pharmacological studies, alongside cloning and sequencing studies, have now determined five families of dopamine receptors: D1-like, which are the D1 and D5 receptors, and D2-like, which are complex entities – the D3 and D4 receptors – both of
which are highly polymorphic. In addition, the D2 receptor is differentially spliced
into two isoforms (for review *see* Shaikh *et al.*, 1997). Most interest so far has fallen
on the D2-like receptor family as a likely candidate for a role in the predisposition of
individuals to schizophrenia, and as a likely therapeutic target for novel antipsychotics.

The D2 receptor

Although clearly the main candidate for antipsychotic action in general, interest still
remains in the possibility that extrastriatal targeting of this receptor can be achieved.
Certainly, long-standing electrophysiological studies have always been able to show
differential pharmacological profiles of firing rates in mesolimbic versus nigrostriatal systems (White and Wang, 1983). Most recent studies have focused on electrophysiological responses in freely moving rats, and the potential for limbic selectivity,
as judged by this effect, is best seen with sertindole which displays an impressive
100-fold selectivity for inhibition of A10 over A9 neurons (Hyttel *et al.*, 1992). It is
hypothesized that the substrate for limbic selectivity arises from the fact that the D2
receptor is differentially spliced into long and short forms and that these show
regional selectivity for striatal and extrastriatal sites. Furthermore, some atypical
antipsychotics, including clozapine, show a small but differential binding preference
to the limbic form (Malmberg *et al.*, 1993). The most interesting drug in this respect
was remoxipride (now withdrawn) whose mechanism of action was puzzling
because of its selective ability only to block dopamine receptors with low affinity.
However, this has the widest differential binding potential at limbic and striatal sites
(Malmberg *et al.* 1993). The most direct evidence for receptor D2 limbic selectivity
comes from SPET studies, in our own group, with the high affinity D2-like ligand
epidepride which show the presence of binding sites outside the striatum. We have

shown conclusively that response to clozapine is limbic-selective, being associated with a high degree of blockade of binding sites in the temporal lobe but low striatal blockade (Pilowsky *et al.*, 1997).

The D3 receptor

The candidacy of the D3 receptor as a novel therapeutic target stems from a number of areas: it has a limbic distribution; it shows affinity to new atypical antipsychotics which also potently increase D3-related mRNA *in vitro* (Buckland *et al.*, 1993); and it is a candidate gene for suscebtibility to schizophrenia. A serine-to-glycine polymorphism at position 9 close to the N-terminal of the protein has been widely studied. Two groups initially reported an excess homozygosity in schizophrenic patients from France and Wales (Crocq *et al.*, 1992) which was replicated by Nimgaonker *et al.* (1993) and Williams *et al.* (1997). Our group was also able to replicate the finding and furthermore meta-analysis of all available data showed an enduring association for an excess of the 1:1 genotype in schizophrenia (Shaikh *et al.*, 1996). D3 receptors have also been found to be reliably increased in post-mortem schizophrenic brains, an effect which seems to be reversed by prior neuroleptic treatment. However, a gene expression study (Schmauss *et al.*, 1993) showed selective loss of D3 receptors in somatosensory areas of cortices and this finding is difficult to relate to the therapeutic potential of this target.

The D4 receptor

Theoretically the D4 receptor is the strongest candidate for an antipsychotic target. It has a very limited and unique localization in limbic regions. It is present in low abundance but quantitative gene expression studies confirm higher levels in the hippocampus and cortex and negligible levels in motor basal ganglia (Matsumoto *et al.*, 1995; Mulcrone and Kerwin, 1997). It also has a distinct high affinity for clozapine and other atypical antipsychotics, including olanzapine, risperidone and ziprasidone, although some typical antipsychotics and some inert compounds also have comparable affinities (*see* Shaikh *et al.*, 1997). Post-mortem studies have been exciting though controversial. Seeman *et al.* (1993) reported a sixfold elevation of D4 receptors in striatal homogenates using a complex double-label subtractive assay. This was in a drug-treated cohort and in a region showing negligible D4 mRNA (Matsumoto *et al.*, 1995; Mulcrone and Kerwin, 1996). However, in a similar study using quantitative autoradiography Murray *et al.* (1995) found a similar but more modest twofold increase. On the other hand Reynolds and Mason (1994) failed to replicate this finding in a more conventional assay and suggested that the previously observed elevated levels were attributable to both D3 and D4 receptors. Gene expression studies of post-mortem tissue should resolve this. One study (Mulcrone and Kerwin, 1996) failed to show an increase in D4 gene expression in the hypothetical cell body region for striatal terminal receptors whereas another study using more sensitive techniques and larger numbers may show a weak elevation of D4 receptor in gene expression (Stefanis *et al.* in press).

Genetic studies have focused on the D4 receptor in two ways. First, as a suscepti-bility gene and second via a pharmacogenetic approach to test if clozapine is acting through this site. Interest has mainly focused upon a polymorphic 48 bp repeat that codes for variation in the third intracytoplasmic loop and may alter clozapine binding *in vitro* (Van Tol *et al.*, 1992). Both linkage and case-control association studies have failed to provide evidence that this variant predisposes individuals to schizophrenia (Kerwin and Owen in press). Furthermore, pharmacological genetic association studies seemed to have ruled out a role for the 48 bp repeat in the third intracytoplasmic loop of the D4 receptor in determining the clozapine response. Shaikh *et al.* (1993; 1995) found no association in variants between 41 responders and 23 non-responders. Kennedy *et al.* (1993, 1994) have performed a number of studies that fail to show any association as do replication studies in larger series (Shaikh *et al.*, 1994).

Despite this uncertainty, receptor D4-selective ligands are being developed as antipsychotics and at least one highly selective drug with an impressive pharmacological and behavioural profile, L-745-570, has been developed, although very early proof of concept through clinical exposure was disappointing (Sodhi and Murray, 1995). This will be an exciting future avenue for research.

The D1 family of receptors

There is much less activity in this area of research which tends to be confined to the D1 receptor. Fundamental interest in the D1 receptor primarily comes from its localization in the prefrontal cortex and its role in working memory. Both *in-vitro* and *in-vivo* PET studies have utilized the selective ligand SCH 23390. Post-mortem studies are sparse and in the main negative. A more definitive finding has been reported using 11C-SCH.23390 and PET where numbers of D1 receptors were reduced in the prefrontal cortex and not in the striatum of patients with schizophrenia (Okubo *et al.*, 1997). Neuropsychologists are interested in this as the neurochemical substrate for negative symptoms and cognitive deficits in schizophrenia and suggest distant potential for selective D1-related drugs in the amelioration of negative symptoms.

The 5HT2 receptor

The 5HT2 receptor is a long-standing candidate for therapeutic targetting in schizophrenia. LSD, a 5HT2 agonist, is a well known psychotomimetic and replicable elevations in levels of 5HT2 receptors in the frontal cortex can be followed back many years (Busatto and Kerwin, 1997). The archetypal antipsychotic chlorpromazine has always been thought to have actions through 5HT2 receptor systems. Clozapine markedly attenuates the neuroendocrine and temperature responses in animals through serotonin-dependent systems (Nash *et al.*, 1988). It inhibits selective 5HT agonist-induced neuronal firing (Wang *et al.*, 1994) and, in clinical neuroendocrine studies, its ability to block 5HT2 receptors may be correlated with its clinical efficacy. All novel antipsychotics block both 5HT2a and 5HT2c receptors. The role of the 5HT2 block in this group of drugs is best illustrated by the highly selective drug ritanserin. This 5HT2 blocker improves both positive and negative symptoms of schizophrenia, either given alone (Wiesel *et al.*, 1994) or in combination with typical antipsychotics (Duinkerke *et al.*, 1993). Its protective effect against extrapyramidal side-effects (EPS) can be seen when the drug is given to patients on conventional neuroleptics (Bersani *et al.*, 1986). Large scale trials of the family of drugs with high

5HT2-blocking potential universally show effects on negative symptoms and protection against EPS, suggesting these may be mediated through serotonergic mechanisms (Meltzer, 1994). The direct effect of 5HT2 systems has been studied with functional receptor imaging and pharmacogenetic studies. Detailed studies have not been possible due to lack of radioligands. Farde *et al.* (1994, 1995) using 11C-N-methylspiperone – a combined D2/5HT2 blocker – have shown equally high levels of blockade for all subtypes of novel neuroleptics, including risperidone and clozapine. We have recently developed and characterized a 5HT2a ligand for use in humans using SPET (Busatto *et al.*, 1997) and recent studies in our group confirm the fact that all novel antipsychotics seem to have indistinguishably high levels of 5HT2 blockade (Travis *et al.*, in press) suggesting indeed that these drugs do block 5HT2 receptors *in vivo* but that their individual clinical differences are not being mediated by differential 5HT effects.

Pharmacogenetic research points to the 5HT2 receptor as a therapeutic site. A range of allelic variants have been described for 5HT2a (Arranz *et al.*, 1995) and 5HT2c receptor genes (Lappaleinen *et al.*, 1995). A number of significant associations have been found. We reported an association between T102C in the 5HT2a receptor gene and clinical response to clozapine (Arranz *et al.*, 1995) with variable replications (Noethen *et al.*, 1995). A further association was found with a structural polymorphism His452Tyr and response to clozapine which has been replicated (Arranz *et al.*, 1996, Badri *et al.*, 1996). One study has been published showing a strong association between possession of a serine, as opposed to a cystine, allele at position 23 and response to clozapine, indicating that the 5HT2c receptor in its own right might mediate antipsychotic response (Sodhi *et al.*, 1995). This pharmacological genetic work is also strengthened by the observation that the T102C polymorphism is also in excess in schizophrenia as a whole compared to controls and contributes quite strongly to the heritability of schizophrenia (Williams *et al.*, 1996). It will be interesting to determine whether allelic variants engineered into cellular expression systems are associated with altered binding or second messenger activation for 5HT ligands. Taken together this work is very strong evidence that 5HT2 receptors mediate therapeutic responses for schizophrenia, possibly with additional advantage for negative symptoms and protection against EPS.

Other newly cloned and sequenced 5HT receptors, notably 5HT3, 5HT6 and 5HT7, are also of emerging theoretical importance because of their limbic distribution and high affinity for atypical drugs, but this work is in its infancy. Thus the present neuropharmacology of schizophrenia is dominated by research into novel dopamine and serotonergic systems.

It is worth at this point examining the pharmacology of the new generation of antipsychotics in order to understand if any of this new knowledge applies to, or is confirmed by, their pharmacology and to see if their pharmacological profiles give clues to the future understanding of the neurochemistry of schizophrenia.

Clozapine

Clozapine (along with thioridazine and sulpiride) is the original atypical antipsychotic which even today has the lowest propensity to produce catalepsy in rats, due to its poor ability to block D2 receptors (Kohler *et al.*, 1981). The drug has a broad spectrum

Table 3.1 Receptor binding profiles of antipsychotics

Drug	Affinity for receptor (K_i (nmol/L))							
	dopamine D1	dopamine D2	dopamine D4	a1 adrenergic	a2 adrenergic	histamine H1	serotonin 5HT2a	serotonin 5HT2c
Existing antipsychotics								
Clozapine	85	126	9	7	8	6	12	8
Haloperidol	25	1	5	46	360	>1000	78	>1000
Remoxipride[a]	>1000	274	>1000	>1000	>1000	>1000	>1000	>1000
Risperidone	75	3	7	3	155	0.6	26	>1000
New antipsychotics								
Olanzapine	31	112	27	19	228	7	4	11
Quetiapine (ICI 204636; Seroquel™)	455	160	NA	7	87	11	220	615
Sertindole[b]	28	41	NA	3.4	350	600	0.39	NA
Ziprasidone	68	8	7.4	7.9	NA	7.3	9	8

[a] Drug withdrawn from the market due to adverse effects.
[b] Values expressed as IC_{50}.
Abbreviations: IC_{50} = concentration of the drug that inhibited binding of a radioligand by 50%; K_i = inhibition constant; NA = no data.

of affinities for the D1, D3, D4 and 5HT2 families of receptors (Kerwin and Taylor, 1996; *see* Table 3.1). Clozapine has particularly high affinity for the D4 receptor as well as for muscarinic, histaminergic and alpha sites. Clozapine has potent neurophysiological effects via 5HT2 block (Ashby and Wang, 1990) and displays high occupancy at 5HT2 receptors in humans (Nordstrom *et al.*, 1993). Its side-effect profile is characterized by a complete lack of EPS (apart from rare myoclonus), weight gain, tachycardia, sedation, sialorrhoea and lowering of the seizure threshold. Due to its haematological toxicity it is restricted to treatment-resistant or treatment-intolerant patients under strict haematological monitoring (Kerwin and Taylor, 1996).

Risperidone

This drug is non-cataleptogenic and EPS-free at lower doses (Jannsen Research Foundation, 1990). It has high affinity for D2 and D4 receptors but not D3 receptors (Leysen *et al.*, 1992). Risperidone is interesting because its high affinity for D2 receptors would suggest that it should be cataleptogenic in animals and produce more neurological side-effects in the clinic. It is, however, truly atypical (Schotte *et al.*, 1989) probably because high affinity 5HT2 blockade counterbalances receptor D2 induced EPS via an inhibitory effect on striatal neurons (Leysen *et al.*, 1992). *In vivo* SPET and PET have confirmed high occupancies at D2 and 5HT2 receptors (Nyberg *et al.*, 1993). Its side-effects are characterized by the emergence of EPS at higher dose ranges.

Olanzapine

This drug's receptor binding profile seems to occupy an intermediate position between clozapine and risperidone. It has greater affinity for 5HT2a and D2 receptors than clozapine but lower affinities than risperidone (Moore *et al.*, 1992). Olanzapine also has appreciable affinities for D3, D4, α1 and α2 receptor sites. It seems also to have an unusual affinity for the M1 muscarinic and H1 histaminic sites (Moore *et al.*, 1992). SPET studies have confirmed that the drug is clozapine-like, having low affinity for D2 receptors *in vivo* (Pilowsky *et al.*, 1996). The side-effect profile is mainly one of first dose sedation, postural hypotension, weight gain and EPS at higher doses.

Sertindole

This atypical drug has a receptor binding profile very similar to that of risperidone, having high affinity for 5HT2 receptors and moderately high affinity for D2 receptors as well as appreciable affinity for D3 and D4 receptors. It has no antimuscarinic activity, but appreciable peripheral alpha activity (Hyttel *et al.*, 1992). In SPET studies, despite its modest affinity for D2 receptors, sertindole is a potent blocker of D2 receptors *in vivo* (Pilowsky *et al.*, 1997). Its side-effect profile is characterized by nasal stuffiness and QT prolongation on the ECG.

It seems that novel drugs help in the evolution of our understanding of the neurochemistry of schizophrenia. Two broad groups emerge. First, clozapine–olanzapine-like drugs with pluripotent pharmacology show that non-dopaminergic treatment is possible, as their rich pharmacology represents a menu of novel candidates of which limbic D2 receptors and 5HT2 receptors may be relevant. Second, risperidone–sertindole-like drugs seem to focus on the possible future potential of biselective D2/5HT2 receptor blockers, whose activity against positive symptoms arises from the D2 block and intrinsic protection from the expected EPS comes from 5HT2 block as well as efficacy against negative symptoms.

As to choosing which drug to use in a clinical setting, the pharmacological profile alone is not informative. One should consider the group as a whole (with the exception of clozapine) as useful broad-spectrum antipsychotics. They should not be serially switched from one to another in a clinical setting as they are not for treatment resistance. If a patient should fail on a single atypical neuroleptic it would be more useful to switch directly to clozapine, which still remains the drug of choice in those patients who are more difficult to treat.

The future

GABA AND GLUTAMATE THEORIES

The previous two sections relate to a neuropharmacology of a mutual evolutionary process, whence primary knowledge came from the drug action which informed neurochemical theories which in turn helped to refine and tune drug discovery. To date there has been no drug discovery in schizophrenia that has arisen *de novo* from a primary and novel finding in schizophrenia. The two areas where this is most likely to be achieved are in the GABA and glutamate receptor systems for which primary experimental evidence for their role in schizophrenia is expanding rapidly. This final section will briefly review progress in these two areas.

GABA (γ-AMINOBUTYRIC ACID)

GABA is the major inhibitory transmitter of both interneuronal and many long pathways including those structurally altered in schizophrenia (Kisvorday *et al.*, 1990) such as the medial temporal lobe (Roberts, 1991) and the anterior cingulate gyrus (Benes, 1993). GABA interneurones have been explicitly shown to be reduced in the cortex in schizophrenia, and secondary modulatory changes in receptors have been demonstrated (Benes *et al.*, 1992). GABA also has a strong modulatory role on dopamine systems (Wood, 1982) and the psychotomimetic actions of GABA drugs are well known (Van Kamman, 1977). There has been a range of post-mortem studies in GABA systems. Both GABA and its synthesizing enzyme have been found to be reduced in schizophrenia, although it is now thought that perimortem artefacts were responsible for these effects (Bird *et al.*, 1977; Spokes *et al.*, 1980). Reynolds *et al.* (1990) have reported reduced uptake of the GABA terminal marker ^{3}H-nipecotic acid in the temporal lobe, which correlates only on the left with the previously reported dopamine reductions in the amygdala. Increased binding of the

GABAa receptor ligand muscimol has been found in association with cell loss in the cingulate gyrus (Benes, 1993). Until recently, there has been no direct *in-vivo* evidence of GABA abnormalities. Our group used ^{123}I-labelled iomazenil which binds with high affinity to the α subunit of the GABAa receptor. Although there were no overall differences between patients and controls a significant negative correlation was found between the severity of psychotic symptoms and iomazenil binding in limbic cortical regions (Busatto *et al.*, 1997). These results are consistent with the previous findings in limbic cortical regions and taken together again support a GABA-deficit hypothesis for schizophrenia, suggesting pharmacological manipulation of this may be useful at some date to explore in schizophrenia.

GLUTAMATE HYPOTHESES FOR SCHIZOPHRENIA

Glutamate receptor hypotheses for schizophrenia have emerged from three broad areas. First, the ability of glutamate to control dopamine release and turnover in a way which would suggest a primary deficit could be hypothesized; second, direct post-mortem abnormalities of glutamate systems; and third, from the pharmacology of the psychotomimetic drug phencyclidine (*see* Kerwin, 1992 for review).

Interaction between glutamate and dopamine

It has long been known that hyperdopaminergic states can arise from abnormal glutamate transmission (Carlsson and Carlsson, 1990). There is a range of studies which suggest a reciprocal relationship between the release and the turnover of these transmitters. This endogenous interaction is supported by the fact that glutamatergic lesions can be restored by nigrostriatal dopamine lesions and vice versa (for review *see* Kerwin, 1992).

Post-mortem studies

A broad consensus is now emerging that in post-mortem brains a reciprocal relationship exists whereby glutamate markers seem to be increased in frontal regions and reduced in temporal regions (Nishikawa *et al.*, 1983; Deakin *et al.*, 1989). We had shown that there is a loss of kainate receptor binding in the medial temporal cortex (Kerwin *et al.*, 1990), and further that gene expression for a range of AMPA receptor genes in post-mortem brains was reduced (Harrison *et al.*, 1991; Eastwood *et al.*, 1995). There is an extensive literature, which is contradictory, on the role of multiple NMDA subunits in schizophrenic brains. However, recent studies have suggested decrements in NMDA receptors that may be correlated with cognitive function (Humphreys *et al.* in press). Several workers have shown a range of abnormalities of gene expression in schizophrenia (Olney and Fibiger, 1995).

The pharmacology of phencyclidine

The sigma phencyclidine receptor is a complex subunit of the NMDA receptor lying within the ion-gated channel which provides allosteric regulation of the activated

NMDA receptor. Agents that bind to this site are all psychotomimetic (Javitt and Zukin, 1991) and many classical antipsychotics bind with high affinity to sigma phencyclidine sites (Tau and Cook, 1984). Large reductions in sigma binding sites were observed in amygdala and hippocampus by Simpson *et al.* (1990), while generalized losses throughout the cortical regions were observed by Weissmann *et al.* (1991). Recently, Olney and Fibiger (1995) have proposed a unifying hypothesis for the role of glutamate in schizophrenia, considering both the excitotoxity and the psychological potential of the NMDA receptor.

There are extensive reasons to suppose that glutamate systems may be abnormal at a number of levels in schizophrenia. The problem is one of non-toxic pharmacological manipulation. Most recent interest has focused on the allosteric glycine regulatory site using glycine or d-cycloserine in clinical trials.

Conclusions

It is likely that the current generation of newly established antipsychotics will dominate therapeutics for several years and draw upon the dual role of dopamine and 5HT in schizophrenia. It is not yet clear whether purely selective drugs are the key to better treatments or whether some degree of pluripotency is required for this complex disease. Clearly, uniselective drugs at some receptors are now only one step away but specific oligoselective drugs will ideally be the overall aim. The roles of GABA and glutamate still remain speculative but information has amassed so quickly that early drug discovery work will soon follow.

References

Arranz, M., Collier, D., Ball, D. *et al.* (1995) Association between clozapine response and allelic variation in the 5HT2a receptor gene. *Lancet*, **346**, 281–2.

Arranz, M.J., Collier, D., Munro, J. *et al.* (1996) Analysis of a structural polymorphism in the 5HT2a receptor and clinical response to clozapine. *Neurosci Lett*, **224**, 95–8.

Ashby, C.R., Jr and Wang, R.Y. (1990) Effect of antipsychotic drugs on 5HT2 receptors in the medial prefrontal cortex; microiontiphoretic studies. *Brain Res*, **506**, 346–8.

Badri, F., Masellis, M., Petronis, A. *et al.* (1996) Dopamine and serotonin system genes may predict clinical response to clozapine. *Am J Human Genet*, **59**, Suppl A247 (abstr).

Benes, F.M. (1993) Neurobiological investigations in cingulate cortex of schizophrenic brain. *Schizophr Bull*, **19**, 537–49.

Benes, F.M., Vincent, S.L., Alsterberg, G. *et al.* (1992) Increase GABAa receptor binding in superficial layers of cingulate cortex in schizophrenics. *J Neurosci*, **12**, 924–9.

Bersani, G., Grispini, A., Marini, S. *et al.* (1986) Neuroleptic induced extrapyramidal side-effects: clinical perspectives with ritanserin (R55667), a new selective 5HT2 receptor blocking agent. *Curr Therapeut Res*, **40**, 492–9.

Bird, E.D., Barnes, J., Iversen, L. L. *et al.* (1977) Increased brain dopamine and reduced glutamic acid decarboxylase and choline acetyl transferase activity in schizphrenia and related psychoses. *Lancet*, **ii**, 1157–9.

Buckland, P.R., O'Donovan, M.C. and McGuffin, P. (1993) Clozapine and sulpiride upregulate D3 receptor mRNA levels. *Psychopharmacology*, **32**, 901–7.

Busatto, G.F. and Kerwin, R.W. (1997) Perspectives on the role of serotonergic mechanisms in the pharmacology of schizophrenia. *J Psychopharmacol*, **11**, 3–12.

Busatto, G.F., Pilowsky, L.S., Costa, D.C. *et al.* (1997) Initial evaluation of ^{123}I 5IR91150 a selective 5HT2a ligand for single photon emission tomography in healthy human subjects. *Eur J Nucl Med*, **24**, 119–24.

Carlsson, A. and Lindqvist, M. (1963) Effect of chlorpromazine and haloperidol on formation of 3-methoxytyramine and normetanephrine in mouse brain. *Acta Pharmacol Toxicol*, **20**, 140–4.

Carlsson, M. and Carlsson, A. (1990) Interactions between glutamatergic and monoaminergic systems within the basal ganglia – implications for schizophrenia and Parkinson's disease. *Trends Neurosci*, **13**, 272–6.

Crocq, M.A., Mant, R., Asherson, P. *et al.* (1992) Association between schizophrenia and homozygosity at the dopamine D3 receptor gene. *J Med Genet*, **29**, 858–60.

Crow, T. J. (1980) Molecular pathology of schizophrenia – more than one disease process. *Br Med J*, **280**, 66–8.

Deakin, J.F.W., Slater, P., Simpson, M.D.C., Gilchrist, A.C. *et al.* (1989) Frontal cortical and left temporal glutamatergic dysfunction in schizophrenia. *J Neurochem*, **52**, 1781–6.

Duinkerke, S.J., Botter, P.A., Jansen, A.A.I. *et al.* (1993) Ritanserin, a selective 5HT2/1c antagonist and negative symptoms in schizophrenia. A placebo controlled double blind trial. *Br J Psychiatry*, **163**, 451–5.

Eastwood, S.L., McDonald, B., Burnet, P. *et al.* (1995) Decreased expression of mRNAs encoding non-NMDA glutamate receptor subunits GluR1 and GluR2 in medial temporal lobe neurones in schizophrenia. *Mol Brain Res*, **29**, 211–33.

Farde, L., Nordstrom, A.L., Wiesel, F.A. *et al.* (1992) Positron emission tomographic analysis of central D1 and D2 receptor occupancy in patients treated with classical neuroleptics and clozapine: relation to extrapyramidal side-effects. *Arch Gen Psychiatry*, **49**, 538–44.

Farde, L., Nordstrom, A.L., Nyberg, S. *et al.* (1994) D1 receptor, D2 receptor and 5HT2 receptor occupancy in clozapine treated patients. *J Clin Psychiatry*, **55**, (suppl B), 67–9.

Farde, L., Nyberg, S., Oxenstierna, G. *et al.* (1995) Positron emission tomography studies on D2 and 5HT2 receptor binding in risperidone-treated schizophrenic patients. *J Clin Psychopharmacol*, **15**, 198–238.

Harrison, P., McLaughlin, D. and Kerwin, R.W. (1991) Decreased hippocampal expression of a glutamate receptor gene in schizophrenia. *Lancet*, **337**, 450.

Hyttell, J., Arnt, J., Costall, B. *et al.* (1992) Pharmacological profile of the atypical neuroleptic sertindole. *Clin Neuropharmacol*, **15** (Suppl 1), 267a–268a.

Hyttell, J., Nielsen, J.B. and Nowak. (1992) The acute effect of sertindole on brain 5HT2, D2 and alpha 1 receptors (*ex-vivo* radioreceptor binding studies). *J Neurol Transmission*, **89**, 61–9.

Jannsen Research Foundation (1990). Risperidone: Investigators brochure.

Javitt, D.C. and Zukin, S.R. (1991) Recent advances in the phencyclidine model of schizophrenia. *Am J Psychiatry*, **148**, 1301–8.

Johnstone, E.C., Crow, T.J., Frith, C.D. *et al.* (1978) Mechanism of the antipsychotic effect in acute schizophrenia. *Lancet*, **i**, 848–51.

Kennedy, J.L., Petronis, A., Gao, J. *et al.* (1994) Genetic studies of DRD4 and clinical response to neuroleptic medication. *Am J Human Genet*, **55**, 3.

Kennedy, J.L., Sidenberg, D.G. and Van Tol H.H.M. (1993). A Hinc II RFLP in the human D4 receptor locus (DRD4). *Nucleic Acid Res*, **19**, 5801.

Kerwin, R.W. (1992). A history of frontal and temporal lobe aspects of the neuropharmacology of schizophrenia. *J Psychopharmacology*, **6**, 230–40.

Kerwin, R.W. (1994). New atypical antipsychotics: The current position. *Br J Psychiatry*, **164**, 141–8.

Kerwin, R.W. and Taylor, D.M. (1996) New antipsychotics – a review of their current status and clinical potential. *CNS Drugs*, **6**, 71–82.

Kerwin, R.W., Patel, S., Meldrum, B. and Reynolds, G.P. (1990) Quantitative autoradiographic analysis of glutamate binding sites in the hippocampal formation in normal and schizophrenic brain post-mortem. *Neuroscience*, **39**, 25–32.

Kiskvarday, Z.F., Gulyas, A., Beroukas, D. *et al.* (1990). Synapses, axonal and dendritic patterns of GABA immunoreactive neurones in human cerebral cortex. *Brain*, **113**, 793–812.

Kohler, C., Haglund, L., Ogren, S.O. and Angeby, T. (1981) Regional blockade by neuroleptic drugs of *in vivo* ³H-spiperone binding in the rat brain. Relation to blockade of apomorphine induced hyperactivity and stereotypes. *J Neurol Trans*, **52**, 163–73.

Lappalainen J., Zhang, L., Dana, M. *et al.* (1995) Identification, expression and pharmacology of a Cys23-Ser23 substitution in the human 5HT2c receptor gene (HTR2c). *Genomics*, **27**, 274–9.

Lee, T., Seeman, P., Tourtelotte, W. *et al.* (1978) Binding of ³H-neuroleptics and ³H-apomorphine in schizophrenic brains. *Nature*, **274**, 897–900.

Leysen, J.E., Gommeron, W.F., Eeens, A. *et al.* (1992) The biochemical profile of risperidone. *J Pharmacol Exp Therapeut*, **24**, 661–70.

Malmberg, A., Jackson, D.M., Eriksson, A. and Monell, N.A. (1993) Unique binding characteristics of neuroleptic agents interacting with human dopamine D2a, D2b and D3 receptors. *Mol Pharmacol* (in press).

Martinot, J.L., Pailliere-Martinot, M.L., Loc'h, C. *et al.* (1991) The estimated denisty of D2 striatal receptors in schizophrenia: a study with positron emission tomography and 76 biomolisuride. *Br J Psychiatry*, **158**, 346–50.

Matsumoto, M., Hidaka, K., Tada, S. *et al.* (1995) Full length cDNA cloning and distribution of human dopamine D4 receptor. *Mol Brain Res*, **29**, 157–62.

Meltzer, H. (1994) Overview of the mechanism of action of clozapine. *J Clin Psychiatry*, **55**, Suppl B, 47–52.

Moore, N.A., Tye, N.E. and Axton, M.S. (1992) The behavioural pharmacology of olanzapine – a novel atypical antipsychotic. *J Pharmacol Exp Therapeut*, **262**, 545–51.

Mulcrone, J. and Kerwin, R.W. (1996) No difference in the expression of the D4 gene in postmortem frontal cortex from controls and schizophrenics. *Neurosci Lett*, **219**, 163–6.

Mulrone, J. and Kerwin, R.W. (1977) The regional pattern of D4 gene expression in human brain. *Neurosci Lett*, **234**, 147–50.

Murray, A.M., Hyde, T.M., Knable, M.B. *et al.* (1995) Distribution of putative D4 dopamine receptors in post mortem striatum from patients with schizophrenia. *J Neurosci*, **15**, 2186–91.

Nash, J.F., Meltzer, H.G. and Gudelsky, G.H. (1988) Antagonism of serotonin receptor mediated neuroendocrine and temperature responses in the rat. *Eur J Pharmacol*, **191**, 463–9.

Nimgaonker, V.L., Zhang, X.R., Caldwell, J.G. *et al.* (1993) Association study of schizophrenia with dopamine D3 receptor gene polymorphism. Probable effect of family history of schizophrenia. *Am J Med Genet*, **48**, 214–17.

Nishikawa, T., Takashima, M. and Toru, M. (1983). Increased ³H-kainic acid binding in the prefrontal cortex in schizophrenia. *Neurosci Lett*, **49**, 245–50.

Noethen, M.M., Rietscel, M., Erdmann, J. *et al.* (1995) Genetic variation of the 5HT2a receptor and response to clozapine. *Lancet*, **346**, 908.

Nordstrom, A.L., Farde, L. and Halldin, C. (1993) High 5HT2 receptor occupancy in clozapine treated patients demonstrated by PET. *Psychopharmacology*, **110**, 365–7.

Nyberg, S., Farde, L., Eriksson, L., Halldin, C. and Eriksson, B. (1993) 5HT2 and D2 dopamine receptor occupancy in the living human brain: a PET study with risperidone. *Psychopharmacology*, **110**, 265–72.

Okubo, Y., Suhara, T., Suzuki, K. *et al.* (1997) Decreased prefrontal dopamine D1 receptors in schizophrenia revealed by PET. *Nature*, **385**, 634–7.

Olney, J.W. and Fibiger, N.B. (1995) Glutamate receptor dysfunction and schizophrenia. *Arch Gen Psychiatry*, **52**, 998–1025.

Owen, F., Crow, T.J., Puulter, M. *et al.* (1978) Increased dopamine receptor sensitivity in schizophrenia. *Lancet*, ii, 223–5.

Pilowsky, L.S., Costa, D.C., Verhoeff, P. and Kerwin, R.W. (1993) Schizophrenia: responders and non-responders to antipsychotic treatments: a SPET study of D2 receptor occupancy. *Psychol Med*, **23**, 791–7.

Pilowsky, L.S., O'Connell, P., Davies, N. *et al.* (1997) In vivo occupancy of striatal dopamine D2 receptors by the novel atypical antipsychotic drug sertindole a ^{123}I IBZM single photon emission tomography (SPET) study. *Psychopharmacology*, **130**, 152–8.

Pilowsky, L.S., Costa, D.C., Ell, P.J. *et al.* (1994) D2 dopamine receptor binding in the basal ganglia of antipsychotic free schizophrenic patients: a ^{123}I IBZM single photon emission tomography study. *Br J Psychiatry*, 16–26.

Pilowsky, L.S., Busatto, G.F., Taylor, M. *et al.* (1996) Dopamine D2 receptor occupancy in vivo by the novel atypical antipsychotic olanzapine a 123 I IBZM single photon emission tomography study. *Psychopharmacology*, **124**, 148–53.

Pilowsky, L.S., Costa, D.C., Ell, P.J., Murray, R.M. and Kerwin, R.W. (1992) Clozapine, single photon emission tomography and D2 dopamine receptor blockade hypothesis of schizophrenia. *Lancet*, **340**, 199–202.

Randrup, A. and Munkvad, I. (1967) Stereotyped activities produced by amphetamine in general animal species and man. *Psychopharmacologia*, **11**, 300–10.

Reynolds, G.P. (1983) Increased concentrations and lateral asymmetry of amygdalor dopamine in schizophrenia. *Nature*, **305**, 527–9.

Reynolds, G.P. (1988) The post-mortem neurochemistry of schizophrenia. *Psychol Med*, **18**, 793–7.

Reynolds, G.P. and Mason, S.L. (1994) Are striatal dopamine D4 receptors increased in schizophrenia. *J Neurochem*, **63**, 1576–8.

Reynolds, G.P., Czudek, C. and Andrews, H.B. (1990) Deficit and hemispheric asymmetry of GABA uptake sites in the hippocampus in schizophrenia. *Biol Psychiatry*, **27**, 1038–44.

Robert, G.A. (1991) Schizophrenia – a neuropathological perspective. *Br J Psychiatry*, **158**, 8–17.

Schmauss, C., Haroutounian, V., Davis, O.O. *et al.* (1993) Selective loss of dopamine D3 type receptor mRNA expression in parietal and motor crotices of patients with chronic schizophrenia. *Proc Natl Acad Sci USA*, **90**, 8942–6.

Schotte, A., De Bruyckere, K., Jannsen, P. and Leysen, J.E. (1989) Receptor occupancy by ritanserin and risperidone measured using *ex-vivo* autoradiography. *Brain Res*, **500**, 295–301.

Seeman, P., Guan, H.C. and Van Tol H.H.M. (1993) Dopamine D4 receptors elevated in schizophrenia. *Nature*, **365**, 441–4.

Shaikh, S., Collier, D., Kerwin, R.W. *et al.* (1993) Dopamine D4 receptor subtypes and response to clozapine. *Lancet*, **341**, 116.

Shaikh, S., Gill, M., Owen, M., Asherson, P. *et al.* (1994) Failure to find linkage between a functional polymorphism in the dopamine D4 receptor gene and schizophrenia. *Am J Med Genet (Neuropsychiat Genet)* **54**, 8–11.

Shaikh, S., Collier, D., Sham, P. *et al.* (1995) An analysis of clozapine response and polymorphisms of the dopamine D4 receptor gene DRD4 in schizophrenic patients. *Am J Med Genet*, **97**, 714–19.

Shaikh, S., Collier, D., Sham, P. *et al.* (1996) Allelic association between a ser-9-gly polymorphism in the dopamine D3 receptor gene and schizophrenia. *J Human Genet*, **97**, 714–19.

Shaikh, S., Makoff, A., Collier, D. and Kerwin, R.W. (1997) Dopamine D4 receptors. Potential therapeutic implications in the treatment of schizophrenia. *CNS Drugs*, **8**, 1–11.

Simpson, M.D.C., Royson, M.C., Slater, P. and Deakin, J.F.W. (1990) Phencyclidine and sigma receptor abnormalities in schizophrenic post-mortem brain. *Schizophr Res*, **3**, 32p.

Snyder, S.H., Bannerjee, S., Yamamura, H. *et al.* (1974) Drugs, neurotransmitters and schizophrenia. *Science*, **184**, 1243–53.

Sodhi, M.S. and Murray, R.M. (1997) Future therapies for schizophrenia. *Expert Opin Therapeut*, **7**, 151–65.

Sodhi, M.S., Arranz, M., Ball, D. *et al.* (1995) Association between clozapine response and allelic variations in the 5HT2c receptor gene. *Neuroreport*, **7**, 169–72.

Spokes, E.G.S., Garrett, N.J. and Rossor, M. N. (1980) Distribution of GABA in post-mortem brain tissue from control, psychotic and Huntington's chorea subjects. *J Neurol Sci*, **48**, 303–13.

Stephanis, N.C., Bresnick, J.N., Kerwin, R.W. *et al.* (1998) Elevation of D4 dopamine receptors mRNA in post-mortem schizophrenic brain. *Mol Brain Res*, **53**, 112–19.

Tau, S.W. and Cook, L. (1984) Sigma opiates and certain antipsychotic drugs mutually inhibit (+) ^{3}H haloperidol binding in guinea pig membranes. *Proc Natl Acad Sci USA*, **81**, 5618–5623.

Travis, M.J., Busatto, G.F., Pilowsky, L.S. *et al.* (1998) 5HT2a receptor blockade in schizophrenic patients treated with risperidone or clozapine. A single photon emission tomography (SPET) study using the novel 5HT2a ligand 123–5–1 R–91150. *Br J Psychiatry*, **173**, 236–241.

Van Kamman, D.P. (1977) γ-aminobutyric acid (GABA) and the dopamine hypothesis of schizophrenia. *Am J Psychiatry*, **134**, 138–43.

Van Tol, H.H.M., Wu, C.M., Ghan, H.C. *et al.* (1992) Multiple dopamine D4 receptor variants in the human population. *Nature*, **358**, 149–52.

Wang, R., Ashby, C.R., Edwards, E. and Zhang, J.Y. (1994) The role of 5HT3 receptors in the action of clozapine. *J Clin Psychiatry*, **55** (Suppl B) 23–6.

Weissmann, A.D., Casanova, M.F., Kleinmann, J.E. *et al.* (1991) Selective losses of cerebral cortical sigma but not PCP binding sites in schizophrenia. *Biol Psychiatry*, **29**, 41–54.

Wiesel, F.A., Nordstrom, A.C., Farde, L. and Eriksson, B. (1994) An open clinical and biochemical study of ritanserin in acute patients with schizophrenia. *Psychopharmacology*, **114**, 31–8.

White, L. and Wang, R. (1983). Differential effects of classical and atypical antipsychotic drugs on A9 and A10 dopamine neurones. *Science*, **221**, 1054–7.

Williams, J., Spurlock, G., Holmans, P. *et al.* (1977) A meta analysis and transmission disequilibrium study of association between the dopamine D3 receptor gene and schizophrenia. *Am J Med Genet*, **74**, 630–7.

Williams, J., Spurlock, G., McGuffin, P. *et al.* (1996) Association between schizophrenia and T102C polymorphism of the 5-hydroxytryptamine type 2a receptor gene. *Lancet*, **347**, 1294–6.

Wolkin, A., Barouche, F., Wolf, A.P. *et al.* (1989) Dopamine blockade and clinical response: evidence for two biological subgroups of schizophrenia. *Am J Psychiatry*, **146**, 905–8.

Wong, D., Wagner, H.N., Tune, L.E. *et al.* (1986) Positron Emission Tomography reveals elevated D2 receptors in drug naïve schizophrenics. *Science*, **234**, 1558–63.

Wood, P.L. (1982) Actions of GABAergic agents on dopamine metabolism in the nigrostriatal pathway of the rat. *J Pharmacol Exp Therap*, **222**, 674–9.

CHAPTER 4

Glutamate, GABA and cortical circuitry in schizophrenia

J.F. WILLIAM DEAKIN

Introduction

The glutamate deficiency theory of schizophrenia has been highly influential and has given rise to a large number of interesting experiments. The hypothesis was originally formulated by Kim *et al.* (1980) on the basis of the finding of reduced glutamate concentrations in cerebrospinal fluid from patients with schizophrenia. This finding has not been replicated (e.g. Perry, 1982) but the hypothesis has been sustained by the ability of antagonists of NMDA glutamate receptors such as phencyclidine to induce psychosis. Phencyclidine psychosis is held to be a model for schizophrenia and this is discussed below (Javitt and Zukin, 1991).

There are two possible mechanisms for reduced glutamate function: deficient release and deficient responsiveness at glutamate receptors. It will be argued that clear evidence for either is wanting. One implication of the glutamate deficiency hypothesis is that symptoms should be improved by drugs that enhance glutamate neurotransmission and the evidence is reviewed below. I have proposed that glutamate neurotransmission is abnormal in schizophrenia only in the sense that there is abnormal cortical wiring or connectivity; this involves glutamate, since glutamate is the efferent neurotransmitter of the cortex. This chapter examines candidate cortical circuits as substrates for pathogenesis.

The glutamate deficiency hypothesis

PHENCYCLIDINE PSYCHOSIS AS A MODEL FOR SCHIZOPHRENIA

NMDA channel antagonists such as phencyclidine (PCP) and ketamine were developed as anaesthetics without hypnotic effects: dissociative anaesthetics. This captures their principal subjective effect: the experience of being cut-off from the outside world; when the drug was prevalent one of its street names was DOA – dead on arrival. Other features of phencyclidine intoxication are listed in Table 4.1.

Table 4.1. Symptoms of phencyclidine and ketamine intoxication

- Dissociation, feeling numb, blank staring
- Body image disturbances
- Tangential and circumstantial thought
- Disorientation, amnesia
- Ataxia, dysarthria, analgesia
- Hallucinations and delusions

That such symptoms can be rated on the Brief Psychiatric Rating Scale (BPRS) has perhaps leant weight to their validity as a model of schizophrenia. The negative symptoms of the BPRS include three sub-scales – 'detached', 'blunted emotion' and 'retardation' – but in schizophrenia these symptoms are not associated with dissociative experiences; in other words the behaviour comes about by different mechanisms. Patients and controls administered phencyclidine, commonly develop body image disturbances and such illusions and distortions can be rated under the positive symptoms of the BPRS, particularly the 'hallucinatory behaviour' sub-scale. Again, however, the relationship between body image disturbances and hallucinations seems distant. Thinking becomes obscured, and patients and controls show tangential and circumstantial thought. These symptoms can be rated under 'conceptual disorganization' on the positive sub-scales of the BPRS. However, this may be true of any intoxicant. Subjects have disorientation, amnesia, ataxia, dysarthria and nystagmus and these are characteristic of organic psycho-syndromes as in delirium, and they are not typical of schizophrenia. Furthermore, few studies report clear-cut hallucinations and delusions following experimental administration of drug. Krystal *et al.* (1994) were suitably cautious in concluding from their study in normal volunteers that 'ketamine does not produce a behavioural state identical to schizophrenia because it is associated with a sense of intoxication, an absence of hallucinations and their dissociative symptoms'.

Investigators of phencyclidine in patients reached similar conclusions. It is instructive to read the original accounts which are often cited in support of the phencyclidine–schizophrenia model. Luby *et al.* (1961) administered PCP to a small number of patients and concluded that the symptoms were a good model of the 'primary' symptoms of schizophrenia. This refers to the primary, Bleulerian, symptoms of schizophrenia – altered associations and altered affect – the Schneiderian, positive symptoms were not mimicked by the drug. Ban *et al.* (1961) gave the drug to 55 patients with schizophrenia and other psychoses. Two became behaviourally disordered for some time afterwards and he concluded that phencyclidine was 'not a psychotomimetic'. Bakker and Amini (1961) gave the drug to five psychiatrists who experienced the characteristic symptoms and were markedly apathetic for some time afterwards. Nevertheless, Bakker concluded that 'comparison with spontaneous psychoses is not fruitful'. Such findings together with the frequent presence of organic features call into question the validity of phencyclidine or ketamine psychosis as a model for schizophrenia. The possibility remains that there are common brain mechanisms of delusions, hallucinations and thought disorder in organic and functional psychoses.

ARE PSYCHOTOMIMETIC EFFECT OF CHANNEL-BLOCKERS MEDIATED BY DECREASED GLUTAMATE FUNCTION?

While NMDA channel blockers interfere with glutamate neurotransmission through NMDA receptors, there is now evidence that glutamate release is increased (Mohghaddam *et al.*, 1997; Breier *et al.*, 1998). Paradoxically, therefore, it is possible that psychotomimetic effects are due to increased glutamate actions through AMPA or kainate receptors. Indeed this was suggested in the seminal glutamate hypofunction paper by Olney and Farber in 1995. They proposed that NMDA receptors which are supposedly hypofunctional in schizophrenia are located on GABA neurons. This would result in failure of activation of GABA inhibitory neurons giving rise to disinhibition of glutamatergic cells in the posterior cingulate thence to glutamatergic cells in the entire limbic system to which these cingulate cells project. Their proposal was in fact a glutamate hyperfunction in theory.

The channel blocking drugs also have the surprising property of selectively activating dopamine release in the mesolimbic system and inducing dopaminergic hyperlocomotion (Bristow *et al.*, 1993; Moghaddam *et al.*, 1997). This may be a consequence of increased glutamate release since the effect is blocked by AMPA antagonists (Moghaddam *et al.*, 1997). Furthermore, in humans raclopride binding to dopamine receptors, detected by PET, was reduced by ketamine (Breier *et al.*, 1998). This suggested that the drug had increased the release of dopamine which then displaced raclopride from its binding sites. Remarkably, antagonists at the glycine site of the NMDA glutamate receptor, block the dopaminergic effects of NMDA channel blockers (Bristow *et al.*, 1993). It is difficult to understand how one kind of NMDA antagonism (through the glycine site) can oppose the actions of another. Nevertheless, this might suggest a therapeutic approach to treatment.

DRUGS WHICH INCREASE GLUTAMATE FUNCTION ARE NOT ANTIPSYCHOTIC

The glutamate hypofunction theory has had the important effect of leading to several attempts to treat the symptoms of schizophrenia by reversing the abnormality. There have been a number of trials of glycine many of which are open label studies. One of the best studies was by Heresco-Levy *et al.* (1996) which demonstrated clinically important improvements of negative symptoms, whereas there was no effect on delusions, hallucinations or thought disorder, supposedly mediated by glutamate hypofunction.

Table 4.2. Trials of glycine treatment in schizophrenia

Author/Year	Dose	Proportion	Change
Adjunct to standard neuroleptic			
● Waziri 1988	5–22 g	4/11	improved negative
● Rosse *et al.* 1989	10 g	3/5	improved
● Costa *et al.* 1990	15 g	2/6	improved; 2 worsened
● Potkin 1998	15 g	2/11	improved negative
● Javitt *et al.* 1994	30 g	15%	improved negative
● Heresco-Levy *et al.* 1996	50 g	7%	improved negative
Adjunct to clozapine			
● Potkin 1998	50 g		worsened
Milacemide – glycine prodrug			
● Rosse *et al.* 1989	1200 mg	5/5	worse
● Rosse *et al.* 1991	400 mg	2/4	worse

Other evidence suggesting enhanced glutamatergic function may actually be counter-productive. There have been two trials of the drug milacemide which is converted into glycine in the brain (Table 4.2). Both of these studies found exacerbation of symptoms in most patients. Some studies of cycloserine, which also works at the glycine site, also contain suggestions that some patients' symptoms are aggravated by the drug (Table 4.3). It seems clear that enhancing glutamatergic function is not therapeutic on the positive symptoms of schizophrenia and may aggravate them. However, the studies suggest that glutamate deficiency may relate to the pathogenesis of the deficit state of schizophrenia.

Table 4.3. Trials of cycloserine in schizophrenia

Author/Year	Dose	Proportion	Change
Adjunct to standard neuroleptics			
● Goff *et al.* 1995	50 mg	20%	improvement negative symptoms
● Cascella *et al.* 1994	250 mg	4/7	worse
● Rosse *et al.* 1996	30 mg	13	no change
● van Berckel *et al.* 1996	50 mg		improvement negative symptoms but 2/10 worse
Adjunct to clozapine			
● Goff *et al.* 1996	<50 mg		worse negative

NO EVIDENCE FOR GENERALIZED GLUTAMATE HYPOFUNCTION IN SCHIZOPHRENIA

One problem for the glutamate hypofunction theory is the lack of biochemical evidence for it in post-mortem brain samples from patients with schizophrenia. A number of studies have measured radioligand binding to the NMDA receptor and expression of NMDA receptor sub-units. In general, normal or increased concentrations have been reported (Table 4.4). One recent study reported reduced expression of the NR1 sub-unit in superior temporal gyrus but not in other regions of the brain and in relation to the cognitive decline shown in ante-mortem assessments (Humphries *et al.*, 1996). This might be in keeping with a role for glutamate deficiency in the deficits of schizophrenia.

Table 4.4. Increased glutamate receptor protein and message in frontal cortex

Ligand	Author
• [^{3}H]-Kainate	(Nishikawa *et al.*, 1983)
• [^{3}H]-Kainate	(Deakin *et al.*, 1989)
• [^{3}H]-Kainate	(Simpson *et al.*, 1992)
• [^{3}H]-TCP	(Simpson *et al.*, 1991)
• [^{3}H]-Glycine	(Ishimaru *et al.*, 1994)
• NMDAR2D mRNA	(Akbarian *et al.*, 1996)

Increased binding to the NMDA receptor complex has often been attributed to an upregulation in compensation for reduced glutamate release, but we found increased rather than reduced radioligand binding to glutamate uptake sites in two series of brains (Deakin *et al.*, 1989; Simpson *et al.*, 1998a). Furthermore, upregulation would

Table 4.5. Hetero-receptors on glutamate cells also increased

Ligand	Region	Author
GABA receptor binding		
• [^{3}H]-Muscimol	DLPFC (BA9)	(Hanada *et al.*, 1987)
• [^{3}H]-Muscimol	Ant cingulate	(Benes *et al.*, 1996)
• [^{3}H]-Muscimol	PFC	(Nakai *et al.*, 1988)
• [^{3}H]-Flunitrazepam	MFC, OFC, OC	(Kiuchi *et al.*, 1989)
5HT1A receptor binding		
• [^{3}H]-8-OH-DPAT	FC Not cingulate	(Hashimoto *et al.*, 1991)
• [^{3}H]-8-OH-DPAT	Cingulate. Not FC	(Joyce *et al.*, 1993)
• [^{3}H]-8-OH-DPAT	OFC (BA11)	(Simpson *et al.*, 1996)
• [^{3}H]-8-OH-DPAT	FC	(Burnet *et al.*, 1996)
• [^{3}H]-LSD	FC	(Whitaker *et al.*, 1981)

Abbreviations:
PFC: pre-frontal cortex; MFC = medial frontal cortex; OFC = orbital frontal cortex; OC = occipital cortex

not explain how other receptors, which are also located on glutamatergic cells, are also increased in schizophrenia. A number of studies have reported increase in binding to the GABA receptor and there are several reports of increased 5HT1A receptor binding (Table 4.5). These have also been attributed to a compensatory upregulation in the face of GABA deficiency and serotonin deficiency. However, such a threefold pathology lacks parsimony. A more simple explanation is that there are more glutamatergic cells and synapses in the frontal cortex as proposed originally by Deakin *et al.* (1989).

INCREASED GLUTAMATERGIC NEURAL ELEMENTS IN FRONTAL CORTEX?

Direct counting of cells corroborates the biochemical evidence for increased glutamate synapses in schizophrenia. Selemon *et al.* (1995) reported increased cell density in frontal cortex and Benes *et al.* (1991) found increased density of pyramidal cells in lamina V of frontal cortex. A recent and unique finding comes from the work of Natalia Uranova in Moscow (Uranova and Orlovskaya, 1996). In an electron microscopic study, the number of axo-dendritic and axo-somatic synapses were increased in frontal cortex. These studies suggest there may indeed be an excess of structural glutamatergic elements, which accounts for the post-mortem brain neurochemical findings in frontal cortex.

DEVELOPMENTAL MECHANISM OF INCREASED CELLULAR MARKERS IN FRONTAL CORTEX

One explanation for increased cell density in cortex, recently proposed by Selemon *et al.* (1995), is that there are fewer dendritic and axonal arborizations, resulting in greater cell packing. We have proposed an alternative, developmental explanation based on the important principle that cells and synapses are overproduced early in development with subsequent elimination of redundant elements. An arrest of this process would result in the increased density of cells and receptors in frontal cortex observed in post-mortem brain studies (Deakin *et al.*, 1989).

Slater working in Manchester, UK has reported a unique study in human infant brain that there is an overproduction of radioligand binding to the glutamate uptake site and to the channel in NMDA receptors in the first two postnatal years (Slater *et al.* 1992, 1993). Adult levels of binding are only reached after year two. This reflects the normal developmental process of neuronal and synaptic overproduction and pruning. On the basis of this finding, we speculated that the putative arrest of development in schizophrenia occurs in the first two postnatal years (Deakin *et al.*, 1989). This suggestion strongly contrasts with the prevailing view that any developmental origins of schizophrenia occur *in utero* in the first trimester (e.g. Fearon *et al.*, this volume).

Candidate circuit abnormalities in schizophrenia

THE PAPEZ CIRCUIT

Entorhinal cortex

Jakob and Beckmann (1986) reported a disruption of cortical neuronal organization in entorhinal cortex. They observed that the characteristic clusters of large cells in lamina II were more diffuse in patients and that large cells were inappropriately located in deeper laminae. They suggested that some cells had failed to migrate to their proper laminar destination. This finding was a major stimulus to the idea that schizophrenia involves an abnormality of cortical development. Other studies have failed to observe dysplasia of entorhinal cortical cells, notably Krimer *et al.* (1997). However, using a quantitative cytoarchitectural approach, Longson *et al.* (1998) found a population of cells in lamina IIA which were larger than those in controls and which were more characteristic of those in laminas I–II. One explanation is that the large cells in lamina II had failed to complete their migration to their appropriate destination in laminas I–II. Further studies using a fully quantitative cytoarchitectural approach should resolve the issue of entorhinal dysplasia in schizophrenia.

Hippocampus

Entorhinal cortex is one of the major sources of afferents to the hippocampus and reports of hippocampal disarray are therefore of considerable interest (Kovelman and Scheibel, 1984; Jonsson *et al.*, 1997). Unfortunately, others have failed to replicate this finding (e.g. Christison *et al.*, 1989; Dwork, 1997). A recent study suggests there may be subtle disorganization of inter-relationships in cell density between sub-regions of hippocampus (Zaidel *et al.*, 1997). Bogerts' report of reductions in hippocampal volume is a landmark in the neuropathology of schizophrenia (Bogerts *et al.*, 1985), but at least one careful study involving complete sectioning of the hippocampus failed to find evidence of cell loss or a statistically significant reduction in volumes (Heckers *et al.*, 1991). It is therefore perplexing that in-vivo MR imaging studies do report hippocampal atrophy rather more consistently (*see* Deakin, 1996).

Neurochemical studies, mainly from one group, report that protein and message for AMPA glutamate receptors and of synaptophysin, a protein associated with synapses, are decreased in hippocampus and this could reflect a loss of cells or of terminals which might underlie MR evidence of atrophy (Eastwood *et al.*, 1995, 1997).

Anterior thalamus and cingulate

There have been almost no neurochemical studies of amino-acid transmitters in the anterior thalamus in schizophrenia. Anterior thalamus projects to anterior cingulate and this structure has been the focus of sustained research interest from the Harvard group (Benes, 1998). They report reduced numbers of small, presumed GABA cells, and increased numbers of vertical axons innervating outer layers of cingulate. Benes *et al.* (1992a, 1992b) propose that developmental loss of GABA cells results in a more exuberant afferent glutamatergic innervation from frontal cortex.

Conclusion

Despite considerable effort, neuropathological and consistent neurochemical changes in the Papez circuit have not been demonstrated in post-mortem brain in schizophrenia. Entorhinal cortex and hippocampus are the focus for the neuropathology of Alzheimer's disease. While psychotic symptoms occur in Alzheimer's disease, they are not a typical early feature and the cardinal sign is forgetfulness. Impairments of memory have been reported in schizophrenia but they are subtle. Dysfunction in the system primarily concerned with long-term memory formation does not seem an especially plausible substrate for psychosis.

DORSAL CORTICO-STRIATAL SYSTEM

Dorsolateral prefrontal cortex

Neuropathological studies of dorsolateral prefrontal cortex are few. Benes *et al.* (1991) reported evidence of reduced densities of small cells, presumed to be GABA interneurons, in Brodmann Area 10 (polar frontal cortex) and increased pyramidal cell densities in laminar V, while Beasley and Reynolds (1997) reported loss of parvalbumin-containing interneurons in dorsolateral prefrontal cortex. However, the latter finding was not confirmed by Woo *et al.* (1997). Selemon *et al.* (1995) reported a generalized increase in neuronal density in the adjacent Brodmann Area 9, which was also seen in visual Area 17. The latter argues in favour of generalized cortical abnormality rather than specific dysfunction in dorsolateral prefrontal cortex. In contrast to Selemon *et al.*'s (1995) finding in fixed tissue, Akbarian *et al.* (1996b) found no changes in cell density in frozen sections of dorsolateral prefrontal cortex.

There are few biochemical studies of glutamate markers in dorsolateral prefrontal cortex. Recently, Akbarian *et al.* (1995) reported that NR2D sub-unit of the NMDA receptor was overexpressed relative to message for other sub-units in dorsolateral prefrontal cortex. However, there were no changes in cell density and this implies some regulatory change in the assembly of NMDA receptors, rather than a structural change.

The principal thalamic afferent to dorsolateral prefrontal cortex is the dorsal medial thalamus. The elegant studies of Pakkenberg, using stereological methodology, found reduced total neuronal numbers in two studies of dorsal medial thalamus (Pakkenberg, 1990, 1992). This finding is in urgent need of replication in both imaging and neuropathological studies. As Jones (1997) points out, the nucleus is highly heterogeneous and the elements that are lost need to be identified.

Akbarian *et al.* (1996a) reported that neurons staining for the enzymes nicotinamide-adenine dinucleotide phosphate-diaphorase (NADPH-D) were abhorrently located in sub-cortical white matter immediately below lamina VI. They suggested that the cortical sub-plate, which is the developmental bridge of the cortex, failed to develop properly or to regress.

In summary, while some imaging studies point to reduced dorsolateral prefrontal cortical volume, the pathological basis for this is unknown. The cell counting studies are contradictory and methodological differences in fixation may be an important part of the discrepancy.

Basal ganglia

Dorsal medial prefrontal cortex projects to dorsal striatum. There is evidence that neuroleptic treatment may be associated with increased basal ganglia volume (Chakos *et al.*, 1994) and this may account for inconsistent reports of volume reduction (*see* Bogerts *et al.*, 1993).

Carlsson has proposed a circuit-based version of the glutamate deficiency theory. It proposes that loss of cortical glutamate afferents to striatum results in failure of activation of inhibitory mechanisms in the thalamus concerned with regulating sensory input into the cortex. Psychotic symptoms are seen as 'cortical sensory overload' due to breakdown of the thalamic sensory filter (Carlsson, 1995). In keeping with the theory, we reported striking reductions in glutamate uptake binding sites (Simpson *et al.*, 1992) but we and others were not able to replicate the finding in three further sets of brains (Noga *et al.*, 1997; Simpson *et al.*, 1998b); nor are we able to explain the original finding. Therefore, it seems unlikely that reports of increases in radioligand binding to NMDA receptors in basal ganglia indicate major structural loss of glutamate afferents (Kornhuber *et al.* 1989; Simpson *et al.*, 1991; Noga *et al.*, 1997; Aparicio-Legarza *et al.*, 1998).

Conclusion

Functional brain imaging studies have long implicated dorsolateral prefrontal cortical hypofunction in schizophrenia and MRI studies suggest there is loss of frontal cortical substance. This has not been documented by stereological or cell-counting studies. Recent reports of increased cell density of dorsolateral prefrontal cortex also report increases in visual cortex pointing to a general cortical abnormality. A single study in a small number of brains suggests an abnormal persistence of cortical subplate cells and this finding is in urgent need of replication, as it would constitute the clearest evidence yet of a neurodevelopmental pathogenesis of schizophrenia. Cytoarchitectural and neurochemical anatomical studies of the dorsal medial thalamus are long overdue. There is evidence for abnormal dopaminergic modulation of the dorsolateral–thalamic–striatal loop.

Dorsolateral prefrontal cortex has been implicated in mechanisms of working memory, attention and locomotor control. Dysfunction in this system has most reliably been linked to the poverty syndrome of schizophrenia (Liddle *et al.*, 1992) rather than with psychotic symptoms of schizophrenia.

BASOLATERAL CIRCUIT

Ventral frontal – ventral striato-limbic systems

Evidence of increased glutamate markers, noted above, occur in ventral frontal cortex. This region is extensively connected with limbic regions of the brain through a prominent tract of white matter, the uncinate fasciculus. There are direct connections with amygdala and anterior temporal cortex. Deakin *et al.* (1989) reported evidence for loss of glutamate uptake sites in these regions. One explanation could be that afferent connections from dysplastic frontal cortex, through the uncinate fasciculus, fail to develop or slowly degenerate (Deakin *et al.*, 1997). Interestingly, the loss of glutamate uptake sites was more marked in left amygdala and this was correlated with increased dopamine content previously assayed in the same brains (Reynolds 1983; Deakin *et al.*, 1989). This suggested that asymmetrically altered glutamatergic innervation of the amygdala might induce secondary and lateralized changes in dopamine function.

There is evidence that the basolateral circuit encodes information about social signals and plans for social acts; it has been proposed as a substrate for the human ability to infer the intentions of other people from their language, gesture and eye gaze – the faculty of social cognition and Theory of Mind (Brothers, 1996; Frith, 1996). Disorganization of neural mechanisms of high-level social information processing seems a plausible substrate for some positive symptoms of schizophrenia. For example, paranoid delusions are almost self-evidently misreadings of the intentions of others (Deakin, 1994; Frith and Corcoran, 1996).

Summary and conclusions

There is compelling evidence that schizophrenia involves a subtle but fairly widespread loss of cortical grey matter and this implies that disturbed cortical wiring is the basis of symptoms rather than a unitary neurochemical lesion such as glutamate deficiency (Schlaepfer *et al.*, 1994; Harvey *et al.*, 1994). Treatment studies with glycine suggest that defective glutamate neurotransmission through NMDA receptors could underlie the negative symptoms of schizophrenia and this would be compatible with the recent studies in post-mortem brain described by Hirsch *et al.* (1997).

Neurochemical and molecular studies in post-mortem brain have yet to reveal a diffuse cortical abnormality that might account for reduced grey matter volumes in schizophrenia. In frontal cortex, there are a number of reports of increased concentrations of markers of glutamatergic cellular elements and there is some corroboration of this from cytoarchitectural studies. Evidence has been summarized that this could come about through an arrest of developmental neural pruning, and that this occurs in the postnatal period. The proposed postnatal date for developmental disturbance in schizophrenia is in contrast to the general view that it occurs *in utero* (Deakin and Simpson, 1997). Increased frontal glutamatergic connectivity predicts that treatments which reduce glutamate neurotransmission, particularly non-NMDA, may have therapeutic potential against positive symptoms. In temporal lobe structures, there is evidence of reduced GABA and glutamate function.

High resolution studies that identify changes in cellular elements in the cortex have the potential to identify abnormalities of large scale wiring, and of microcircuitry which earlier studies suggested. Front-runners currently include loss of frontotemporal cortical connectivity (Weinberger *et al.*, 1992; Woodruff *et al.*, 1997; Deakin and Simpson, 1997), increased interhemispheric frontal connectivity (Deakin *et al.*, 1989) or decreased temporal connectivity (Woodruff *et al.*, 1993), increased glutamate innervation of cingulate cortex (Benes *et al*, 1992b), and, loss of frontal neuropil (Selemon *et al.*, 1995).

References

Akbarian, S., Huntsman, M.M., Kim, J.J., Tafazzoli, A., Potkin, S.G., Bunney, Jr W.E. and Jones, E.G. (1995) GABA(A) receptor subunit gene expression in human prefrontal cortex: comparison of schizophrenics and controls. *Cerebral Cortex*, **5**, 550–60.

Akbarian, S., Kim, J.J., Potkin, S.G., Hetrick, W.P., Bunney, Jr W.E. and Jones, E.G. (1996) Maldistribution of interstitial neurons in prefrontal white matter of the brains of schizophrenic patients. *Arch Gen Psychiatry*, **53**, 425–36.

Akbarian, S., Kim, J.J., Potkin, S.G., Hagman, J.O., Tafazzoli, A., Potkin, S.G., Bunney, Jr W.E. and Jones, E.G. (1996b) Gene expression for glutamic acid decarboxylase is reduced without loss of neurons in prefrontal cortex of schizophrenics. *Arch Gen Psychiatry*, **52**, 258–66.

Aparicio-Legarza, M.I., Davis, B., Hutson, P.H. and Reynolds, G.P. (1998) Increased density of glutamate/N-methyl-D-aspartate receptors in putamen from schizophrenic patients. *Neuroscience Lett*, **241**, 143–6.

Bakker, C.B. and Amini, F.C. (1961) Observations on the psychotomimetic effect of Serenyl. *Comp Psychiatry*, **2**, 269–80.

Ban, T.A., Lohrenz, J.J. and Lehmann, H.E. (1961) Observations on the action of Serenyl – a new psychotropic drug. *Canadian Psychiatric Assoc J*, **6**, 150–7.

Beasley, C.L. and Reynolds, G.P. (1997) Parvalbumin-immunoreactive neurons are reduced in the prefrontal cortex of schizophrenics. *Schizophr Res*, **24**, 349–55.

Benes, F.M., McSparren, J., Bird, E.D., SanGiovanni, J.P. and Vincent, S.L. (1991) Deficits in small interneurons in prefrontal and cingulate cortices of schizophrenic and schizoaffective patients. *Arch Gen Psychiatry*, **48**, 996–1001.

Benes, F.M., Vincent, S.L., Alsterberg, G., Bird, E.D. and SanGiovanni, J.P. (1992a) Increased GABAA receptor binding in superficial layers of cingulate cortex in schizophrenics. *J Neurosci*, **9**, 24–9.

Benes, F.M., Sorensen, I., Vincent, S.L., Bird, E.D. and Sathi, M. (1992b) Increased density of glutamate-immunoreactive vertical processes in superficial laminae in cingulate cortex in schizophrenic brain. *Cerebral Cortex*, **2**, 503–12.

Benes, F.M., Vincent, S.L., Marie, A. and Khan, Y. (1996) Up-regulation of GABA(A) receptor binding on neurons of the prefrontal cortex in schizophrenic subjects. *Neuroscience*, **75**, 1021–31.

Benes ,F.M. (1998) Model generation and testing to probe neural circuitry in the cingulate cortex of postmortem schizophrenic brain. *Schizophr Bull*, **24**, 219–30.

Bogerts, B., Meertz, E. and Schonfeldt-Bausch, R. (1985) Basal ganglia and limbic system pathology in schizophrenia. A morphometric study of brain volume and shrinkage. *Arch Gen Psychiatry*, **42**, 784–91.

Bogerts, B., Falkai, P., Greve, B., Schneider, T. and Pfeiffer, U. (1993) The neuropathology of schizophrenia: past and present. *J Hirnforsch*, **34**, 193–205.

Breier, A., Adler, C.M., Weisenfeld, N., Su, T.P., Elman, I., Picken, L., Malhotra, A.K. and Pickar, D. (1998) Effects of NMDA antagonism on striatal dopamine release in healthy subjects: application of a novel PET approach. *Synapse*, **29**, 142–7.

Bristow, L.J., Hutson, P.H., Thorn, L. and Tricklebank, M.D. (1993) The glycine/NMDA receptor antagonist, R-(+)-HA-966, blocks activation of the mesolimbic dopaminergic system induced by phencyclidine and dizocilpine (MK-801) in rodents. *Br J Pharmacol*, **108**, 1156–63.

Brothers, L. (1996) Brain mechanisms of social cognition. *J Psychopharmacol*, **10**, 2–8.

Burnet, P.W., Eastwood, S.L. and Harrison, P.J. (1996) 5HT^{1A} and 5HT^{2A} receptor mRNAs and binding site densities are differentially altered in schizophrenia. *Neuropsychopharmaco,* **15**, 442–55.

Carlsson, A. (1995) Neurocircuitries and neurotransmitter interactions in schizophrenia. *Int Clin Psychopharmacol*, **10**, 21–8.

Cascella, N.G., Macciardi, F., Cavallini, C. and Smeraldi, E. (1994) D-cycloserine adjuvant therapy to conventional neuroleptic treatment in schizophrenia: an open-label study. *J Neural Transm Gen Sect*, **95**, 105–11.

Chakos, M.H., Lieberman, J.A., Bilder, R.M., Borenstein, M., Lerner, G., Bogerts, B., Wu, H., Kinon, B. and Ashtari, M. (1994) Increase in caudate nuclei volumes of first-episode schizophrenic patients taking antipsychotic drugs. *Am J Psychiatry*, **151**, 1430–6.

Christison, G.W., Casanova, M.F., Weinberger, D.R., Rawlings, R. and Kleinman, J.E. (1989) A quantitative investigation of hippocampal pyramidal cell size, shape and variability of orientation in schizophrenia. *Arch Gen Psychiatry*, **46**, 1027–32.

Costa, J., Khaled, E., Sramek, J., Bunney, Jr W. and Potkin, S.G. (1990) An open trial of glycine as an adjunct to neuroleptics in chronic treatment-refractory schizophrenics. *J Clin Psychopharmacol*, **10**, 71–2.

Deakin, J.F.W., Slater, P., Simpson, M.D.C., Gilchrist, A.C., Skan, W.J., Royston, M.C., Reynolds, G.P. and Cross, A.J. (1989) Frontal cortical and left temporal glutamatergic dysfunction in schizophrenia. *J Neurochem*, **52**, 1781–6.

Deakin, J.F.W. (1994) Neuropsychological implications of brain changes in schizophrenia: an overview. *Psychopathol*, **27**, 251–4.

Deakin, J.F.W. (1996) Neurobiology of schizophrenia. *Current Opinion in Psychiatry* **9**, 50–6.

Deakin, J.F.W. and Simpson, M.D.C. (1997) A two-process theory of schizophrenia: evidence from studies in post-mortem brain. *J Psychiatry Res*, **31**, 277–95.

Deakin, JF.W., Simpson, M.D.C., Slater, P. and Hellewell, J.S.E. (1997) Familial and developmental abnormalities of frontal lobe function and neurochemistry in schizophrenia. *J Psychopharmacol*, **11**, 133–42.

Dwork, A.J. (1997) Postmortem studies of the hippocampal formation in schizophrenia. *Schizophr Bull*, **23**, 385–402.

Eastwood, S.L., McDonald, B., Burnet, P.W., Beckwith, J.P., Kerwin, R.W. and Harrison P.J. (1995) Decreased expression of mRNAs encoding non-NMDA glutamate receptors GluR1 and GluR2 in medial temporal lobe neurons in schizophrenia. *Brain Res Mol Brain Res*, **29**, 211–23.

Eastwood, S.L. and Harrison, P.J. (1995b) Decreased synaptophysin in the medial temporal lobe in schizophrenia demonstated using immunoautoradiography. *Neuroscience*, **69**, 339–43.

Eastwood, S.L., Kerwin, R.W. and Harrison, P.J. (1997) Immunoautoradiographic evidence for a loss of alpha-amino-3-hydroxy-5-methyl-4-isoxazole propionate-preferring non-N-methyl-D-aspartate glutamate receptors within the medial temporal lobe in schizophrenia. *Biol Psychiatry*, **41**, 636–43.

Frith, C.D. (1996) Brain mechanisms for 'having a theory of mind'. *J Psychopharmacol*, **10**, 9–15.

Frith, C.D. and Corcoran, R. (1996) Exploring 'theory of mind' in people with schizophrenia. *Psychol Med* **26**, 521–30.

Goff, D.C., Tsai, G., Manoach, D.S. and Coyle, J.T. (1995) Dose-finding trial of D-cycloserine added to neuroleptics for negative symptoms in schizophrenia. *Am J Psychiatry*, **152**, 1213–15.

Goff, D.C., Tsai, G., Manoach, D.S., Flood, J., Darby, D.G. and Coyle, J.T. (1996) D-cycloserine addeed to clozapine for patients with schizophrenia. *Am J Psychiatry*, **153**, 1628–30.

Hanada, S., Mita, T., Nishino, N., and Tanaka, C. (1987) [^{3}H]muscimol binding sites increased in autopsied brains of chronic schizophrenics. *Life Sciences*, **40**, 259–66.

Harvey, I., Persaud, R., Ron, M.A., Baker, G. and Murray, R.M. (1994) Volumetric MRI measurements in bipolars compared with schizophrenics and healthy controls. *Psychol Med*, **24**, 689–99.

Hashimoto, T., Nishino, N., Nakai, H. and Tanaka, C. (1991) Increase in serotonin 5-HT1A receptors in prefrontal and temporal cortices of brains from patients with chronic schizophrenia. *Life Sciences*, **48**, 355–63.

Heckers, S., Heinsen, H., Geiger, B. and Beckmann, H. (1991) Hippocampal neuron number in schizophrenia. A stereological study. *Arch Gen Psychiatry*, **48**, 1002–8.

Heresco-Levy, U., Javitt, D.C., Ermilov, M., Mordel, C., Horowitz, A. and Kelly, D. (1996) Double-blind, placebo-controlled, crossover trial of glycine adjuvant therapy for treatment-resistant schizophrenia. *Brit J Psychiatry*, **169**, 610–17.

Hirsch, S.R., Das, I., Garey, L.J. and de Belleroche, J. (1997) A pivotal role for glutamate in the pathogenesis of schizophrenia, and its cognitive dysfunction. *Pharmacol Biochem Behav*, **56**, 797–802.

Humphries, C., Mortimer, A., Hirsch, S. and De Belleroche, J. (1996) NMDA receptor mRNA correlation with antemortem cognitive impairment in schizophrenia. *NeuroReport*, **7**, 2051–5.

Ishimaru, M., Kurumaji, A. and Toru, M. (1994) Increases in strychnine-insensitive glycine binding sites in cerebral cortex of chronic schizophrenics: evidence for glutamate hypothesis. *Biol Psychiatry*, **35**, 84–95.

Jakob, H. and Beckmann, H. (1986) Prenatal development disturbances in the limbic allocortex in schizophrenics. *J Neural Transmiss*, **65**, 303–26.

Javitt, D.C. and Zukin, S.R. (1991) Recent advances in the phencyclidine model of schizophrenia. *Am J Psychiatry*, **148**, 1301–8.

Javitt, D.C., Zylberman, I., Zukin, S.R., Heresco-Levy, U. and Lindenmayer, J.P. (1994) Treatment of negative symptoms in schizophrenia by glycine. *Am J Psychiatry*, **151**, 1234–6.

Jones, E.G. (1997) Cortical development and thalamic pathology in schizophrenia. *Schizophr Bull*, **23**, 483–501.

Jonsson, S.A., Luts, A., Guldberg-Kjaer, N. and Brun, A. (1997) Hippocampal pyramidal cell disarray correlates negatively to cell number: implications for the pathogenesis of schizophrenia. *Eur Arch Psychiatry Clin Neurosci*, **247**, 120–7.

Joyce, J.N., Shane, A., Lexow, N., Winokur, A., Casanova, M.F. and Kleinman, J.E. (1993) Serotonin uptake sites and serotonin receptors are altered in the limbic system of schizophrenics. *Neuropsychopharmacol*, **8**, 315–36.

Kim, J.S., Kornhuber, H.H., Schmid-Burgk, W. and Holzmuller, B. (1980) Low cerebrospinal fluid glutamate in schizophrenia patients and a new hypothesis on schizophrenia. *Neuroscience Letts*, **20**, 379–82.

Kiuchi, Y., Kobayashi, T., Takeuchi, J., Shimizu, H., Ogata, H. and Toru, M. (1989) Benzodiazepine receptors increase in post-mortem brain of chronic schizophrenics. *Eur Arch Psychiatry Neurol Sci*, **239**, 71–8.

Kornhuber, J., Mack-Burkhardt, F., Riederer, P., Hebenstreit, G.F., Reynolds, G.P., Andrews, H.B. and Beckmann, H. (1989) [³H]MK-801 binding sites in postmortem brain regions of schizophrenic patients. *J Neural Transmiss*, **77**, 231–6.

Kovelman, J.A. and Scheibel, A.B. (1984) A neurohistological correlate of schizophrenia. *Biol Psychiatry*, **19**, 1601–21.

Krimer, L.S., Herman, M.M., Saunders, R.C., Boyd, J.C., Hyde, T.M., Carter, J.M., Kleinman, J.E. and Weinberger, D.R. (1997) A qualitative and quantitative analysis of the entorhinal cortex in schizophrenia. *Cerebral Cortex*, **7**, 732–9.

Krystal, J.H., Karper, L.P., Seibyl, J.P., Freeman, G.K., Delancy, R., Bremner, J.D., Heninger, G.R., Bowers, Jr M.B. and Charney, D.C. (1994) Subanesthetic effects of the noncompetitive NMDA antagonist, ketamine, in humans. Psychotomimetic, perceptual, cognitive and neuroendocrine responses. *Arch Gen Psychiatry*, **51**, 199–214.

Liddle, P.F., Friston, K.J., Frith, C.D., Hirsch, S.R., Jones, T. and Frackowiak, R.S. (1992) Patterns of cerebral blood flow in schizophrenia. *Brit J Psychiatry*, **160**, 179–86.

Longson, D., Longson, C.M., Deakin, J.F.W. and Benes, F.M. (1998) Specific increase in size of lamina II pyramidal cells in the entorhinal cortex in schizophrenia. *Schizophr Res*, **29**, 87.

Luby, E.D., Gotlieb, J.S., Cohen, B.D., Rosenbaum, G. and Domino, E.F. (1961) Model psychoses and schizophrenia. *Am J Psychiatry*, **119**, 61–7.

Moghaddam, B., Adams, B., Verma, A. and Daly, D. (1997) Activation of glutamatergic neurotransmission by ketamine: a novel step in the pathway from NMDA receptor blockade to dopaminergic and cognitive disruptions associated with the prefrontal cortex. *J Neurosci*, **17**, 2921–7.

Nakai, T., Hashimoto, T., Kitamura, N., Nishino, N., Shirakawa, O., Hanada, S., Mita, T. and Tanaka, C. (1988) Alterations of neurotransmitter receptors in schizophrenic patients. *Psychopharmacol*, **96** (suppl), 187.

Nishikawa, T., Takashima, M. and Toru, M. (1983) Increased [3H]kainic acid binding in the prefrontal cortex in schizophrenia. *Neuroscience Letts*, **40**, 245–50.

Noga, J.T., Hyde, T.M., Herman, M.M., Spurney, C.F., Bigelow, L.B., Weinberger, D.R. and Kleinman, J.E. (1997) Glutamate receptors in the postmortem striatum of schizophrenic, suicide and control brains. *Synapse*, **27**, 168–76.

Olney, J.W. and Farber, N.B. (1995) Glutamate receptor dysfunction and schizophrenia. *Arch Gen Psychiatry* **52**, 998–1007.

Pakkenberg, B. (1990) Pronounced reduction of total neuron number in mediodorsal thalamic nucleus and nucleus accumbens in schizophrenics. *Arch Gen Psychiatry*, **47**, 1023–8.

Pakkenberg, B. (1992) The volume of the mediodorsal thalamic nucleus in treated and untreated schizophrenics. *Schizophr Res* **7**, 95–100.

Perry, T.L. (1982) Normal cerebrospinal fluid and brain glutamate levels in schizophrenia do not support the hypothesis of glutamatergic neuronal dysfunction. *Neuroscience Letts*, **28**, 81–85.

Potkin, S. (1998) Personal communication.

Reynolds, G.P. (1983) Increased concentrations and lateral asymmetry of amygdala dopamine in schizophrenia. *Nature*, **305**, 527–9.

Rosse, R.B., Theut, S.K., Banay-Schwartz, M., Leighton, M., Scarcella, E., Cohen, C.G. and Deutsch, S.I. (1989) Glycine adjuvant therapy to conventional neuroleptic treatment in schizophrenia: an open-label, pilot study. *Clin Neuropharmacol*, **12**, 416–24.

Rosse, R.B., Schwartz, B.L., Davis, R.E. and Deutsch, S.I. (1991) An NMDA intervention strategy in schizophrenia with 'low dose' milacemide. *Clin Neuropharmacol*, **14**, 268–72.

Rosse, R.B., Fay-McCarthy, M., Kendrick, K., Davis, R.E. and Deutsch, S.I. (1996) D-cycloserine adjuvant therapy to molindone in the treatment of schizophrenia. *Clin Neuropharmacol*, **19**, 444–50.

Schlaepfer, T.E., Harris, G.J., Tien, A.Y., Peng, L.W., Lee, S., Federman, E.B., Chase, G.A., Barta, P.E. and Pearlson, G.D. (1994) Decreased regional cortical gray matter volume in schizophrenia. *Am J Psychiatry*, **151**, 842–8.

Selemon, L.D., Rajkowska, G. and Goldman-Rakic, P.S. (1995) Abnormally high neuronal density in the schizophrenic cortex. A morphometric analysis of prefrontal area 9 and occipital area 17. *Arch Gen Psychiatry*, **52**, 805–18.

Simpson, M.D.C., Slater, P., Royston, M.C. and Deakin, J.F.W. (1991) Alterations in phencyclidine and sigma binding sites in schizophrenic brains. Effects of disease process and neuroleptic medication. *Schizophr Res*, **6**, 41–8.

Simpson, M.D.C., Slater, P., Royston, M.C., Deakin, J.F.W. (1992) Regionally selective deficits in uptake sites for glutamate and gamma-aminobutyric acid in the basal ganglia in schizophrenia. *Psychiatry Res*, **42**, 273–82.

Simpson, M.D.C., Lubman, D., Slater, P. and Deakin, J.F.W. (1996) Autoradiography with [³H]8-OH-DPAT reveals increases in 5–HT¹ᴬ receptors in ventral prefrontal cortex in schizophrenia. *Biol Psychiatry*, **39**, 919–28.

Simpson, M.D.C., Slater, P. and Deakin, J.F.W. (1998a) Comparison of glutamate and gamma-aminobutyric acid uptake binding sites in frontal and temporal lobes in schizophrenia. *Biol Psychiatry*, **44**, 423–7.

Simpson, M.D.C., Slater, P., Deakin, J.F.W., Gottfries, C.G., Karlsson, I., Grenfeldt, B. and Crow, T.J. (1998b) Absence of basal ganglia amino acid neuron deficits in schizophrenia in three collections of brains. *Schizophr Res*, **31**, 167–75.

Slater, P., McConnell, S., D'Souza, S.W., Barson, A.J., Simpson, M.D.C. and Gilchrist, A.C. (1992) Age-related changes in binding to excitatory amino acid uptake site in temporal cortex of human brain. *Dev Brain Res*, **65**, 157–60.

Slater, P., McConnell, S.E., D'Souza, S.W. and Barson, A.J. (1993) Postnatal changes in N-methyl-D-aspartate receptor binding and stimulation by glutamate and glycine of [³H]-MK-801 binding in human temporal cortex. *Brit J Pharmacol*, **108**, 1143–9.

Uranova, N.A. and Orlovskaya, D.D. (1996) Ultrastructural pathology of neuronal connectivity in post-mortem brains of schizophrenic patients. *Ann Psychiatry*, **6**, 55–72.

van Berckel, B.N., Hijman, R., van der Linden, J.A., Westenberg, H.G., van Ree, J.M. and Kahn, R.S. (1996) Efficacy and tolerance of D-cycloserine in drug-free schizophrenic patients. *Biol Psychiatry*, **40**, 1298–1300.

Waziri, R. (1988) Glycine therapy of schizophrenia. *Biol Psychiatry*, **23**, 210–11.

Weinberger, D.R., Berman, K.F., Suddath, R. and Torrey, E.F. (1992) Evidence of dysfunction of a prefrontal-limbic network in schizophrenia: a magnetic resonance imaging and regional cerebral blood flow study of discordant monozygotic twins. *Am J Psychiatry*, **149**, 890–7.

Whitaker, P.M., Crow, T.J. and Ferrier, I.N. (1981) Tritiated LSD binding in frontal cortex in schizophrenia. *Arch Gen Psychiatry*, **38**, 278–0.

Woo, T.U., Miller, J.L. and Lewis, D.A. (1997) Schizophrenia and the parvalbumin-containing class of cortical local circuit neurons. *Am J Psychiatry*, **154**, 1013–15.

Woodruff, P.W.R., Pearlson, G.D., Geer, M.J., Barta, P.E. and Chilcoat, H.D. (1993) A computerized magnetic resonance imaging study of corpus callosum morphology in schizophrenia. *Psychol Med*, **23**, 45–56.

Woodruff, P.W.R., Wright, I.C., Shuriquie, N., Russouw, H., Rushe, T., Howard, R.J., Graves, M., Bullmore, E.T. and Murray, R.M. (1997b) Structural brain abnormalities in male schizophrenics reflect fronto-temporal dissociation. *Psychol Med*, **27**, 1257–66.

Zaidel, D.W., Esiri, M.M. and Harrison, P.J. (1997a) Size, shape and orientation of neurons in the left and right hippocampus: investigation of normal asymmetries and alterations in schizophrenia. *Am J Psychiatry*, **154**, 812–18.

CHAPTER 5

Molecular genetics of schizophrenia

PAUL R. BUCKLAND AND PETER MCGUFFIN

Genetics and environment

That there is a genetic contribution to the aetiology of schizophrenia is not in doubt. Both Kraepelin, who first described *dementia praecox,* and later Bleuler, who introduced the term *schizophrenia* both agreed that they were dealing with a familial illness. However, the familiality does not necessarily mean that genes are involved and teasing apart genetic and environmental influences is a complex task.

The evidence favouring a familial basis for schizophrenia has been collated by Gottesman (1991). He showed that the lifetime risk of a member of the general population is slightly lower than 1%. This increases to 3–4% in second degree relatives and to around 10% in the first degree relatives of schizophrenics. The risk also increases with the number of affected relatives, so that the lifetime risk for someone who has both a schizophrenic parent and sibling is about 16%. In addition, there have been many twin studies of schizophrenia, all of which have shown the same pattern of findings, with higher concordance in monozygotic (MZ) than dizygotic (DZ) twins, typically just under 50% for MZ and 10% for DZ twins (Farmer *et al.,* 1987; Onstad *et al.,* 1991).

Taking all the evidence together from family, adoption and twin studies, there is a consistent pattern of results favouring an important genetic contribution to schizophrenia, albeit not a simple Mendelian one. Typically in biometric models, environmental factors are considered to have two component parts, shared environment which contributes to the aggregation of a trait within families, and non-shared, or residual environment that does not. When such models have been applied to schizophrenia data, typically the finding is of a heritablity, or genetic contribution of around

70% (McGuffin *et al.*, 1994). Furthermore, it is usually possible to drop the shared environmental component from the model entirely. This is in keeping with the results of adoption studies and findings on MZ twins reared apart, which suggest that the environment in which an individual is raised has little or no effect on his or her susceptibility to schizophrenia (Gottesman, 1991).

It is clear therefore that although there is a major genetic contribution to schizophrenia, what is inherited is a predisposition to the illness. The idea of a liability/threshold model to explain the transmission of common familial disorders was first applied to schizophrenia by Gottesman and Shields (1967). The assumption is that liability to develop the disorder is normally distributed in the population and that this distribution reflects the additive effects of several different genes plus environmental factors. Only those individuals whose liability at some time exceeds a certain threshold manifest the disease. Relatives of schizophrenics have on average an increased liability compared with the general population, and hence more relatives lie beyond the threshold for manifesting the disorder. This is usually referred to as the polygenic threshold model (implying many genes), but the same pattern could result from oligogenic inheritance (a few genes) .

By contrast, other workers have put forward single-gene explanations of schizophrenia, invoking the notion of incomplete penetrance to explain the lack of Mendelian segregation ratios. However, single-gene models do not resist rigorous statistical scrutiny, and the data from twin and family studies have been shown to be incompatible either with the hypothesis that schizophrenia can be accounted for by a mutation in a single gene, or that it represents a collection of single-gene disorders each with a similar clinical manifestation (McGue and Gottesman, 1989)

In addition to being statistically more satisfactory, liability/threshold models in which schizophrenia results from the combined action of several different genes offer explanations of several observed phenomena. First, such models fit with the observation that the risk of schizophrenia increases with the number of other relatives affected. Second, they account for the finding in some (but not all) family studies of higher concentrations of schizophrenia among relatives of severe, early onset cases. Third, a model involving several genes is easier than a single-gene model to reconcile with the fact that schizophrenia persists at high rates in the population despite being associated with reduced reproductive fitness.

An alternative explanation of schizophrenia transmission that has not been excluded by statistical studies is the mixed model of inheritance in which there is a gene of major effect acting in combination with a background of polygenes. Attempts to test a mixed model have yielded inconclusive results (Vogler *et al.*, 1991). A further complication is that although multi-locus models have traditionally assumed that genes contributing to schizophrenia act in a mainly additive way, family data can be interpreted as showing epistasis – that is, two or more loci have a multiplicative interaction, where the final result is greater than the sum of the effects of individual loci (Risch, 1990).

Another reason for the inconclusive results of statistical model fitting is that most studies have sought a unitary explanation for the transmission of schizophrenia. Bleuler originally wrote about 'the group of schizophrenias', with the implication that he was describing a collection of phenotypically similar but perhaps genotypically distinct conditions. If this were true we might expect schizophrenia sub-types to show homotypia, that is to breed true within families. Some older studies of pairs of affected relatives have shown a tendency toward homotypia with statistically significant (albeit incomplete) concordance for Kraepelinian sub-types (e.g. paranoid, hebephrenic, and catatonic schizophrenia) but more recent studies have been more equivocal (McGuffin *et al.*, 1987). A further difficulty is that separation of schizophrenia into sub-types shows instability over time with a tendency, for example, for paranoid schizophrenics to progress to hebephrenic or undifferentiated types.

A more straightforward suggestion is that schizophrenia can be divided into genetic and common non-genetic types (phenocopies) and that this explains both the absence of family history in most cases and the inconclusive results of genetic modelling. This might also account for phenomena such as discordance in monozygotic (MZ) twins. However, Gottesman and Bertelsen (1989) have shown in a study of offspring of discordant MZ twins that the risk of schizophrenia to children of normal MZ co-twins is the same as that in children of the affected proband. This result, together with the findings of earlier studies that there is little difference in rates of schizophrenia in first-degree relatives of discordant versus concordant MZ twins, argues against the notion that non-genetic phenocopies constitute a substantial proportion of those with schizophrenia.

Finally, modern genetics has revealed several mechanisms that may give rise to complex patterns of inheritance and phenotypic variability. They include genomic imprinting and the discovery that some diseases are caused by mutations involving unstable DNA sequences in the form of expanded trinucleotide repeats. Imprinting refers to the differential expression of a gene or set of genes, according to whether it is of maternal or paternal origin. Trinucleotide repeats can form dynamic mutations that expand from one generation to the next, resulting in alterations in disease severity between generations and also irregular patterns of transmission due to the fact that expansion may depend upon the sex of the parent. One phenomenon especially associated with dynamic mutations is that of anticipation, in which there is a progressively earlier age of onset and increasing disease severity in successive generations. The discovery of dynamic mutations has re-awakened interest in anticipation in mental illness and recently claims have been made that it can be observed in schizophrenia (Asherson *et al.*, 1994). Such studies should be interpreted cautiously since it is extremely hard to rule out ascertainment bias, but a role for dynamic mutations in schizophrenia remains a real possibility (O'Donovan *et al.*, 1995)

Molecular genetic approaches

Despite uncertainties about the mode of transmission and the implausibility of a simple single-gene explanation for schizophrenia, much current effort is directed at locating schizophrenia genes by linkage analysis in large families with multiple affected members. This is based on the assumption that heterogeneity exists and that such multiplex families, or at least a proportion of them, are segregating genes of major effect. Focusing research on highly familial sub-forms has proved to be a successful approach in other complex disorders such as Alzheimer's disease, non-insulin dependent diabetes, and breast cancer. Furthermore, the recent availability of large numbers of highly polymorphic genetic markers based on simple sequence repeat polymorphisms has increased the feasibility of systematic searches for linkage. The aim is to study about 300 DNA markers evenly spread throughout the genome. By examining their co-segregation with the disorder within families, one can then infer the position of the disease gene. This is the first step in what is now known as positional cloning, where the goal is to move from finding linked markers to identifying the gene itself.

Several groups have already conducted fairly extensive searches of a substantial proportion of the genome and there has been partial confirmation of linkages on chromosomes 6, 8 and 22 (e.g. Morris *et al.*, 1995; Gill *et al.*, 1996; Levinson *et al.*, 1997). However, given the possibility that there is more than one major locus involved in the causation of schizophrenia, the best hope for this approach probably lies in large collaborative studies that can provide sufficient sample size to detect major gene effects despite the presence of heterogeneity. Such studies are currently in progress in Europe under the auspices of the European Science Foundation and in the USA by the National Institute of Mental Health. We can be confident that, if genes of major effect are involved reasonably commonly in the aetiology of schizophrenia, they will be detected and localized during the next few years.

However, there are several reasons why a systematic search with conventional linkage analysis may not be successful. The most important is that the existence of multiplex families does not necessarily indicate the operation of major gene effects, and such families can occur even under conditions of polygenic transmission. Indeed the most frequently replicated linkage result to date, with markers on chromosome 6p, is probably detecting a gene of only small effect (Levinson *et al.*, 1997). Another difficulty with large families is that of diagnostic instability. For example, in a well-known study of bipolar affective disorder, highly promising results suggesting linkage to markers on chromosome 11 proved to be a probable false positive when family members initially classified as unaffected became ill. This is inevitably a hazard in any study attempting to find linkage in a functional psychosis where the age of risk for a first episode of illness extends into middle or even later life.

Diagnostic difficulties also arise when the index case satisfies a narrow definition of schizophrenia but several relatives have other disorders that may or may not be genetically related. The common solution to this problem is to conduct analyses with several definitions which vary in relation to the breadth of the affected category. Unfortunately, this method involves multiple testing and again may produce false positive results. For instance, the results suggesting linkage between a schizophrenia susceptibility gene and markers on chromosome 5 were most positive for a very broad definition of the disorder (Sherrington *et al.*, 1988) and could not be replicated by other groups (McGuffin *et al.*, 1990).

Even if the search for markers linked to schizophrenia is successful, the question arises as to whether the results will be relevant to the more common cases of the disorder where there are few or no affected relatives. Alternatively, if linkage is not detected this suggests that schizophrenia is entirely dependent for its transmission on several or perhaps many genes each having only a small effect. The question then becomes: how can such genes be detected?

Both of these difficulties have a common solution, which is to conduct studies among pairs of affected relatives using allele-sharing methods to detect linkage. Studies of affected sibling pairs are the simplest approach and the aim is to determine whether the alleles of any marker are shared more often than would be expected by chance. For example, for a particular locus, in the absence of linkage, affected siblings sharing two, one, or no marker alleles would be expected to occur in the ratio of $1:2:1$. Any statistically significant departure from this ratio suggests a relation between the marker locus and the disease. A further advantage of concentrating on sibling pairs is that this allows a focus on purely core diagnoses of schizophrenia, whilst relatives who may have fringe phenotypes can be ignored. By contrast with conventional methods of detecting linkage in large families, sibling-pair methods do not require any knowledge about the mode of transmission of the disorder and so avoid errors due to mis-specification of the mode of transmission. The main disadvantage of the general approach is that although robust, power is relatively low, and so large sample sizes are required. Nevertheless, the feasibility of accomplishing a complete genome scan in sibling pairs has been demonstrated in a study of type 1 diabetes where it now seems probable that at least five different susceptibility loci are involved. Similar studies involving 200 or more sib-pairs affected by schizophrenia are currently underway.

A variation on the sib-pair approach is not to consider schizophrenia as a simple dichotomy – affected and unaffected – but to attempt to measure the liability to schizophrenia in siblings of schizophrenics. One way in which this might be achieved is to use schizotypy scores. The usefulness of this so-called quantitative trait locus (QTL) approach has recently been demonstrated in the study of reading disability indicating a locus on the short arm of chromosome 6 (Cardon *et al.*, 1994).

A further method that is also able to detect and localize genes with comparatively small effects is to search for allelic association. The most common and straightforward design is simply to compare the frequency of marker alleles in a sample of patients with ethnically matched controls. A significantly higher frequency of the marker allele in the patient group suggests either that the marker itself has some direct influence on susceptibility to the disease, or that it is in linkage disequilibrium with a susceptibility locus. Before the discovery of DNA polymorphisms, many allelic association studies were conducted with classic markers in schizophrenia (e.g. HLA and red blood cell types). Although there was a suggestion from several studies of a weak association between HLA A9 and paranoid schizophrenia, the status of these results remains uncertain and has not been confirmed. Current interest in association studies focuses on functionally significant variations in candidate genes, that is, genes coding for proteins that might plausibly be involved in pathogenesis of the disorder.

Candidate genes

Candidate genes for schizophrenia come from two main sources: studies of either living or post-mortem brains or the effects of antipsychotic and psychotogenic drugs. If the gene in question has been identified and cloned, polymorphisms within the gene may be used for genetic studies, including linkage analysis and association studies. No candidate gene has so far proved positive in the former but several have shown positive results in association studies. These include the dopamine D2 (Arinami *et al.*, 1997) and D3 receptors (Crocq *et al.*, 1992) and the serotonin

5HT2A receptor (Williams *et al.*, 1996). A polymorphism within the 5HT2C receptor has been shown to be associated with efficacy of drug treatment (Sodhi *et al.*, 1996).

Most known causes of genetic illnesses involve a mutation or abnormality within a gene, leading to either abnormal protein functioning due to a mutation in the coding region of the gene or abnormal protein expression due to a mutation in the 5' flanking or promoter region of the gene which could affect the rate of initiation of transcription. Gene expression can be controlled by any one of a cascade of mechanisms leading from the gene to the functional protein. These can be roughly put into three categories: changes in the functional state of the protein, changes in the abundance of the protein, and changes in the abundance of the encoding mRNA. These changes occur naturally in response to a perturbation of the system in order to maintain homeostasis in the short, medium and long term, respectively.

The associations reported to date with polymorphisms at dopamine or serotonin receptors do not suggest major alterations in the receptor proteins. It has been suggested that in both receptors, dopamine D3 and 5HT2A, findings may indicate linkage disequilibrium with other polymorphisms in the 5' flanking region of the genes, and that the latter are the real modulators of susceptibility to schizophrenia. If this were so, these promoter region mutations would be expected to exert their effect by changing the rate of initiation of transcription, producing more or less mRNA and encoded protein. The abundance of these receptors rather than their ligand binding ability may therefore be what confers susceptibility to schizophrenia, and any drug-induced regulation of receptor mRNA levels may be central to the effects of antipsychotics rather than merely a side-effect. Other polymorphisms have recently been found in the promoter region of the 5HT2A receptor, including one in linkage disequilibrium with the T102C polymorphism. However, Burnet *et al.*, (1996a) have presented data which suggest that the 5HT2A polymorphism (T102C) does not give rise to differential mRNA levels. Other recent research has shown that in transfected cells the promoter region polymorphism does not differentially affect gene transcription and also the expression of the two variants is not altered in lymphocytes expressing only one or the other allele (M.J. Owen *et al.* unpublished data). An alternative explanation is that the dopamine D3 and/or 5HT2 polymorphisms may affect the ability of the control mechanisms for receptor density to respond appropriately and adapt to external or internal stimuli.

Below we discuss briefly the neurochemical and pharmacological evidence relating to a number of potential candidate genes with an emphasis on those studies reporting polymorphisms associated with schizophrenia.

STUDIES OF SCHIZOPHRENIC BRAINS

Neurochemical abnormalities reported to be found in schizophrenic brains include: a reduction of glutamic acid decarboxylase mRNA in prefrontal cortex (Akbarian *et al.*, 1995); selective alterations in gene expression for NMDA receptor sub-units in prefrontal cortex (Akbarian *et al.*, 1996); a reduction of synaptophysin mRNA in CA4, CA3, subiculum and parahippocampal gyrus (Eastwood *et al.*, 1995a); a decrease in cholecystokinin mRNA in frontal cortex and superior temporal cortex (Virgo *et al.*, 1995); and decreased expression of mRNAs encoding non-NMDA glutamate receptors GluR1 and GluR2 in medial temporal lobe neurons (Eastwood *et al.*, 1995b).

Of the above perhaps the glutamate system is of most interest. The basal ganglia and limbic systems receive inputs from both glutamate and dopamine neuronal projections. These are normally in balance, and overstimulation or blocking of the dopaminergic system can be counteracted respectively by blockade of, or increased stimulation of, the glutamatergic system. The opposite is also true and blockade of the glutamatergic system gives rise to functional effects similar to overstimulation of the dopaminergic system. Phencyclidine (PCP) is an NMDA antagonist which can cause psychosis with similarities to both the positive and negative symptoms of schizophrenia. It causes increased dopamine release but both its biochemical and psychological effects can be blocked by haloperidol. An aberrant glutamatergic system could therefore give rise to psychosis which would be ameliorated by dopaminergic drugs. However, no genetic associations have so far been found with any glutamatergic system components.

PHARMACOLOGICAL STUDIES

There have been many studies on the effects of acute and chronic antipsychotic drug treatment on protein abundance/activity or mRNA levels in animal brains. Most of these have been carried out with haloperidol, frequently compared with clozapine. It has long been established that dopamine D2 receptors are upregulated but few other changes have been confirmed. Recently, many studies on mRNA abundance have been reported. Changes reported include: a downregulation of gonadotrophin-releasing hormone (Li and Pelletier, 1992), preprotachykinin A (Lindefors, 1992) and neuropeptide Y mRNA (Herman, 1996), but upregulation of enkephalin (Delfs *et al.*, 1994), pro-opiomelanocortin (Oyarce *et al.*, 1996), carboxypeptidase E (Grigoriants *et al.*, 1993), glutamate decarboxylase (Delfs *et al.*, 1995) and secretogranin II mRNA (Kroesen *et al.*, 1995).

NEUROTENSIN

Neurotensin is an endogenous tridecapeptide with a wide spectrum of biological activity in the central and peripheral nervous systems with effects including hypotension, hyperglycaemia, hypothermia, antinociception, and regulation of intestinal motility and secretion (Liégeois *et al.*, 1995). In addition it functions either as a modulator of neurotransmission or as a transmitter in its own right having its own receptor. It is widely distributed throughout the CNS, predominantly in regions enervated by, or associated with, dopaminergic neurons, i.e. ventral tegmentum, substantia nigra, septum, amygdala and nucleus accumbens (Liégeois *et al.*, 1995). In the prefrontal cortex (studied because there are few dopaminergic neurons) dopamine and neurotensin co-localize to the same neurons and have a complex relationship (Elsworth and Roth, 1997). Neurotensin has been shown to act as a positive modulator of ligand binding (7-OH-DPAT) at the dopamine D3 receptor (Liu *et al.*, 1994). There is now a large body of biochemical, behavioural and electrophysiological evidence showing that neurotensin interacts with dopaminergic transmission (Bean *et al.*, 1992).

In laboratory animals centrally administered neurotensin has a remarkably similar effect to peripherally administered antipsychotics (Nemeroff *et al.*, 1992; Liégeois *et al.*, 1995). Neurotensin induces catalepsy, decreases locomotor activity, increases dopamine turnover, antagonizes amphetamine-induced hyperactivity, potentiates barbiturate-induced sedation, induces hypothermia, decreases response in a conditioned avoidance paradigm, and produces several other effects similar to those caused by antipsychotic drugs (Liégeois *et al.*, 1995). Specifically, neurotensin has similar effects to 'atypical' neuroleptics and neurotensin agonists are being developed as potential 'atypical' antipsychotic drugs (Liégeois *et al.*, 1995).

From the above discussion, it is not surprising that neurotensin has been described as an endogenous 'antipsychotic' and it has been postulated that decreased expression of the gene or a defective neurotensin protein may result in psychosis (Nemeroff *et al.*, 1992). This hypothesis is indirectly supported by the observation that all clinically efficacious antipsychotics selectively increase neurotensin mRNA in the shell of the nucleus accumbens while 'typical' but not 'atypical' antipsychotics also increase neurotensin mRNA in the dorsolateral striatum (Kinkead and Nemeroff, 1994). More direct evidence comes from a report that drug-free schizophrenic patients have low levels of neurotensin in cerebrospinal fluid, which increases on treatment with antipsychotic drugs (Nemeroff *et al.*, 1992). Therefore on theoretical as well as empirical grounds, neurotensin is a strong candidate gene for psychosis.

The neurotensin receptor (NTR) couples to G-protein and second messengers including cGMP, inositol 1,4,5-triphosphate and Ca^{2+}. This receptor is found in pre- and post-synaptic and also somatodendritic neuronal locations. High affinity binding sites for neurotensin parallel the distribution of the peptide with the exception of the caudate nucleus where the neurotensin receptor density is low (Liégeois *et al.*, 1995).

Ligand binding studies of post-mortem brain have revealed a 44% reduction in neurotensin binding in layer II cell clusters of the entorrhinal cortex where cytoarchitectural abnormalities have also been reported in schizophrenia (Wolf *et al.*, 1995). However, this may have due to downregulation of neurotensin receptor expression or loss of neurons. In addition the mRNA encoding the NTR has been shown to be upregulated in the substantia nigra/ventral tegmental area following chronic treatment with haloperidol (Watson-Bolden *et al.*, 1993).

2-PHENYLETHYLAMINE

A very similar situation to that of neurotensin is found for the enzyme aromatic L-amino acid decarboxylase (AADC) and we have previously described the evidence for AADC being a candidate gene for schizophrenia (Buckland *et al.*, 1992a, 1996, 1997b). This enzyme is rate limiting in the production of two potentially psychotogenic amines, tryptamine and 2-phenylethylamine (2PE). These monoamines act as positive modulators of serotonin and dopamine respectively but may have their own receptors. It has been postulated that 2PE is an endogenous psychotogen and that aberrant expression of AADC may be associated with schizophrenia. 2-PE is found in excess in the serum of schizophrenics, and the activity of the enzyme AADC is increased in the brains of living schizophrenics. When given to rats, 2PE has a similar effect to that of amphetamine, and indeed the two compounds have a similar structure and may act at the same site. Two psychotogenic drugs, lysergic acid diethylamide (LSD) and phencyclidine (PCP) upregulate AADC mRNA and presumably therefore, increase the production of 2PE. Both antipsychotic drugs and amphetamine effect the production of AADC and 2PE but in the opposite way than might at first be expected (Buckland *et al.*, 1992a, 1996, 1997b). Neuroleptics antagonize the effect of 2PE and amphetamine agonizes it, and so homeostatic compensation results in upregulation of AADC by the former and downregulation by the latter. Again, however, no genetic polymorphisms or associations have so far been reported.

DOPAMINE RECEPTORS

It has long been known that a common property of antipsychotic drugs is that they all act as antagonists at dopamine receptors. Much research has been carried out in this area and dopamine receptors remain prime candidate genes for schizophrenia. A number of studies in the past have suggested that dopamine D2 receptor numbers were increased in drug-naïve schizophrenics. However, several recent studies using either positron emission tomography to look at living brains or ligand binding of post-mortem tissue have found no change in D2 receptor numbers (Knable *et al.*, 1994; Sedvall *et al.*, 1995 and refs. cited). Nevertheless, the controversy still has not been decided as other workers are still reporting an increase (Roberts *et al.*, 1994). Other workers have shown a decrease in D1 receptors in the basal ganglia (Sedvall *et al.*, 1995) and prefrontal cortex (Okubo *et al.*, 1997). Sceman *et al.* (1993) claim dopamine D4 receptors are increased in schizophrenic brains. However, Reynolds and Mason (1994) dispute this. In fact there are no generally accepted abnormalities in the dopaminergic system of schizophrenic brains.

One difficulty in the above work is the lack of specificity of ligands for different receptor sub-types. Since the discovery of the five sub-types of dopamine receptor and the advent of molecular technology, each receptor mRNA can be measured with a theoretical 100% specificity. A large number of researchers have addressed the effect of chronic antipsychotic treatment on dopamine D1, D2 and D3 receptor mRNA levels in rodents, but surprisingly disparate results appear to have been obtained.

One problem is the variation in drug dosages given to animals in different studies. Other variations in research protocols include different times of administration and different brain regions studied. Buckland *et al.* (1997a) and D'Souza *et al.* (1998) have recently carried out a survey of the effects of six antipsychotic drugs on dopamine and 5HT2 receptor mRNAs in rat brain using different dosages and time points and also, in the case of three representative drugs, a number of different brain regions encompassing the entire brain (Buckland *et al.*, 1997a; D'Souza *et al.*, 1998).

D1 Receptor

Relatively little work has been carried out on the expression of this receptor in relation to chronic antipsychotic treatment. Buckland *et al.* (1992b) have shown that 32 days treatment with haloperidol and loxapine resulted in D1 receptor mRNA increases of 100 and 400% respectively in whole brain but no other antipsychotic drug has the same effect (D'Souza *et al.*, 1998). This rise has been localized to the striatum and prefrontal cortex (D'Souza *et al.*, 1998). Damask *et al.* (1996) treated rats with haloperidol for 14 days and also found a rise in D1 mRNA in striatum and prefrontal cortex. However, Jaber *et al.* (1994) and Xu *et al.* (1992), using similar protocols, found no change in striatum.

D'Souza *et al.* (1998) have recently shown that chronic treatment with haloperidol, sulpiride or clozapine elicited a 25–50% downregulation of the D1 mRNA in hippocampus, whilst the former two drugs also downregulated it in cerebellum by similar amounts. The levels of D1 mRNA are at their lowest in these brain regions, which are usually associated with the serotonergic system. However, these changes may have major significance. Buckland *et al.* (1997a) have previously shown that in the same brain samples, drug treatment causes a significant drop in 5HT2A receptor mRNA in the hippocampus and a significant drop in 5HT2C receptor mRNA in the cerebellum (*see* below). An interaction between the dopaminergic and serotonergic systems in the therapeutic effects of antipsychotic drugs have frequently been postulated and this may be seen as direct evidence for this.

D2 receptor

In comparison to D1 receptors, a large amount of work has been carried out on D2 receptor expression. At least 24 research reports have addressed the question of upregulation of dopamine D2 receptor mRNA; 15 report upregulation of varying degrees following chronic treatment with antipsychotic drugs, mainly haloperidol, whilst seven report no changes, RNA being measured in either whole brain or striatum, in either rats or mice (D'Souza *et al.*, 1998 and refs. cited). An additional paper reports an upregulation in the anterior cingulate cortex but not striatum. D'Souza *et al.* (1998) looked at a number of regions encompassing most of the brain. Changes following haloperidol treatment were only found in the striatum and prefrontal cortex, in parallel with the changes found in D1 mRNA above.

D'Souza *et al.* (1997) have shown that three factors all affect the finding of an increase in D2 mRNA: the drug dosage, the time of administration, and the drug in question. Seven of the eight reports which found no change used either a low dosages or short times of administration; under comparative conditions D'Souza *et al.* (1998) also found no changes. Only one of these negative papers uses a comparable protocol to that of D'Souza *et al.* (1998) but reports inconsistent results. However, on the reverse side, of the papers reporting an increase in D2 mRNA, five of these used low dosages or short times of administration. Nevertheless, the increases in each case were small and similar to those reported after 16 days treatment by D'Souza *et al.* (1998). The evidence strongly suggests therefore, that upregulation of dopamine D2 receptor mRNA requires a relatively high dose and prolonged time of administration of haloperidol.

With the exception of a very small increase in the mid-brain region, D'Souza *et al.* (1998) found no significant changes in the D2 mRNA levels of any brain region following clozapine or sulpiride treatment. This confirms the lack of any changes found in whole brain samples by Buckland *et al.* (1992b). These results are supported by Zhang *et al.* (1995), who found no change in D2 mRNA following 21 days infusion of clozapine in mice, but differ from Damask *et al.* (1996) who report small drops in D2 mRNA in cortical regions and also the striatum and nucleus accumbens following clozapine treatment. However, it is clear that clozapine and sulpiride do not upregulate D2 mRNA levels whilst haloperidol does.

The lack of any effect by both sulpiride and clozapine in any brain region and by other drugs in whole brain on either dopamine D1 or D2 mRNA has led several groups to postulate that the upregulation by haloperidol may be related to its propensity to cause side-effects such as tardive dyskinesia. However, the work of Arinami *et al.* (1997) showing an association between schizophrenia and a D2 receptor promoter region polymorphism suggests otherwise. What is clear is that upregulation of D2 receptors is not essential for antipsychotic action.

D3 receptor

Gerevich *et al.* (1997) found that dopamine D3 receptors were elevated in the limbic striatum and its efferents in the brains of untreated schizophrenics, but not in treated patients compared to controls, suggesting that drug treatment lowers D3 receptor binding. In contrast, Schmauss *et al.* (1993) reported that there was a decrease in dopamine D3 receptor mRNA in parietal and motor cortices of schizophrenic patients, and this may be due to enhanced mRNA cleavage, giving rise to a protein that does not appear to be a G-protein coupled receptor (Schmauss, 1996). Compared to the dopamine D2 receptor, the D3 receptor has a low affinity for antipsychotics and a high affinity for dopamine, so at typical antipsychotic dosages, the D3 receptor is not blocked. Any regulation of this receptor by such drugs may therefore have a functional effect.

Several papers have looked at the effects of chronic antipsychotic treatment on D3 receptor mRNA levels. Four reports have shown upregulation of dopamine D3 receptor mRNA whilst three have shown no change (D'Souza *et al.*, 1998, and refs. cited). However, as in the case for the D2 receptor mRNA above, D'Souza *et al.* (1998) only found upregulation at higher dosages and longer times of administration, which were not used in the negative studies.

D'Souza *et al.* (1998) have shown that six structurally different antipsychotic drugs upregulate D3 receptor mRNA levels if given at high enough dosages and for long enough. Five drugs: haloperidol, loxapine, pimozide, flupenthixol and sulpiride, all upregulate D3 mRNA after 32 days treatment whereas clozapine upregulates D3 mRNA after 4 days (Buckland *et al.*, 1992b, 1993). These changes were only found in the nucleus accumbens and olfactory tubercles but not striatum or elsewhere (D'Souza *et al.*, 1998) and concurs with Wang *et al.* (1996). D'Souza and coworkers have also shown that clozapine upregulated dopamine D3 receptor ligand binding in the nucleus accumbens but not the striatum (unpublished data). This confirms the mRNA results.

Upregulation of D3 receptor mRNA, therefore, unlike that of D1 or D2 receptors appears to be common to all antipsychotic drugs. The human D3 receptor promoter region has not yet been sequenced or studied, but in light of the above and the already discovered association between a coding region polymorphism and schizophrenia, this must be a prime target of speculation.

5HT RECEPTORS

The role of serotonin in the aetiology of schizophrenia has been given much attention in recent years following the re-emergence of clozapine and the introduction of new antipsychotics thought to have an important serotonergic action. Most if not all antipsychotic drugs, as well as being dopamine D2 antagonists are also 5HT2 type antagonists. It has long been known that chronic treatment with antipsychotic drugs causes a downregulation of 5HT receptors in rats and possibly humans.

Clozapine acts as a competitive antagonist at 5HT2A and 5HT2C receptors and other 'older' antipsychotics act similarly but are less potent (Canton *et al.*, 1994). It has been postulated that 5HT2A antagonism is important, conferring 'atypical' status on drugs in that this effect to some extent counterbalances excessive dopamine D2 blockade (Kapur, 1996). However, the evidence for this is far from conclusive. It has also been postulated that 5HT2A antagonism may be contributory to amelioration of the negative symptoms of schizophrenia and there is some evidence of this (Schmidt *et al.*, 1995).

Serotonergic axons originate primarily from neuronal cell bodies in the dorsal and medial raphe nuclei in the mid-brain. The former project principally to the striatum, substantia nigra and frontal cortex, whereas the latter project to the hippocampus and limbic structures; both have projections to the neocortex. However, many other brain areas also receive serotonergic axons.

5HT2A receptor

Several studies have been carried out to determine if 5HT2A receptor binding is changed in schizophrenic patients. These have all been carried out on post-mortem tissue which introduces theoretical problems and the results have been mixed, possibly because many of the patients studied were on antipsychotic medication prior to death (Burnet *et al.*, 1996a; Kahn and Van Pragg, 1996; Meltzer and Faterni, 1996). Of seven studies looking at 5HT2A receptor binding in the frontal cortex, four have reported a decrease and three have reported no change (Burnet *et al.*, 1996a; Kahn and Van Pragg, 1996; Meltzer and Faterni, 1996, and refs. cited).

Burnet *et al.* looked at 5HT2A receptor mRNA levels and receptor binding in the same schizophrenic and normal control brain samples (Burnet *et al.*, 1996a). They found downregulation of binding in the prefrontal cortex and parahippocampal gyrus but no change in striate cortex. However, the mRNA was downregulated not only in prefrontal cortex but also in several regions of the cortex. In addition they was no change in parahippocampal gyrus. These studies suggest a complex relationship between mRNA and receptor abundance in schizophrenia. They also highlight the apparent paradoxical nature of regulation by some antipsychotic drugs which seem to lower 5HT2A receptor abundance whilst schizophrenia itself is associated with lower receptor numbers, and 5HT agonists also downregulate 5HT receptors.

Acute treatment with several antipsychotics including both clozapine and the 'typical' drug loxapine causes a downregulation in 5HT2A receptor binding in rat cortex, although treatment with some other drugs do not (Matsubara and Meltzer, 1989). Chronic treatment has been more consistently shown to downregulate 5HT2A receptor binding. Downregulation of 5HT2A binding in the frontal cortex has been shown to occur following treatment with drugs, including loxapine (Lee and Tang, 1984), clozapine (Burnet *et al.*, 1996b) and chlorpromazine, but not risperidone (Kuoppamäki *et al.*, 1995). Cortical 5HT2A binding is downregulated by drugs, including clozapine (Reynolds *et al.*, 1983), chlorpromazine (Mikuni and Meltzer, 1984) and flupenthixol (Andree *et al.*, 1986). However, several studies have shown that haloperidol and sulpiride do not downregulate 5HT2A receptor binding in rat cortex (Andree *et al.*, 1986; O'Dell *et al.*, 1990; Wilmot and Szczepanik, 1989; Burnet *et al.*, 1996b). Burnet *et al.* (1996b) have found that chronic clozapine treatment downregulates 5HT2A receptor mRNA in cingulate and frontal cortex but that haloperidol does not have the same effect. Buckland *et al.* (1997a) have found no significant decrease in mRNA abundance in the frontal or temporal cortex with chronic clozapine treatment, although a lower dose of clozapine was used. They have, however, found modest (13–39%) downregulation of 5HT2A mRNA following treatment with clozapine, sulpiride and haloperidol in three regions of the brain (hippocampus, mid-brain and brain stem).

5HT2C receptor

Both the 5HT2C receptor (Abramowski *et al.*, 1995) and its encoding mRNA (Hoffman and Mezey, 1989; Molineaux *et al.*, 1989; Wright *et al.*, 1995; Buckland *et al.*, 1997a) have been shown to be widespread in both human and rat brain.

The affinity of clozapine for the 5HT2C receptor is three orders of magnitude greater than that of haloperidol and therefore clozapine might be expected to have a different effect on the 5HT2C receptor than does haloperidol. Kuoppamäki *et al.* (1992, 1995, and refs. cited) have reported that 5HT2C receptor binding is downregulated in the choroid plexus by 14 days treatment with clozapine, but not haloperidol, chlorpromazine, or risperidone. Burnet *et al.* (1996b) have not found a change in 5HT2C mRNA levels in choroid plexus or other areas following similar clozapine and haloperidol treatment and suggest that the results of Kuoppamäki *et al.* (1992, 1995) can be explained by post-transcriptional regulation. Buckland *et al.* (1997a) have found no change in mid-brain (containing choroid plexus cells) 5HT2C mRNA levels after chronic (32 day) clozapine treatment, in agreement with Burnet *et al.* (1996b) but there was an increase after 4 days. It is possible that initial antagonism of the receptor by clozapine causes a classical compensatory upregulation of the 5HT2C receptor by increasing its rate of transcription, but then other effects predominate and the levels return to normal. This secondary effect may well be related to dopaminergic effects and the relatively rapid changes suggest that 5HT2C receptors in the choroid plexus are highly regulated.

Among antipsychotic drugs available, until the recent launch of new atypicals, clozapine had a unique clinical profile and might be expected to have had a different effect on brain biochemistry to other antipsychotics. The rise in 5HT2C mRNA at day four followed by a drop back to base line mirrors the pattern of change seen in the dopamine D3 mRNA (Buckland *et al.*, 1993). Neither change can be easily explained, nor is it easy to relate these two changes to clinical effect. However, it is clear that they may be linked and these data may be seen as further evidence of the interdependence of the two neurotransmitter systems.

The most robust and consistent effect that Buckland *et al.* (1997a) have found is the downregulation of the 5HT2C receptor mRNA in both cortex and cerebellum by haloperidol, sulpiride and clozapine of 28–44%. Unfortunately, no other studies have looked at the effect of antipsychotic drugs on 5HT2C receptors in these brain areas, as they contain few 5HT2C receptors and the cerebellum is not usually associated with schizophrenia or antipsychotic drug effects. However, the fact that these areas do have relatively few 5HT2C receptors or their mRNA may imply that these changes have little overall effect. Further studies are required to answer these questions.

Overall, a complex pattern of changes has been reported and downregulation of 5HT2 receptors does not appear to correlate with either 'atypicality' or the drugs' abilities to ameliorate negative symptoms. Nevertheless, association studies and other evidence suggest that the 5HT2 type receptors do play a role in the treatment of schizophrenia.

Conclusion

For many years the dopaminergic system has been the prime candidate in the aetiology of schizophrenia with the serotonergic system being close behind. Recent allelic associations studies have supported a role for these systems, not as major pathological factors but more likely as contributors to susceptibility. There are other, as yet undiscovered, genetic abnormalities which play a role in the pathogenesis of schizophrenia, although it is unlikely that there is a gene of major effect even in familial sub-groups. There must also be environmental effects and some of these may be ubiquitous, although they may not be enviromental risk factors of the type easily identified by standard epidemiological approaches (McGuffin *et al.*, 1994). Candidate gene analysis is a way forward but a strong case needs to be found to justify the work as almost any known gene could not be ruled out with present knowledge. It is clear therefore that research over a wide front still needs to be carried out in order to find the genes that contribute to schizophrenia.

References

Abramowski, D., Rigo, M., Duc, D., Hoyer, D. and Staufenbiel, M. (1995) Localization of the 5-hydroxytryptamine2c receptor protein in human and rat brain using specific antisera. *Neuropharmacology,* **34,** 1635–45.

Akbarian, S., Kim, J.J., Potkin, S.G. *et al.* (1995) Gene expression for glutamic acid decarboxylase is reduced without loss of neurons in prefrontal cortex of schizophrenics. *Arch Gen Psychiatry,* **52,** 258–66.

Akbarian, S., Sucher, N.J., Bradley, D. *et al.* (1996) Selective alterations in gene expression for NMDA receptor subunits in prefrontal cortex of schizophrenics. *J Neurosci,* **16,** 19–30.

Andree, T.H., Mikuni, M., Tong, C.Y. *et al.* (1986) Differential effect of subchronic treatment with various neuroleptic agents on serotonin 2 receptors in rat cerebral cortex. *J Neurochem,* **46,** 191–7.

Arinami, T., Gao, M., Hamaguchi, H. and Toru, M. (1997) A functional polymorphism in the promoter region of the dopamine D2 receptor gene is associated with schizophrenia. *Human Mol Genet*, **6**, 577–82.

Asherson, A., Walsh, C., Williams J. *et al.* (1994) Imprinting and anticipation. Are they relevant to genetic studies of schizophrenia? *Br J Psychiatry*, **164**, 619–24.

Bean, A.J., Dagerlind, A., Hökfelt, T. and Dobner, P.R. (1992) Cloning of human neurotensin/neuromedin N genomic sequences and expression in the ventral tegmental mesencephalon of schizophrenics and age/sex matched controls. *Neuroscience*, **50**, 259–68.

Buckland, P.R., O'Donovan, M.C. and McGuffin, P. (1992a) Changes in dopa decarboxylase mRNA but not tyrosine hydroxylase mRNA levels in rat brain following antipsychotic treatment. *Psychopharmacology*, **108**, 98–102.

Buckland, P.R., O'Donovan, M.C. and McGuffin, P. (1992b) Changes in dopamine D_1, D_2 and D_3 receptor mRNA levels in rat brain following antipsychotic treatment. *Psychopharmacology*, **106**, 479–83.

Buckland, P.R., O'Donovan, M.C. and McGuffin, P. (1993) Clozapine and sulpiride up-regulate dopamine D3 receptor mRNA levels. *Neuropharmacology*, **32**, 901–907.

Buckland, P.R., Spurlock, G. and McGuffin, P. (1996) Amphetamine and vigabatrin down regulate aromatic L-amino acid decarboxylase mRNA levels. *Mol Brain Res*, **35**, 69–76.

Buckland, P.R., D'Souza, U., Maher, N.A. and McGuffin, P. (1997a) The effects of antipsychotic drugs on the mRNA levels of serotonin $5HT_{2A}$ and $5HT_{2C}$ receptors. *Mol Brain Res*, **48**, 45–52.

Buckland, P.R., Marshall, R., Watkins, P. and McGuffin, P. (1997b) Does phenylethylamine have a role in schizophrenia?: LSD and PCP up-regulate aromatic L-amino acid decarboxylase mRNA levels. *Mol Brain Res*, **49**, 266–70.

Burnet, P.W.J., Eastwood, S.L. and Harrison, P.J. (1996a) 5-HT1A and 5-HT2A receptor messenger-RNAs and binding site densities are differentially altered in schizophrenia. *Neuropsychopharmacology*, **15**, 442–55.

Burnet, P.W.J., Chen, C.PL.-H., McGowan, S. *et al.* (1996b) The effects of clozapine and haloperidol on serotonin-1A, -2A and -2C receptor gene expression and serotonin metabolism in the rat forebrain. *Neuroscience*, **73**, 531–40.

Canton, H., Verriele, L. and Millan, M.J. (1994) Competitive antagonism of serotonin (5-HT)2C and 5-HT2A receptor-mediated phosphoinositide (PI) turnover by clozapine in the rat: a comparison to other antipsychotics. *Neurosci Lett*, **181**, 65–8.

Cardon, L.R., Smith, S.D., Fulker, D.W. *et al.* (1994) Quantitative trait locus for reading disability on chromosome 6. *Science*, **266**, 276–9.

Crocq, M.-A., Mant, R., Asherson, P. *et al.* (1992) Association between schizophrenia and homozygosity at the dopamine D3 receptor gene. *J Med Genet*, **29**, 858–60.

Damask, S.P., Bovenkerk, K.A., de la Pena, G. *et al.* (1996) Differential effects of clozapine and haloperidol on dopamine receptor mRNA expression in rat striatum and cortex. *Mol Brain Res*, **41**, 241–9.

Delfs, J.M., Yu, L., Ellison, G.D. *et al.* (1994) Regulation of mu-opioid receptor mRNA in rat globus pallidus: effects of enkephalin increases induced by short- and long-term haloperidol administration. *J Neurochem*, **63**, 777–80.

Delfs, J.M., Anegawa, N.J. and Chesselet, M.F. (1995) Glutamate decarboxylase messenger RNA in rat pallidum: comparison of the effects of haloperidol, clozapine and combined haloperidol-scopolamine treatments. *Neuroscience*, **66**, 67–80.

D'Souza, U., McGuffin, P. and Buckland, P.R. (1998) Antipsychotic regulation of dopamine D_1, D_2 and D_3 receptor mRNA. *Neuropharmacology*, **36**, 1689–96.

Eastwood, S.L., Burnet, P.W. and Harrison, P.J. (1995a) Altered synaptophysin expression as a marker of synaptic pathology in schizophrenia. *Neuroscience*, **66**, 309–19.

Eastwood, S.L., McDonald, B., Burnet, P.W. *et al.* (1995b) Decreased expression of mRNAs encoding non-NMDA glutamate receptors GluR1 and GluR2 in medial temporal lobe neurons in schizophrenia. *Mol Brain Res,* **29,** 211–23.

Elsworth, J.D. and Roth, R.H. (1997) Dopamine autoreceptor pharamcology and function. In K.A. Neve and R.L. Neve (eds), *The Dopamine Receptors*. New Jersey: Humana Press, 223–66.

Farmer, A.E., McGuffin,P. and Gottesman, I.I. (1987). Twin concordance for DSM-III schizophrenia: scrutinising the validity of the definition. *Arch Gen Psychiatry,* **44,** 634–1.

Gerevich, E.V., Bordelon, Y., Shapiro, R.M. *et al.* (1997) Mesolimbic dopamine D₃ receptors and use of antipsychotics in patients with schizophrenia. *Arch Gen Psychiatry,* **54,** 225–32.

Gill, M., McGuffin, P., Parfitt, E. *et al.* (1993). A linkage study of schizophrenia with DNA markers from the long arm of chromosome II. *Psychol Med,* **23,** 27–44.

Gottesman, I.I. (1991) *Schizophrenia genesis*. New York: W.H. Freeman.

Gottesman, I.I. and Shields J. (1967) A polygenic theory of schizophrenia. *Proc Natl Acad Sci USA,* **58,** 199–205.

Gottesman, I.I and Bertelsen, A. (1989) Confirming unexpressed genotypes for schizophrenia: risks in the offspring of Fischer's Danish identical and fraternal discordant twins. *Arch Gen Psychiatry,* **46,** 867–72.

Grigoriants, O., Devi, L. and Fricker, L.D. (1993) Dopamine antagonist haloperidol increases carboxypeptidase E mRNA in rat neurointermediate pituitary but not in various other rat tissues. *Mol Brain Res,* **19,** 161–4.

Herman, Z.S. (1996) Neuropeptide Y (NPY) and its mRNA in discrete brain areas after subchronic administration of neuroleptics. *Acta Neurobiol Exp,* **56,** 55–61.

Hoffman, B.J. and Mezey, E. (1989) Distribution of serotonin 5-HT1c receptor mRNA in adult rat brain. *FEBS Lett,* **247,** 453–62.

Jaber, M., Tison, F., Fournier, M.C. *et al.* (1994) Differential influence of haloperidol and sulpiride on dopamine and peptide mRNA levels in the rat striatum and pituitary. *Mol Brain Res,* **23,** 14–20.

Kahn, R.S. and Van Praag, H.M. (1996) Dopamine, serotonin, and their interactions in schizophrenia. In J.M. Kane, H.-J. Moller and F.A. Wouters (eds), *Serotonin in antipsychotic treatment*, New York: Dekker, 131–52.

Kapur, S. (1996) 5HT2 antagonism and EPS benefits: is there a causal connection? *Psychopharmacology,* **124,** 35–9.

Knable, M.B., Hyde, T.M., Herman, M.M. *et al.* (1994) Quantitative autoradiography of dopamine-D1 receptors, D2 receptors, and dopamine uptake sites in post-mortem striatal specimens from schizophrenic patients. *Biol Psychiatry,* **36,** 827–35.

Kinkead, B. and Nemeroff, C.B. (1994) The effects of typical and atypical antipsychotic drugs on neurotensin-containing neurons in the central nervous system. *J Clin Psychiatry,* **55,** 30–2.

Kroesen, S., Marksteiner, J., Mahata, S.K. *et al.* (1995) Effects of haloperidol, clozapine and citalopram on messenger RNA levels of chromogranins A and B and secretogranin II in various regions of rat brain. *Neuroscience,* **69,** 881–91.

Kuoppamäki, M., Palvinaki, E.-P., Hietala, J. and Syvalaḥti, E. (1995) Differential regulation of rat 5HT2A and 5HT2C receptors after chronic treatment with clozapine, chlorpromazine and three putative atypical antipsychotic drugs. *Neuropsychopharmacology,* **13,** 139–50.

Kuoppamäki, M., Seppala, T., Syvalahti, E. and Hietala, J. (1992) Chronic clozapine treatment decreases 5-hydroxytryptamine 1c receptor density in the rat choroid plexus: comparison with haloperidol, *J Pharmacol Exp Therap,* **264,** 1262–7.

Lee, T. and Tang, S.W. (1984) Loxapine and clozapine decrease serotonin (S2) but do not elevate dopamine (D2) receptor numbers in the rat brain. *Psychiatry Res,* **12,** 277–85.

Levinson, D.F., Wildenauer, D.B., Schwab, S.G. *et al.* (1996) Additional support for schizophrenia linkage on chromosomes 6 and 8: A multicenter study. *Am J Med Genet Neuropsychiatr Genet,* **67,** 580–94.

Li, S. and Pelletier, G. (1992) Role of dopamine in the regulation of gonadotropin-releasing hormone in the male rat brain as studied by in situ hybridization. *Endocrinology*, **131**, 395–9.

Liégeois, J-F., Bonaventure, P., Delarge, J. and Damas, J. (1995) Antipsychotics and neuropeptides: the atypical profile of CI-943 and its relationship to neurotensin. *Neurosci Biobehav Rev*, **19**, 519–31.

Lindefors, N. (1992) Amphetamine and haloperidol modulate preprotachykinin A mRNA expression in rat nucleus accumbens and caudate-putamen. *Mol Brain Res*, **13**, 151–4.

Liu, Y., Hillefors-Berglund, M. I. and von Euler, G. (1994) Modulation of dopamine D_3 receptor binding by N-ethylmaleimide and neurotensin. *Brain Res*, **643**, 343–8.

McGue, M., and Gottesman, I.I. (1989) Genetic linkage in schizophrenia, perspectives from genetic epidemiology. *Schizophr Bull*, **15**, 453–64.

McGuffin, P., Sargeant, M., Hett, G. *et al*. (1990) Exclusion of a schizophrenia gene from chromosome 5q11-q13 region: new data and a re-analysis of previous reports. *Am J Human Genet*, **47**, 524–35.

McGuffin, P., Farmer, A.E. and Gottesman, I.I. (1987). Is there really a split in schizophrenia? The genetic evidence. *Br J Psychiatry*, **150**, 581–92.

McGuffin, P., Asherson, P., Owen, M. *et al*. (1994) The strength of the genetic effect – is there room for an environmental influence in the aetiology of schizophrenia? *Br J Psychiatry*, **164**, 593–9.

McGuffin, P., Owen, M.J., O'Donovan, M.C. *et al*. (1994) *Seminars in psychiatric genetics*. London: Gaskell.

Matsubara, S. and Meltzer, H.Y. (1989) Effect of typical and atypical antipsychotic drugs on 5-HT2 receptor density in rat cerebral cortex. *Life Sci*, **45**, 1397–406.

Meltzer H.Y. and Fatemi, S.H. (1996) The role of serotonin in schizophrenia and the mechanisms of action of antipsychotic drugs. In J.M. Kane, H.-J. Moller and F. Awouters (eds), *Serotonin in antipsychotic treatment*. New York: Dekker, 77–107.

Mikuni, M. and Meltzer, H.Y. (1984) Reduction of serotonin2 receptors in rat cerebral cortex after subchronic administration of imipramine, chlorpromazine, and the combination thereof. *Life Sci*, **34**, 87–92.

Molineaux, S.M., Jessell, T.M., Axel, R. and Julius, D. (1989) 5-HT1c receptor is a prominent serotonin receptor subtype in the central nervous system. *Proc Natl Acad Sci USA*, **86**, 6793–7.

Morris, A.G., Gaitonde, E., McKenna, P.J., Mollon, J.D. and Hunt, D.M. (1995) GAG repeat expansions and schizophrenia associations with disease in females and with early age-at-onset. *Human Mol Genet*, **4**, 1957–61.

Nemeroff, C.B., Levant, B., Myers, B. and Bissette, G. (1992) Neurotensin, antipsychotic drugs, and schizophrenia. *Ann New York Acad Sci*, **668**, 146–56.

O'Dell, S.J., La Hoste, G.J., Widmark, C.B. *et al*. (1990) Chronic treatment with clozapine or haloperidol differentially regulates dopamine and serotonin receptors in rat brain. *Synapse*, **6**, 146–53.

O'Donovan, M.C., Guy, C., Craddock, N. *et al*. (1995). Expanded CAG repeats in schizophrenia and bipolar disorder. *Nature Genet*, **10**, 380–1.

Okubo, Y., Suhara, T., Suzuki, K. *et al*. (1997) Decreased prefrontal dopamine receptors in schizophrenia revealed by PET. *Nature*, **385**, 634–6.

Onstad, S., Skre, I., Torgersen, S. *et al*. (1991) Twin concordance for DSM-III-R schizophrenia. *Acta Psychiat Scand*, **83**, 395–401.

Oyarce, A.M., Hand, T.A., Mains, R.E. and Eipper, B.A. (1996) Dopaminergic regulation of secretory granule-associated proteins in rat intermediate pituitary. *J Neurochem*, **67**, 229–41.

Reynolds, G.P., Garrett, N.J., Rupniak, N. *et al*. (1983) Chronic clozapine treatment of rats down-regulates cortical 5-HT2 receptors. *Eur J Pharmacol*, **89**, 325–6.

Reynolds, G.P. and Mason, S.L. (1994) Are striatal dopamine D4 receptors increased in schizophrenia? *J Neurochem*, **63**, 1576–7.

Risch, N. (1990). Linkage strategies for genetically complex traits. III. The effect of marker polymorphism analysis on affected relative pairs. *Am J Human Genet*, **46**, 242–53.

Roberts, D.A., Balderson, D., Pickering-Brown, S.M. *et al.* (1994) The abundance of mRNA for dopamine D2 receptor isoforms in brain tissue from controls and schizophrenics. *Mol Brain Res*, **25**, 173–5.

Schmauss, C., Haroutunian, V., Davis, K.L. and Davidson, M. (1993) Selective loss of dopamine D3-type receptor mRNA expression in parietal and motor cortices of patients with chronic schizophrenia. *Proc Natl Acad Sci USA*, **90**, 8942–6.

Schmauss, C. (1996) Enhanced cleavage of an atypical intron of dopamine D_3 receptor premRNA in chronic schizophrenia. *J Neurosci*, **16**, 7902–9.

Schmidt, C.J., Sorensen, S.M., Kehne, J.H. *et al.* (1995) The role of 5HT2A receptor in antipsychotic activity. *Life Sci*, **56**, 2209–22.

Sedvall, G., Pauli, S., Karlsson, P. *et al.* (1995) PET imaging of neuroreceptors in schizophrenia. *Eur Neuropsychopharmacol*, **5**(Suppl), 25–30.

Seeman, P., Guan, H.C. and Van Tol, H.H. (1993) Dopamine D4 receptors elevated in schizophrenia. *Nature*, **365**, 441–5.

Sherrington, R., Brynjolffson, J., Petursson, H. *et al.* (1988) Localization of a susceptibility locus for schizophrenia on chromosome 5. *Nature*, **336**, 164–7.

Sodhi, M.S., Arranz, M.J., Ball, D.M. *et al.* (1996) Association between clozapine response and allelic variation in the 5HT2A and 5HT2C receptor genes. *Schizophr Res*, **18**, 3.

Virgo, L., Humphries, C., Mortimer, A. *et al.* (1995) Cholecystokinin messenger RNA deficit in frontal and temporal cerebral cortex in schizophrenia. *Biol Psychiatry*, **37**, 694–701.

Vogler, G.P., Gottesman, I.I., McGue, M.K. *et al.* (1991) Mixed model segregation analysis of schizophrenia in the Lindelius Swedish pedigrees. *Behav Genet*, **20**, 461–72.

Wang, W., Hahn, K-H., Bishop, J. *et al.* (1996) Up-regulation of D_3 dopamine receptor mRNA by neuroleptics. *Synapse*, **23**, 232–5.

Watson-Bolden, C., Watson, M.A., Murray, K.D. *et al.* (1993) Haloperidol but not clozapine increases neurotensin receptor mRNA levels in rat substantia nigra. *J Neurochem*, **61**, 1141–3.

Williams, J., Spurlock, G., McGuffin, P. *et al.* (1996) Association between schizophrenia and T102C polymorphism of the 5–hydroxytryptamine type 2A-receptor gene. *Lancet*, **347**, 1294–6.

Wilmot, C.A. and Szczepanik, A.M. (1989) Effects of acute and chronic treatments with clozapine and haloperidol on serotonin (5–HT2) and dopamine (D2) receptors in the rat brain. *Brain Res*, **487**, 288–98.

Wolf, S.S., Hyde, T.M., Saunders, R.C. *et al.* (1995) Autoradiographic characterisation of neurotensin receptors in the entorhinal cortex of schizophrenic patients and control subjects. *J Neur Transmis*, **102**, 55–65.

Wright, D.E., Seroogy, K.B., Lundgren, K.H. *et al.* (1995) Comparative localization of serotonin1A, IC and 2 receptor subtype mRNAs in rat brain. *J Comp Neurol*, **351**, 357–73.

Xu, S., Monsma, F.J., Sibley, D.R. and Creese, I. (1992) Regulation of D_{1A} and D_2 dopamine receptor mRNA during ontogenesis, lesion and chronic antagonist treatment. *Life Sci*, **50**, 383–96.

Zhang, S.P., Connell, T.A., Price, T., Simpson, G.M., Zhou, L.W. and Weiss, B. (1995) Continuous infusion of clozapine increases mu and delta opioid receptors and proenkephalin in mouse brain. *Biol Psychiatry*, **37**, 496–503.

CHAPTER 6

Structural imaging and treatment response in schizophrenia

CALUM G. CROSTHWAITE AND MICHAEL A. REVELEY

Introduction

The seemingly anomalous idea that schizophrenia, a so-called 'functional' psychosis, should be associated with neuroanatomical changes is not a new one. Indeed Kraepelin attributed dementia praecox to cerebral pathology, stating that 'diffuse loss of cortical cells could be established' (1896). As long ago as 1871 Hecker reported ventricular enlargement (VE) in schizophrenic patients in post-mortem studies, a finding replicated consistently since (for review *see* Arnold and Trojanowski, 1996). But with the advent of in-vivo imaging techniques the study of structural brain abnormalities in schizophrenia became greatly facilitated, allowing the visual assessment of brain structure without the confounding effects of neuroleptic treatment, ageing, fixing and other factors present in post-mortem studies.

Imaging techniques and findings

Introduced by Dandy in 1919, pneumoencephalography (PEG) was the first technique to allow visual imaging of brain structure during life. Air introduced into the ventricles via a spinal tap served to act as a contrast medium allowing X-ray images to be taken. An early study using PEG by Jacobi and Winkler (1927) found that there was 'hydrocephalus internus' and 'unquestionable atrophy' in 95% of the schizophrenic patients tested. This expansion of the cerebroventricular system and the cortical sulci could not be explained by common causes of cerebral atrophy such as ageing or substance abuse and so prompted interest from other researchers. More than 30 studies published subsequently were generally consistent in substantiating the significant findings that enlarged ventricles are found more frequently in schizophrenic patients than controls, and that cortical atrophy (CA) is also a factor in a significant proportion of schizophrenic patients (Cazzullo, 1963; Asano, 1967).

Computerized tomography (CT) was a breakthrough in structural brain imaging, as it enabled images to be obtained without the need for the painful, invasive and somewhat dangerous procedures involved in PEG, so permitting the use of normal controls for comparison with patient groups. CT imaging involves an X-ray source which rotates in a specified plane around the circumference of the skull. The voltages of the X-rays that transverse the brain substance are measured and reconstructed into an image. Johnstone *et al.* (1976) conducted the first study employing CT scans in schizophrenia and found that, similar to PEG findings, patients with schizophrenia had larger lateral ventricles when compared to control subjects, a finding replicated soon after by Weinberger *et al.* (1979) in a larger and younger sample. More than 50 studies later, in a review of the field, Lewis (1990) concluded that a significant proportion of schizophrenic patients demonstrate 'relative enlargement of the third and lateral ventricles, and cortical sulci'.

Though still commonly used, CT has been surpassed technically by magnetic resonance imaging (MRI) which gives higher resolution images, better tissue contrast and also has multiplanar abilities. MRI relies on the fact that positively charged hydrogen nuclei, the most abundant nuclei in biological tissue, rotate around an axis. By the use of a transient external radio frequency signal these protons can be brought into phase, after which time they return or 'relax' to their original direction of spin. The rate at which this relaxation process occurs can be detected, and differs among tissues, and so can be used to confer contrast to the resulting image. Recent MRI studies have reached conclusions consonant with those derived from the PEG and CT studies, that when compared to normal controls, patients with schizophrenia are shown to possess larger lateral ventricles and demonstrate signs of CA (Lawrie *et al.* 1997).

Relationship between brain structural abnormalities and treatment response/outcome

In a PEG study Cazzullo (1963) found that VE in schizophrenia was related to both a chronic disease course and a poorer response to antipsychotic treatment. The potential significance of this finding becomes clear when it is considered that up to 30% of patients have a less than adequate response to neuroleptic treatment of acute symptomatology (Kane, 1989), and that 6–8% fail to respond to months or years of intensive drug therapy (May *et al.*, 1988). It is clear that drug resistance phenomena further complicate the management of the disorder and may have a detrimental effect on outcome. If, however, the predictive validity of abnormal brain morphology with respect to treatment response can be established, clinicians might be able to select the most appropriate and beneficial treatment regimens in advance. This might result in the reduction of the time to symptom remission, and prevent the needless administration of high doses of neuroleptics, with accompanying serious side-effects, frequently used to combat refractory symptoms.

Not until almost twenty years later, did Weinberger *et al.* (1980) replicate the finding of Cazzullo (1963) that marked brain abnormality in schizophrenic patients seemed to be a marker for a poorer response to neuroleptic medication. Many studies over the years utilizing CT and more recently MRI have endeavoured to establish beyond reasonable doubt the relationship between structural brain abnormalities and short-term treatment response or long-term outcome. Studies have generally employed one of three designs: (i) grouping participants according to the presence of brain abnormalities and comparing the groups' response to neuroleptic medication (*see* Table 6.1); (ii) assessing the degree of brain abnormality in groups of patients who show different levels of response to medication (*see* Table 6.2); or (iii) carrying out correlational tests to determine whether a relationship exists between treatment response and degree of brain abnormality (*see* Table 6.3).

All relevant studies have been included in the tables presented here, simply for completeness. For the sake of brevity, we will limit our discussion only to those studies that employ a prospective design. The use of a retrospective study design has been shown to give rise to selection bias, as demonstrated by Luchins *et al.* (1984) who subsequently scanned patients who had been excluded as they had not met the inclusion criteria of five weeks prior treatment. The excluded patients were found to show a larger ventricle : brain ratio (VBR) and less psychopathology on the Global Assessment Scale (GAS) than those included in the study. Thus, if the ability to remain drug-free for a specified period is a factor related to ventricular size then retrospective studies employing such pre-set requirements might give rise to selection bias. Indeed, in an unpublished prospective study Weinberger *et al.* (1982) failed to replicate the findings of their original retrospective study (Weinberger *et al.*, 1980) of an inverse relationship between VE and treatment response, and those patients unable to tolerate the drug-free period had, against prediction, smaller ventricles. The prospective studies reported here (Naber *et al.*, 1985; Losonczy *et al.*, 1986; Pandurangi *et al.*, 1986; Silverman *et al.*, 1987; Smith *et al.*, 1987; Nimgaonkar *et al.*, 1988; Shelton *et al.*, 1988; Wolkowitz *et al.*, 1988; MacDonald and Best, 1989; Kaplan *et al.*, 1990; Friedman *et al.*, 1991; Katsanis *et al.*, 1991; Vita *et al.*, 1991; Breier *et al.*, 1992; DeLisi *et al.*, 1992; Lieberman *et al.*, 1993; Schroder *et al.*, 1993; Bersani *et al.*, 1994; Honer *et al.*, 1995) which recruit consecutive admissions and follow patients' progress for the duration of the study, have a methodological advantage over those taking a retrospective approach.

Brain abnormalities as a prediction of treatment response

The overall findings of the studies included in Table 6.1 are that VE is associated with treatment response, but that CA is not. Though many of the studies presented imply otherwise, methodological considerations suggest their findings may be compromised.

Table 6.1. Studies where patients were grouped according to the presence or absence of abnormality.

Author, year	Abnormality investigated	N	Controls	Duration	Response/outcome criteria	Significance level P
Studies reporting an inverse relationship between abnormality and treatment response/outcome						
Weinberger et al. (1980)	VE	20	Yes	56 days	BPRS	0.003
Schulz et al. (1983)	VE	12	Yes	14–42 days	BPRS	< 0.05
Smith et al. (1983)	VE, CA (P, O)	30	Yes	24 days	BPRS & NHSI	< 0.01
Luchins et al. (1983)	VE	35	Yes	35 days	GAS, SADS-C	< 0.04
Luchins et al. (1984)	VE	35	Yes	35 days	GAS, SADS-C	< 0.04
Gattaz et al. (1987)	3rd VE, CA (F,T,P)	10	Yes	21 days	BPRS	Unreported
Gattaz et al. (1988)	3rd VE, CA (F,T,P)	30	Yes	21 days	BPRS	0.01
Buckman et al. (1990)	VE	31	No	14–64 days	BPRS	0.038
Katsanis et al. (1991)	VE	36	No	18 months	SCL-90–R, GAS, OFAS	< 0.01
Vita et al. (1991)	VE, CA (F,T,P)	18	Yes	2 years	Strauss–Carpenter Scale	< 0.04
Jewart et al. (1991)*	VE	29	No	214 days	BPRS	Unreported
Lieberman et al. (1993)*	VE, 3rd VE	70	No	6–52 weeks	SADS-C+PD, CGI	< 0.047
Mauri et al. (1994)	VE	24	Yes	28 days	BPRS	< 0.01
Studies reporting no relationship between abnormality and treatment response/outcome						
Nasrallah et al. (1983a)	VE	55	Yes	Not specified	3 point classification	N/S
Nasrallah et al. (1983b)	CA (F,T,P)	55	Yes	Not specified	3 point classification	N/S
Boronow et al. (1985)	3rd VE, CA (P, O)	30	Yes	28 days	BPRS	N/S
Pandurangi et al. (1986)	VE, CA (F,T,P,O)	23	Yes	2–19 years	Clinical judgement	N/S
Smith et al (1987)	CA (P, O)	39	Yes	24 days	NHSI, BPRS	N/S
Shelton et al (1988)	VE, 3rd VE, CA (F)	40	Yes	42 days	BPRS	N/S
Nimgaonkar et al (1988)	CA (F,T,P)	36	No	42 days	GAS, MSS	N/S
Vita et al. (1988)	CA (F,T,P)	124	No	30–180 days	BPRS	0.085
MacDonald and Best (1989)	CA (F,T,P)	34	Yes	42 days	Krawiecka	N/S
Buckman et al. (1990)	CA (F,T,P,O)	31	No	14–64 days	BPRS	N/S
Lieberman et al. (1993)*	CA (F,P)	70	No	6–52 weeks	SADS-C+PD, CGI	N/S

Studies reporting a positive relationship between abnormality and treatment response/outcome

Smith et al. (1983)	VE, CA (P, O)	30	Yes	24 days	BPRS & NHSI	< 0.01
Boronow et al. (1985)	VE	30	Yes	28 days	BPRS	0.04
Smith et al. (1985)	VE	39	Yes	21 days	BPRS	< 0.1
Wilms et al. (1992)	VE	42	Yes	84 days	PANSS	0.07

* = MRI study; all others = CT studies.
N/S, not significant.

The issue of control subjects is an important one in relation to the studies presented in Table 6.1. From the earliest of these studies, patients have been considered to have abnormalities if their brain measures are more than two standard deviations above the control mean. However, Smith and Iacono (1986) found that studies finding VE and those which did not find VE differed, not in the mean ventricle size of the patient sample, but in the mean ventricle size of the control groups. Therefore, those studies which use only control subjects whose scans have been rated as 'normal' (Luchins and Meltzer, 1983; Schulz *et al.*, 1983; Smith *et al.*, 1983; Luchins *et al.*, 1984; Boronow *et al.*, 1985; Pandurangi *et al.*, 1986; Wilms *et al.*, 1992) might exclude controls with brain measures at the upper limit of what is considered to be normal, leading to possible underestimation of the mean control brain measure and so an overestimation of the patient/control difference. Similarly, studies using scans of patient controls with possible neurological illness for comparison to those of schizophrenic patients (Luchins and Meltzer, 1983; Smith *et al.*, 1983; Luchins *et al.*, 1984; Gattaz *et al.*, 1987, 1988; Nasrallah *et al.*, 1983a, 1983b; Smith *et al.*, 1985; Pandurangi *et al.*, 1986; Wilms *et al.*, 1992) might overestimate the mean control brain measure and so underestimate the patient/control difference. The ideal therefore would appear to be healthy volunteers matched on several demographic variables such as age and sex (Shelton *et al.*, 1988; MacDonald and Best, 1989; Vita *et al.*, 1991).

A number of the studies in Table 6.1 use other means by which to define brain measures as abnormal. Of those studies that outline their methods, Katsanis *et al.* (1991) use a median split and Lieberman *et al.* (1993) and Nimgaonkar *et al.* (1988) use a three-category classification employing reference images to which they compare their patients' scans. The discussion of Table 6.1 will therefore be limited to these three studies along with those control studies that employ suitable controls as defined above.

Nimgaonkar *et al.* (1988) assessed the role of brain damage on pharmacological response in 36 first episode or chronic schizophrenic patients after six weeks of conventional antipsychotic medication. Response to treatment was found not to be different between the two groups when defined as possessing normal or abnormal frontal, temporal or parietal cortical measures. A subsequent analysis found no statistically significant difference in mean VBR between responders and non-responders, and correlational analyses failed to find any significant relationships between response to conventional antipsychotics and VE or CA. However, Nimgaonkar *et al.* (1988) failed to take advantage of their prospective design by neglecting to report data on those patients excluded from their analysis due to protocol violation (i.e. subjects who did not require 600 mg chlorpromazine equivalents for at least six weeks after recruitment). This potentially undermines their findings, as the better response in these patients may be a factor related to the morphological measures of interest. Also, no wash-out period was employed, further compromising the reliability of their findings, as a drug wash-out period is necessary for the accurate estimation of the degree of symptom change brought about by treatment.

Shelton *et al.* (1988) addressed these shortcomings in a rigorous design, by including a six-week wash-out period and reporting data on patients unable to complete the protocol. They found that patients with abnormalities in lateral ventricle, third ventricle or frontal cortex measures did not differ significantly in their response to neuroleptics from those with normal measures. Correlational analyses also failed to find any significant associations. Kaplan *et al.* (1990) suggested that the patients included in this study be considered neuroleptic non-responsive, and Shelton *et al.* (1988) themselves admitted that the very small range of improvement in these patients, and the relatively small number of patients demonstrating VE, suggested that their chronic in-patient sample may not have been representative of the schizophrenic population as a whole.

Studies of patient samples consisting predominantly of chronic patients (Losonczy *et al.*, 1986; Smith *et al.*, 1987; Shelton *et al.*, 1988; Friedman *et al.*, 1991; Vita *et al.*, 1991; Breier *et al.*, 1992; Schroder *et al.*, 1993; Honer *et al.*, 1995) are more likely to find a narrower range of response, simply because by definition chronic patients are less responsive. This treatment resistance in research samples may be due to the possible effects of cumulative treatment exposure or changing symptomatology, or may simply be due to a preponderance of severely ill patients in the populations from which such samples are drawn. Whatever the reason, this imposes limitations on the interpretation of the findings of such studies. Studies involving first episode patients, on the other hand, (Macdonald and Best, 1989; Katsanis *et al.*, 1991; DeLisi *et al.*, 1992; Lieberman *et al.*, 1993) would be expected to show a wider range of responsiveness to treatment, allowing a more meaningful interpretation of their results with respect to structural abnormalities. It has, however, been suggested that CT scan abnormalities may be epiphenomena, associated with pharmacological or physical aspects of treatment in chronic patients (Marsden, 1976). Studies of drug-naïve first episode patients have, however, found scan abnormalities in a significant proportion of patients (Schulz *et al.*, 1983; Gattaz *et al.*, 1988; Katsanis *et al.*, 1991; DeLisi *et al.*, 1992; Lieberman *et al.*, 1993), suggesting that 'structural brain abnormalities are not secondary to the disease process itself or its treatment, but instead, are already present in a subset of patients at the onset of the illness' (Gattaz *et al.*, 1988, p. 301).

The study of MacDonald and Best (1989) drew a sample of first-episode patients from multiple sources, thus minimizing the possibility of recruiting an unrepresentative sample, and maximizing the potential for a wider range of responses. They also recruited healthy age- and sex-matched controls. The fact that they found no significant difference between controls and patients with respect to VBR, third ventricle width and the maximum widths of cortical fissures is worthy of comment. The large degree of overlap between the scans of patient and control samples, acknowledged for some years now (*see* Lewis, 1990 for review), emphasizes the subtle nature of any atrophy found in schizophrenia. The studies by Reveley *et al.* (1982) and Suddath *et al.* (1990), who compared monozygotic twins discordant for schizophrenia, have demonstrated that almost every affected individual was characterized by *subtle* abnormalities which were not always easily distinguished when compared to normal controls. When patients were compared to their unaffected sibling, however, the abnormalities became apparent.

MacDonald and Best (1989) found that treatment response after six weeks of conventional antipsychotics was not related to frontal, temporal or parietal sulcal enlargement, the only brain measure they found to distinguish patients from controls. The use of two different scanners in this study is potentially significant as differences in machines and settings are potentially confounding variables. However, these factors were controlled for in the subsequent analyses. Other potentially confounding variables not assessed were alcohol intake and history of perinatal trauma, which have both been shown to have an effect on CT scan results (Gurling *et al.*, 1984; Reveley, 1985). Whilst acknowledging these limitations, the rigorous design of this study makes its findings compelling.

The findings of Vita *et al.* (1991) suggest that lateral VE and frontal, temporal and parietal cortical measures may have some influence on clinical outcome in chronic schizophrenic patients after two years. The data with respect to CA are more persuasive than those for ventricular atrophy, as only one (useful employment) of the six outcome scales was predicted by VE. Individual VBR values were not found to correlate significantly with any of the outcome scale scores. CA, on the other hand, significantly differentiated patients' outcome on five of the six scales utilized, indicating a poorer outcome with respect to useful employment, hospital stay, social contacts, total Strauss–Carpenter score, and intimacy of interpersonal contacts. The same scales gave significant negative correlations between outcome values and atrophy scores. However, it seems unlikely that brain atrophy in these cortical areas exerts an influence on drug response, as the 'severity of symptoms' element of the Strauss–Carpenter scale was the only measure on which no association was found. Furthermore, the omission of data on pre-morbid functioning raises the important issue of whether the chronic schizophrenic patients with abnormal cortical measures may have exhibited poorer premorbid functioning, a deficit which was still present after two years.

Katsanis *et al.* (1991) assessed premorbid functioning and controlled for this factor in their subsequent analyses. They assessed the effect of VE on outcome measures in a broadly based sample of 88 newly medicated patients who had experienced their first episode of psychosis. Patients with large ventricles (i.e. above the median) were found not to be characterized by poorer premorbid adjustment. However, at follow-up (9 and 18 months) schizophrenic patients with ventriculomegaly had a poorer outcome, which was statistically significant on the SCL-R-90, but which was a non-significant trend on the Occupational Functioning Assessment Scale and the GAS. Schizophreniform patients demonstrated no significant differences with regard to follow-up variables, though trends similar to those in schizophrenic patients were observed on all three scales used. This well-designed study would seem to suggest that in schizophrenia the degree of VE is in some way related to the patients' level of occupational and global functioning, and the number and severity of their symptoms. Interestingly, whilst patients with psychotic mood disorder did not differ significantly from schizophrenic patients in ventricular size, they demonstrated an absence of association between VBR and outcome. This would suggest that ventricular size may have a different significance for these two groups.

The findings of Lieberman *et al.* (1993) using MRI, mirror those of Katsanis *et al.* (1991) with respect to VE, and MacDonald and Best (1989) with respect to CA. Seventy consecutively admitted, first-episode, neuroleptic-free patients participated in a conventional antipsychotic treatment protocol in accordance with a standard algorithm. Stringent response criteria were set according to scores on the Schedule for Affective Disorders and Schizophrenia Change and Psychosis + Disorganization Scale (SADS-C + PD), and the Clinical Global Impression (CGI) scale. This study found that lateral and third ventricular abnormalities predicted longer time to remission, whereas cortical and medial temporal lobe abnormalities did not. A similar pattern of association emerged in relation to level of remission. Despite the rigorous response criteria, 83% of patients recovered from their first episode of psychosis, a statistic consistent with the findings of other first episode studies (MacDonald and Best, 1988). However, the length of time to remission for the patients in the present study (mean = 42 weeks) is well beyond the usual duration of clinical treatment trials (Lieberman *et al.*, 1993). This may be due to the strict response criteria set, or because these unmedicated patients were exhibiting symptoms of a severity not seen in chronic patients who have been receiving maintenance treatment. Although neuroleptics begin to work pharmacologically in the first or second week, and clinical improvement occurs in the first few weeks of treatment, this study demonstrates that many patients show additional improvement up to one year after treatment commenced. The finding that evidence of atrophy predicts a poorer level of recovery and a duration of treatment to symptom remission sometimes as long as 54 weeks, throws into question the adequacy of studies with a treatment duration of only a few weeks. These studies may therefore only be serving to gauge the influence of brain measures on *acute* response to neuroleptics, neglecting the possibility that patients with structural brain abnormalities may simply respond more slowly than those without such abnormalities.

The findings of Lieberman *et al.* (1993) and others in Table 6.1 with respect to brain morphologic features and treatment response are strengthened by the use of MRI, which permits easier delineation of ventricle borders and enhanced definition of other structures of interest. Therefore, the conclusions that can be drawn from those studies in Table 6.1 which comply with those study design elements identified as requisite are that ventriculomegaly can determine treatment response, and that CA is not related to response.

Treatment response as an indicator of brain abnormalities

In Table 6.2, since treatment-responsive and unresponsive patients are compared on the degree of cerebral abnormality exhibited, the definition of responsiveness is clearly important. As can be seen, the techniques which have been employed to gauge response have been diverse, from three and four factor classifications based on symptom change, to length of hospitalizations, and to improvement on various rating scales. Even when the same rating scale is used, different criteria may be set. This makes meaningful comparisons between studies difficult, a fact which should be borne in mind when interpreting the studies in Table 6.2. This said, the studies in Table 6.2 seem to suggest that there is no relationship between VE and response, but that CA may exert some influence.

Losonczy *et al.* (1986) and Silverman *et al.* (1987), whose patient samples overlap, found that there was no significant relationship between lateral VE and treatment response (though Losonczy *et al.* (1986) did find that three of the four patients with VBR higher than 2 SD above the control mean were non-responsive). There was a relative absence of response to conventional neuroleptics in these small samples of

Table 6.2. Studies where patients were grouped according to their response to neuroleptics

Author, year	Abnormality investigated	N	Controls	Duration	Response/outcome criteria	Significance level P
Studies reporting an inverse relationship between abnormality and treatment response/outcome						
Nasrallah et al. (1980)	VE	7	No	21 days	IBRS	Unreported
Jeste et al. (1982)	VE	20	No	56 days	BPRS	< 0.03
Kolakowska et al. (1985)	VE	77	No	3 months	3 point classification	< 0.05
Williams et al. (1985)	VE	40	No	28 days	4 point classification	< 0.05
Luchins et al. (1986)	VE	22	No	Not specified	% of illness in hospital	0.001
Johnstone et al. (1989)*	VE	21	No	Not specified	Coopers Scale	< 0.05
Kaiya et al. (1989)	CA (F,T,P)	80	No	90 days	3 point classification	< 0.01
Kaplan et al. (1990)	3rd VE	24	No	7–47 days	NHSI	0.03
Friedman et al. (1991)	CA (F)	34	No	42 days	BPRS	0.004
Honer et al. (1995)	CA (F,T)	42	No	4–28 weeks	CGI	< 0.05
Lawrie et al. (1997)*	CA (P, O)	40	No	Not specified	Krawiecka	0.06
Studies reporting no relationship between abnormality and treatment response/outcome						
Losonczy et al. (1986)	VE	19	No	42 days	BPRS, CGI	N/S
Smith et al. (1987)	CA (P, O)	39	No	24 days	NHSI, BPRS	N/S
Silverman et al. (1987)	VE	27	No	28–42 days	BPRS, CGI	N/S
Nimgaonkar et al.(1988)	VE	36	No	42 days	GAS, MSS	N/S
Wolkowitz et al. (1988)	VE, 3rd VE,CA(P,O)	12	No	14–28 days	B-H Global Rating Scale	N/S
Kaiya et al. (1989)	VE	80	No	90 days	3 point classification	N/S
Miller et al. (1991)*	VE	44	No	28–42 days	Not specified	N/S
Friedman et al. (1991)	VE	34	No	42 days	BPRS	N/S
Harvey et al. (1993)*	CA (F,T)	48	No	Not specified	DAS, NSRS	N/S
Honer et al. (1995)	VE, 3rd VE	42	No	4–28 weeks	CGI	N/S
Lawrie et al. (1995)*	CA (F,T)	40	No	Not specified	Krawiecka	N/S
Studies reporting a positive relationship between abnormality and treatment response/outcome						
Wolkowitz et al. (1988)	CA (F)	12	No	14–28 days	B-H Global Rating Scale	< 0.05

* = MRI study; all others = CT studies.
N/S, not significant.

chronic patients who, as Silverman *et al.* (1987) acknowledge, may not be a representative sample of schizophrenic patients. Wolkowitz *et al.* (1988) found a significantly *positive* relationship between frontal CA and treatment response, suggesting that greater atrophy is associated with better response. They also found that parieto-occipital CA, third ventricle width, and VE were not associated with response. Their study, however, assessed the effectiveness of alprazolam, a benzodiazepine used as an adjunct to neuroleptics, and not the relationship between antipsychotic treatment response and brain atrophy. Their findings are also compromised by a very small sample (*n* = 12).

Kaplan *et al.* (1990) addressed the issue of whether patients with structural brain abnormalities may simply respond more slowly than those without such abnormalities. They compared treatment-responsive or new-onset mood incongruent psychotic patients, defined as rapid- or delayed-responders to haloperidol, on the degree of third ventricle abnormality that they exhibited, an index they claimed to be more stable than lateral ventricular measures. All patient and control scans were judged as normal, though the schizophrenic patient means were significantly larger than age- and gender-matched controls, a fact emphasizing the subtlety of abnormality in patients. Delayed-responders were found to have significantly greater third ventricle area and width than either rapid-responders or controls. There was also a positive correlation between age and duration of illness, and the area and width of the third ventricle only in the delayed-responders. However, since the presence of affective symptoms is believed to be associated with good outcome (Kolakowska *et al.*, 1985), the inclusion of mood-incongruent patients in this and other studies (Smith *et al.*, 1987; Pandurangi *et al.*, 1989; Friedman *et al.*, 1991; Katsanis *et al.*, 1991; DeLisi *et al.*, 1992; Lieberman *et al.*, 1993; Honer *et al.*, 1995) may be significant.

Friedman *et al.* (1991) and Honer *et al.* (1995) found results strikingly similar to one another from their studies of clozapine, an atypical antipsychotic, on schizophrenic patients resistant to conventional antipsychotics. Friedman *et al.* (1991) assessed their patients' response over a period of six weeks. They found a highly significant linear trend indicating that non-responders to clozapine have the greatest degree of frontal cortical atrophy, moderate responders have an intermediate degree, and good responders have a small degree according to total Brief Psychiatric Rating Scale (BPRS) scores. When the five BPRS sub-scales were analysed separately, the linear trend was statistically significant for Thought Disorder, Positive Symptoms, Negative Symptoms, and Paranoid Disturbance, but not Anxiety/Depression. Multiple regression analysis also found that frontal cortical atrophy was a significant predictor of BPRS-Total at six weeks, and also of Thought Disorder, Positive Symptoms and Negative Symptoms sub-scales. No significant relationships were evident for VBR, emphasizing the independence of CA and VE. However, as Friedman *et al.* (1991) themselves warned, their findings should be interpreted with caution as the inter-rater reliability for frontal cortical atrophy was only acceptable (Intraclass Correlation Coefficient (ICC) = 0.69).

The questions of whether the association between response to atypical-antipsychotics and CA endures beyond six weeks, and whether other cortical areas might also be implicated were addressed by Honer *et al.* (1995). They obtained CT scans from patients undergoing up to 18 weeks of treatment on which the size of nine regions of interest were assessed according to a 1 to 7 rating of severity using over

40 reference scans obtained from normal controls and schizophrenic patients. The size of cortical sulcal spaces was found to be increased in responders to clozapine relative to non-responders, but no such difference was observable with respect to ventricular spaces. Multiple regression analyses revealed statistically significant results only for the posterior frontal and lateral temporal sulci. Again no significant association was found between the size of the lateral or third ventricles and treatment response.

In addition to the potentially confounding influence of the diverse response criteria employed in those studies in Table 6.2, it has also to be remembered that by design most of these studies recruit samples unrepresentative of the schizophrenic population, i.e. those who are treatment-resistant, making generalization of their conclusions hazardous. Acknowledging these limitations, the more robust of the studies in Table 6.2 contrast with those in Table 6.1 and seem to suggest that CA, but not VE, is associated with treatment response.

Correlation between brain abnormalities and treatment response

The requirement to define morphological abnormality, and good or poor treatment response, necessitates the setting of arbitrary boundaries. In the light of the above reported finding of Smith and Iacono (1986), studies, such as those in Table 6.1, which split their patient sample into normal and ventricle-enlarged groups on the basis of control mean measures must be viewed with caution. Likewise, those studies in Table 6.2 which set response criteria must also be regarded with scepticism due to the arbitrary nature of these criteria, and their diversity. The studies in Table 6.3, however, which carry out correlational tests to determine the relationship between brain measures and treatment response do not suffer from such shortcomings.

Naber *et al.* (1985), using a correlational design to assess the relationship between VE or CA and psychopathological changes, found no significant association between brain measures and response to withdrawal from conventional antipsychotics. However, interpretation of this study is problematic as symptoms were rated after neuroleptic withdrawal rather than subsequent to treatment commencement, and thus the phenomena observed may be more reflective of withdrawal than a drug-free state. Smith *et al.* (1987) assessed response to conventional antipsychotics after a one to three week wash-out period in 39 schizophrenic patients partially responsive to typical antipsychotics. They found no significant correlations between response and mean sulcal width, global atrophy or mean white matter density. Neither did patients defined as good- or poor-responders on the basis of their BPRS scores show significantly different brain morphology measures. The relatively short duration of treatment in this study (24 days) also should signal caution.

Pandurangi *et al.* (1989) also employed a relatively short period of treatment duration and a small sample in their study. The main focus of their study was the relationship between lateral ventricle size and symptomatic response to the Amphetamine Challenge Test (ACT), but they also gauged the patients' symptomatic response to haloperidol and thiothixene. Their correlational analysis found that

Table 6.3. Studies investigating the correlation between abnormalities and treatment response/outcome

Author, year	Abnormality investigated	N	Controls	Duration	Response/outcome criteria	Significance level P
Studies reporting an inverse relationship between abnormality and treatment response/outcome						
Pandurangi et al. (1989)	VE	19	No	13–45 days	BPRS	< 0.03
Vita et al. (1991)	CA (F,T,P)	18	No	2 years	Strauss-Carpenter Scale.	< 0.04
DeLisi et al. (1992)*	VE	29	No	2 years	BPRS	< 0.02
Schroder et al. (1993)	3rd VE, CA (F,T,P)	50	No	30 days	BPRS	< 0.05
Studies reporting no relationship between abnormality and treatment response/outcome						
Naber et al. (1985)	VE, CA (F,T,P)	36	No	3 months	BPRS	N/S
Smith et al. (1987)	CA (P, O)	39	No	24 days	NHSI, BPRS	N/S
Shelton et al. (1988)	VE, CA (P, O, F)	40	No	42 days	BPRS	N/S
Nimgaonkar et al. (1988)	VE, CA (F,T,P)	36	No	42 days	GAS, MSS	N/S
Vita et al. (1991)	VE	18	No	2 years	Strauss-Carpenter Scale	N/S
Breier et al. (1992)	VE, CA (P, O, F)	30	No	Not specified	GAS, BPRS, SANS, S-C	N/S
Schroder et al. (1993)	VE	50	No	30 days	BPRS	N/S
Studies reporting a positive relationship between abnormality and treatment response/outcome						
Smith et al. (1985)	VE	39	No	21 days	BPRS	< 0.1
Bersani et al. (1994)	VE	18	No	1 year	PANSS	Unreported

* = MRI study; all others = CT studies.

N/S, not significant.

treatment response had an inverse correlation with VBR. However, the group of patients considered for the ACT and whose treatment response was analysed were those patients ready for discharge from hospital, and may therefore represent only a sub-group of treatment-responsive schizophrenic patients.

In an MRI study DeLisi *et al.* (1992) examined the relationship between brain morphology and outcome after two years in 29 first episode patients newly medicated with typical antipsychotics. Outcome was assessed according to the total number of hospitalizations, duration of hospital stay, the GAS, the Strauss–Carpenter outcome sub-scale, and the total BPRS. They found that the larger the lateral ventricles at onset, the poorer the outcome as measured by the number of hospitalizations, the duration of hospital stay, and the total BPRS. Correlations of ventricular size with the GAS, and the Strauss–Carpenter scales were not found to be significant. The better resolution of MRI compared to CT, and the recruitment of first episode newly medicated patients bolster the findings of this study, though the researchers maintain that first episode hospitalized patients may represent a select group of acute onset, relatively good premorbid history patients and therefore may not be a representative sample.

Breier *et al.* (1992) also assessed outcome in a long-term study of chronic schizophrenic patients treated with typical antipsychotics. The morphological indices of interest were the VBR, third ventricular width, frontal lobe atrophy, and general cortical atrophy. The principal outcome measures were the GAS, the BPRS, the Strauss–Carpenter scale, the Scale for the Assessment of Negative Symptoms (SANS), and total time spent in hospital between index admission and follow-up. No significant correlations between brain morphological indices and outcome measures were found, though poor premorbid functioning predicted unfavourable outcome. Breier *et al.* (1992) suggested that in the light of their own previous research reporting functional but not structural impairment of the frontal cortex related to poor outcome, any deficit may be relatively subtle. The variable duration of follow-up in this study (from 2–12 years) is a matter worthy of consideration. Long-term outcome as assessed in this study is the result of the interaction of many uncontrolled environmental or intrapsychic factors affecting patients to differing degrees; therefore, we should not expect to find variables that alone have a high prognostic value. Allied with that is the observation by Friedman *et al.* (1992) who suggested that 'structural brain abnormalities may have greatest impact on earlier, rather than later, response' (pp. 50–51). These factors should encourage caution when interpreting outcome studies such as this.

Schroder *et al.* (1993) used two indices to assess the early response to treatment of 50 consecutively admitted schizophrenic patients. Absolute improvement was the change in BPRS score between admission and discharge, and relative improvement related the degree of improvement to the score at admission. From CT scans five indices were obtained; frontal horn ratio, ventricular ratio, width of third ventricle, VBR, width of frontal interhemispheric fissure, and the average width of the three largest cortical sulci. Most patients were maintained on conventional neuroleptics, though unresponsive patients or those experiencing extrapyramidal side-effects were given clozapine. Only correlations between absolute improvement and VBR, and relative improvement and frontal horn ratio proved *not* to be significant. Improvement on the BPRS sub-scales was correlated with the CT variables, with

Thought Disorders, which the authors state represents the core symptomatology of schizophrenia, showing the strongest correlation, especially with third ventricle width. Neither treatment response nor any of the CT variables differed significantly between patients receiving clozapine and those receiving typical neuroleptics. These findings, it is suggested, support the conclusion that treatment response is not regulated by one specific site, and that neither does it depend only on alterations in regions rich in dopamine D2 receptors.

Though these studies have the advantage over those previously discussed in not requiring the setting of arbitrary definitions of normal brain measures, or of quality of response, because of the diversity of methodology they do not give rise to unanimous conclusions. However, consideration of individual studies in the light of the conclusions drawn from Tables 6.1 and 6.2 may prove enlightening.

Conclusion

As is demonstrated by the discussion of those well designed studies outlined above, the literature on the relationship between structural abnormalities and treatment response is anything but straightforward, with the differing methodology employed and the influence of many potentially confounding factors making interpretation difficult. However, tentative conclusions can be drawn with respect to the influence that cerebral atrophy has on treatment response. The studies of Katsanis et al. (1991); Lieberman et al. (1993); Kaplan et al. (1990) and DeLisi et al. (1992) all suggested that in first episode patients, or patients with a history of treatment response, VE is inversely related to response to conventional antipsychotic medication, i.e. the greater the degree of VE the worse the response. None of the well designed studies contradicts this interpretation other than Nimgaonkar et al. (1988), whose interpretation is made difficult by the use of a mixed sample of chronic and first episode patients. There is also substantial support for the conclusion that CA does not have a significant influence on response to conventional antipsychotics in either first episode patients (MacDonald and Best, 1989; Lieberman et al., 1993) or in chronic or treatment-resistant patients (Naber et al., 1985; Smith et al., 1987; Nimgaonkar et al., 1988; Shelton et al., 1988; Breier et al., 1992). Two studies do find an association between response to antipsychotics and CA; however, the class of neuroleptic used by Vita et al. (1991) is not detailed, and Schroder et al. (1993) recruited a sample of patients who were taking either conventional neuroleptics or clozapine.

The literature suggests that, in treatment-resistant patients, the degree of VE is unrelated to response to conventional antipsychotics (Losonczy et al., 1986; Silverman et al., 1987; Shelton et al., 1988) or atypical antipsychotics (Friedman et al., 1991; Honer et al., 1995). This inability of VE to predict response to neuroleptics in treatment-resistant patients might arguably be attributed to two factors. First, patients who are treatment-resistant may have VE above some threshold over which the degree of VE is no longer predictive of response to conventional antipsychotics. In support of this are the findings reported above that larger VE predicts treatment-resistance, and the observation that those treatment resistant patients participating in the studies of Losonczy et al. (1986), Silverman et al. (1987), and Shelton et al. (1988) had VBRs significantly higher than controls. Second, VE might demonstrate no association with response to atypical antipsychotics because response to these drugs is mediated via mechanisms unrelated to VE. Support for this conclusion comes from the studies of Friedman *et al.* (1991) and Honer *et al.* (1995) who found that patients unresponsive to conventional antipsychotics responded to atypical antipsychotics, suggesting that it is the non-dopaminergic aspects of atypical antipsychotics that are effective in treatment-resistant cases. Also, as the studies of Friedman *et al.* (1991) and Honer *et al.* (1995) found, in those patients unresponsive to conventional antipsychotics, response to atypical drugs is somehow influenced by the degree of CA which they display (the question of whether CA or VE might also predict response to atypical antipsychotics in patients who are *responsive* to conventional antipsychotics remains to be explored).

What might be the role of CA be in preventing the amelioration of symptoms via atypical antipsychotic medication in those patients resistant to the antipsychotic effects of typical neuroleptics? In addition to dopamine receptors, atypical antipsychotic drugs have the ability to block other neurotransmitter receptors. The frontal cortex is replete with 5HT2 (serotonin) receptors, which clozapine and other atypicals target extensively (Lundberg *et al.*, 1986). The density of these receptors is reported to be decreased in the frontal cortex of schizophrenic patients, and clinical response to clozapine was found to be related to the magnitude of the clozapine-induced reduction of cortical metabolism in this area (Meltzer, 1991; Potkin *et al.*, 1993). It seems plausible, therefore, that frontal CA in some schizophrenic patients may reflect the reduced availability of 5HT2 receptors, which serves to circumscribe the potential for symptom improvement. Reduction of prefrontal cortical neurons which project to the basal ganglia and limbic regions, regulating dopamine activity, may also be a limiting factor in the amelioration of positive symptoms (Leccesse and Lyness, 1987). The findings of Honer *et al.* (1995) that lateral temporal lobe sulci are also related to poor response are supported by a study which reported an increased density of serotonin receptors in the limbic system of schizophrenic patients, with the number of re-uptake sites unchanged (Joyce *et al.*, 1993). However, caution must be exercised in the interpretation of these findings, as no conclusions can yet be drawn about any causal involvement of the frontal lobes in the genesis of these symptoms.

Numerous factors conspire to obscure the truth about the influence of cerebral atrophy on response to treatment. However, it is fair to say that the existence of structural brain abnormalities in some patients with schizophrenia is now beyond reasonable doubt. Frontal and temporal brain areas would seem to be the focus of these abnormalities reflected by VE and CA. These areas of dysfunction are compatible with the symptoms characteristic of the disorder. A body of evidence exists which suggests that the aetiology of these lesions is probably neurodevelopmental in origin, with genetic and environmental factors playing a role. From the investigations considered herein we can see that difficulties arise when comparisons are attempted between those studies that are methodologically different. However, the literature supports the conclusion that VE is associated with response to conventional antipsychotics, and that CA in some way mediates the effects of atypical drugs. The application of magnetic resonance imaging should provide a more detailed analysis of brain structures, with the studies above suggesting that frontal and temporal areas are worthy of most attention.

References

Arnold, S. and Trojanowski, J. Q. (1996) Recent advances in defining the neuropathology of schizophrenia. *Acta Neuropath*, **3**, 217–31.

Asano, N. (1967) Pneumoencephalographic study of schizophrenia. In N. Mitsuda (ed.), *Clinical genetics in psychiatry*. Tokyo: Igaku-Shoin, 209–19.

Bersani, G., Venturi, P., Tanfani, G.and Pancheri, P. (1994) Ventricular size and response to a long-term treatment with risperidone in chronic schizophrenia. *Schizophr Res*, **11**(2), 135.

Boronow, J., Pickar, D., Ninan, P. T. *et al.* (1985) Atrophy limited to the third ventricle in chronic schizophrenic patients. *Arch Gen Psychiatry*, **42**, 266–71.

Breier, A., Schreiber, J. L., Dyer, J. and Pickar, D. (1992) Course of illness and predictors of outcome in chronic schizophrenia: Implications for pathophysiology. *Br J Psychiatry*, **161** (suppl. 18), 38–43.

Buckman, T. D., Kling, A., Sutphin, M. S., Steinberg, A. and Aiduson, S., (1990). Platelet glutathione peroxidase and monoamine oxidase activity in schizophrenics with CT scan abnormalities: relation to psychosocial variables. *Psychiat Res*, **31**, 1–14.

Cazzullo, C. L. (1963). Biological and clinical studies on schizophrenia related to pharmacological treatment. *Rec Adv Biol Psychiatry*, **5**, 114–43.

Dandy, W. E. (1919). Roentgenography of the brain after injection of air into the cerebral ventricles. *Am J Roentgen*, **6**, 26.

DeLisi, L., Stritzke, P., Riordan, H. *et al.* (1992). The Timing of brain morphological changes in schizophrenia and their relationship to clinical outcome. *Biol Psychiatry*, **31**, 241–54.

Friedman, L., Knutson, L., Shurell, M. and Meltzer, H. Y. (1991) Prefrontal sulcal prominence is inversely related to response to clozapine in schizophrenia. *Biol Psychiatry*, **29**, 865–77.

Friedman, L., Lys, C. and Schultz, S. C. (1992) The relationship of structural imaging parameters to antipsychotic treatment response: a review . *J Psychiat Neurosci*, **17** (2), 42–54.

Gattaz, W. F., Kohlmeyer, K. and Gasser, T. (1987) Structural brain abnormalities in schizophrenia: an integrative model. In H. Hafner, W. F. Gattaz, and W. Janzarik, (eds), *Search for the causes of schizophrenia*. Heidelberg: Springer-Verlag, 250.

Gattaz, W. F., Rost, W., Kohlmeyer, K., Bauer, K., Hubner, C. and Gasser, T. (1988) CT scans and neuroleptic response in schizophrenia: a multidimensional approach. *Psychiat Res*, **26**, 293–303

Gurling, H. M. D., Reveley, M. A. and Murray, R. M. (1984) Increased cerebral ventricular volume in monozygotic twins discordant for alcoholism. *Lancet*, i, 986–8.

Harvey, I., Ron, M. A., Du Boulay, G., Wicks, D., Lewis, S. W. and Murray, R. M. (1993) Reduction of cortical volume in schizophrenia on magnetic resonance imaging. *Psychol Med*, **23**, 591-604.

Honer W. G., Smith, G. N., Lapointe, J. S., MacEwan, G. W., Kopala, L. and Altman, S. (1995) Regional cortical anatomy and clozapine response in refractory schizophrenia. *Neuropsychopharmacology*, **13** (1), 85–7.

Jacobi, W. and Winkler, H. (1927) Encephalographische studien an chronisch schizophrenen. *Archiv Psychiat Nervenkrankheiten*, **81**, 299–332.

Jeste, D. V., Kleinman, J. E., Potkin, S. G., Luchins, D. J., S. and Weinberger, D. R., (1982) Ex, Uno, Multi: subtyping the schizophrenic syndrome. *Biol Psychiatry*, **17**, 199–222.

Jewart, R. D., Lewine, R. J., Manning, D. E. *et al.* (1991) MRI findings as a predictor of clozapine response. *Schizophr Res*, **4**, 406.

Johnstone, E. C., Crow, T. J., Frith, C. D., Husband, D. and Kreel, L. (1976) Cerebral ventricular size and cognitive impairment in chronic schizophrenia. *Lancet*, **ii**, 924–6.

Joyce, J. N., Shane, A., Lexow, N, Winokur, A., Casanova, M. F. and Kleinman, J. E. (1993) Serotonin uptake sites and serotonin receptors are altered in the limbic system of schizophrenics. *Neuropsychopharmacology*, **8**, 315–36.

Kaiya, H., Uemetsu, M., Ofuji, M., Nishida, A., Morikiyo, M. and Adachi, S. (1989) Computerised tomography in schizophrenia: familial versus non-familial forms of illness. *Br J Psychiatry*, **155**, 444–50.

Kane, J. (1989) The current status of neuroleptics. *J Clin Psychiatry*, **50**, 322–8.

Kaplan, M. J., Lazoff, M., Kelly, K., Lukin, R. and Garver, D. L. (1990) Enlargement of cerebral third ventricle in psychotic patients with delayed response to neuroleptics. *Biol Psychiatry*, **27**, 205–14.

Katsanis, J., Iacono, W. G. and Beiser, M., (1991) Relationship of lateral ventricular size to psychophysiological measures and short-term outcome. *Psychiat Res*, **37**, 115–29.

Kolakowska, T., Williams, A. O., Ardern, M. *et al.* (1985). Schizophrenia with good and poor outcome. I: Early clinical features, response to neuroleptics and signs of organic dysfunction. *Br J Psychiatry*, **146**, 229–46.

Kraepelin, E. (1896) *Psychiatrie*, 5th Edition. Leipzig: Barth.

Lawrie, S. M., Ingle, G. T., Santosh, C. G. *et al.* (1995) Magnetic resonance imaging and single photon emission tomography in treatment responsive and treatment resistant schizophrenia. *Br J Psychiatry*, **167**, 202–10.

Lawrie, S. M., Abukmeil, S. S., Chiswick, A., Egan, V., Santosh, C. G. and Best, J. J. K. (1997) Qualitative cerebral morphology in schizophrenia; a magnetic resonance imaging study and systematic literature review. *Schizophr Res*, **25**, 155–66.

Leccesse, A. P. and Lyness, W. H. (1987) Lesions of dopamine neurons in the medial prefrontal cortex: Effects on self-administration of amphetamine and dopamine synthesis in the brain of the rat. *Neuropharmacology*, **26**, 1303–8.

Lewis, S. W. (1990) Computerised tomography in schizophrenia 15 years on. *Br J Psychiatry*, **157** (suppl. 9), 16–24.

Lieberman, J., Jody, D., Geisler, S. *et al.* (1993) Time course and biologic correlates of treatment response in first-episode schizophrenia. *Arch Gen Psychiatry*, **50**, 369–76.

Losonczy, M. F., Song, I. S., Hohs, R. C. *et al.* (1986) Correlates of lateral ventricular size in chronic schizophrenia. I: Behavioural and treatment response measures. *Am J Psychiatry*, **143** (8), 976–81.

Luchins, D. J. and Meltzer, H. Y. (1983) A blind, controlled study of occipital cerebral asymmetry in schizophrenia. *Psychiat Res*, **10**, 87–95.

Luchins, D. J., Lewine, R. R. J. and Meltzer, H. Y. (1984) Lateral ventricular size, psychopathology, and medication response in the psychoses. *Biol Psychiatry*, **19**, 29–43.

Lundberg, T., Lindstrom, L. H., Hartvig, P. *et al.* (1986) Striatal and frontal cortex binding of ^{11}C-labelled clozapone visualized by positron emission tomography (PET) in drug-free schizophrenics and healthy volunteers. *Psychopharmacology*, **99**, 8–12.

Macdonald, H. L. and Best, J. J. K., (1988) The Scottish first episode schizophrenia study. V: One year follow-up. *Br J Psychiatry*, **153**, 470–6.

Macdonald, H. L. and Best, J. J. K. (1989) The Scottish first episode schizophrenia study. VI: Computerised tomography brain scans in patients and controls. *Br J Psychiatry*, **154**, 492–8.

Marsden, C. D. (1976) Cerebral atrophy and cognitive impairment in chronic schizophrenia. *Lancet*, ii, 1079.

Mauri, M. C., Vita, A., Giobbio, G. M. *et al.* (1994) Prediction of response to haloperidol in schizophrenia: neuroendocrine, neuromorphological and clinical variables. *Int Clin Psychopharmacol*, **9**, 3–7.

May, P. R. A., Dencker, S. J., Hubbard, J. W. *et al.* (1988) A systematic approach to treatment resistance in schizophrenic disorders. In S. J. Denzker and F. Kulhaneck (eds), *Treatment resistance in schizophrenia*. Braunschweig/Wiesbaden: Vieweg Verlag, 22–33.

Meltzer, H. Y. (1991) The mechanism of action of novel anti-psychotic drugs. *Schizophr Bull*, **17**, 263–87.

Miller, D. D., Flaum, M. A. and Andreasen, N. C. (1991) A magnetic resonance imaging study comparing treatment-refractory and treatment-responsive schizophrenics. *Schizophr Res*, **4**, 406.

Naber, D., Albus, M., Burke, H. *et al.* (1985). Neuroleptic withdrawal in chronic schizophrenia: CT and endocrine variables relating to psychopathology. *Psychiat Res*, **16**, 207–19.

Nasrallah, H. A., Kleinman, J. E., Weinberger, D. R. *et al.* (1980) Cerebral ventricular enlargement and dopamine synthesis inhibition in chronic schizophrenia (letter). *Arch Gen Psychiatry*, **37**, 1427.

Nasrallah, H. A., Kuperman, S., Hamra, B. J. and McCalley-Whitters, M. (1983a) Clinical differences between schizophrenic patients with and without large cerebral ventricles. *J Clin Psychiatry*, **44**, 407–9.

Nasrallah, H. A., Kuperman, S., Jacoby, C. G., McCalley-Whitters, M. and Hamra, B. (1983b) Clinical correlates of sulcal widening in chronic schizophrenia. *Psychiatry Res*, **10**, 237–42.

Nimgaonkar, V. L., Wessley, S., Tune, L. E. and Murray, R. M. (1988) Response to drugs in schizophrenia: the influence of family history, obstetric complications and ventricular enlargement. *Psychol Med*, **18**, 583–92.

Pandurangi, A. K., Dewan, M. J., Boucher, M. *et al.* (1986) A comprehensive study of chronic schizophrenic patients. II: Biological, neuropsychological, and clinical correlates of CT abnormality. *Acta Psychiat Scand*, **73**, 161–71.

Pandurangi, A. K., Goldberg, S. C., Brink, D. D., Hill, M. H., Gulati, A. N. and Hamer, R. M. (1989) Amphetamine challenge test, response to treatment, and lateral ventricle size in schizophrenia. *Biol Psychiatry*, **25**, 207–14.

Potkin, S. G., Buchsbaum, M. S., Jin, Y. *et al.* (1993) Clozapine markedly affects glucose metabolic rate in the striatum and cortex. *Schizophr Res*, **9**, 207.

Reveley, A. M., Reveley, M. A., Clifford, C. A. and Murray, R. M. (1982) Cerebral ventricular size in twins discordant for schizophrenia. *Lancet*, ii, 540–1.

Reveley, M. A. (1985) CT scans in schizophrenia. *Br J Psychiatry*, **146**, 367–71.

Schroder, J., Gieder, F. J. and Sauer, H. (1993) Can computerised tomography be used to predict early treatment response in schizophrenia. *Br J Psychiatry*, **163** (Suppl. 21), 13–5.

Schulz, S. C., Conley, R. R., Kahn, E. M. and Alexander, J. (1983) Treatment response and ventricular brain enlargement in young schizophrenic patients. *Psychopharmacol Bull*, **19**, 510–12.

Shelton, R. C., Karson, C. N., Doran, A. R., Pickar, D., Bigelow, L. B. and Weinberger, D. R. (1988) Cerebral structural pathology in schizophrenia: evidence for a selective prefrontal cortical defect. *Am J Psychiatry*, **145**, 154–63.

Silverman, J. M., Mohs, R. C., Davidson, M. *et al.* (1987) Familial schizophrenia and treatment response. *Am J Psychiatry*, **144** (10), 1271–7.

Smith, R. C., Largen, J., Calderon, M., Schoolar, J., Shvartburd, A. and Ravichandran, G. K. (1983) CT scans and neuropsychological tests as predictors of clinical response in schizophrenia. *Psychopharmacol Bull*, **19**, 505–9.

Smith, R. C., Baumgartner, R., Ravichandran, G. K. *et al.* (1985) Lateral ventricular enlargement and clinical response in schizophrenia. *Psychiat Res*, **14**, 214–53.

Smith, R. C. and Iacono, W. G., (1986). Lateral ventricular size in schizophrenia and choice of control group. *Lancet*, June 21, 1450.

Smith, R. C., Baumgartner, R., Ravichandran, G. K. *et al.* (1987) Cortical atrophy and white matter density in the brains of schizophrenics and clinical response to neuroleptics. *Acta Psychiat Scand*, **75**, 11–19.

Suddath, R. L., Christison, G. W., Torrey, E. F., Casanova, M. F. and Weinberger, D. R. (1990) Anatomical abnormalities in the brains of monozygotic twins discordant for schizophrenia. *New Engl J Med*, **322**, 789–94.

Vita, A., Sacchetti, E., Calzeroni, A. and Cazzullo, C. L. (1988) Cortical atrophy in schizophrenia: prevalence and associated features. *Schizophr Res*, **1**, 329–37.

Vita, A., Dieci, M., Giobbio, G. M. *et al.* (1991) CT scan abnormalities and outcome of chronic schizophrenia. *Am J Psychiatry*, **148**(11), 1577–9.

Weinberger, D. R., Torrey, E. F., Neophytides, A. N. and Wyatt, R. J. (1979) Lateral cerebral ventricular enlargement in chronic schizophrenia. *Arch Gen Psychiatry*, **36**, 733–9.

Weinberger, D. R., Bigelow, L. B., Kleinman, L. E., Klein, S. T., Rosenblatt, J. E. and Wyatt, R. J. (1980) Cerebral ventricular enlargement in chronic schizophrenia. *Arch Gen Psychiatry*, **37**, 11–13.

Weinberger, D. R., DeLisi, L. E., Perlman, G. P., Targum, S. and Wyatt R. J. (1982) Computed tomography in schizophreniform disorder and other acute psychiatric disorders. *Arch Gen Psychiatry*, **39**, 778.

Williams, A. O., Reveley, M. A., Kalakowska, T., Ardern, M. and Mandelbrote, B. M. (1985) Schizophrenia with good and poor outcome. II: Cerebral ventricular size and its clinical significance. *Br J Psychiatry*, **147**, 239–46.

Wilms, G., Van Ongeval, C., Baert, A. L. *et al.* (1992) Ventricular enlargement, clinical correlates and treatment outcome in chronic schizophrenic inpatient. *Acta Psychiat Scand*, **85**, 306–12.

Wolkowitz, O. M., Breier, A., Doran, A. *et al.* (1988) Alprazolam augmentation of the antipsychotic effects of Fluphenazine in schizophrenic patients. *Arch Gen Psychiatry*, **45**, 664–72.

CHAPTER 7

Functional brain imaging of schizophrenia

PETER F. LIDDLE

Introduction

The clinical features of schizophrenia include not only defective evaluation of reality, which is the defining feature of psychosis, but also disabling disorders of the initiation and organization of voluntary behaviour, thought, and emotion. In addition to these symptoms, there are a multiplicity of neuropsychological impairments. A full understanding of the illness demands an understanding of the way in which the illness affects the function of the diverse neural pathways involved. Functional imaging techniques such as Positron Emission Tomography (PET), Single Photon Emission Tomography (SPET) and functional Magnetic Resonance Imaging (fMRI) measure the changes in local cerebral perfusion associated with neural activity, and thereby offer the possibility of mapping the diverse patterns of aberrant cerebral activity in schizophrenia.

For the purpose of designing and interpreting studies of the cerebral activity in schizophrenia, it is important to distinguish between unconstrained, self-generated mental activity, and constrained mental activity associated with the performance of an externally specified task. Studies of the cerebral activity associated with unconstrained mental activity are potentially informative about the brain processes involved in the expression of schizophrenic symptoms. Studies of cerebral activity during specified neuropsychological tests might allow the identification of malfunction in circuits serving specified cognitive processes.

Many of the functional imaging studies of schizophrenia performed in the decade following the pioneering study of regional Cerebral Blood Flow (rCBF) in schizophrenia by Ingvar and Franzen (1974) were studies of unconstrained ('resting state') mental activity. In any functional imaging study, interpretation is difficult unless it is possible to compare images of a brain state of interest with images of a reference brain state that differs in a well-defined manner from the state of interest. In studies of unconstrained, self-generated mental activity it is necessary to ensure that any systematic differences between images can be attributed to definable differences in mental state. In most of the studies of schizophrenia performed in the 1970s, that first decade of functional imaging, the differences in mental state that accounted for the observed differences between images were inadequately defined. Consequently, these studies resulted in conflicting findings: some confirmed Ingvar and Franzen's (1974) original observation of relative underactivity of the frontal lobes, while others did not (Early *et al.*, 1987).

Meanwhile, neuropsychological challenge techniques for measuring the pattern of cerebral activity associated with externally specified tasks were developed. In the mid-1980s, Weinberger and colleagues demonstrated that the increases in frontal lobe rCBF associated with performance of the Wisconsin Card Sorting Test (Weinberger *et al.*, 1986) were smaller in schizophrenic patients than in healthy subjects. Since that time, studies employing neuropsychological challenge have demonstrated that schizophrenic patients exhibit aberrant cerebral activity in a variety of different brain areas during a variety of tasks, ranging from simple motor acts to relatively demanding planning tasks.

The challenge of measuring unconstrained mental activity in an informative manner was not addressed systematically until the beginning of the 1990s, when Liddle *et al.* (1992) introduced a strategy based on the observation that the characteristic clinical features of schizophrenia can be assigned to three orthogonal dimensions, at least during stable phases of illness. The orthogonality of the dimensions makes it possible to measure correlations between rCBF and severity of each symptom dimension, with minimal confounding arising from the presence of symptoms from different dimensions. Liddle and colleagues succeeded in determining the patterns of cerebral activity associated with each of the three major dimensions of persistent schizophrenic symptoms. Subsequently, strategies based on the variation of severity of symptoms over time within a single individual have been employed to delineate the pattern of cerebral activity associated with individual symptoms.

In this chapter, we will begin with a brief account of imaging techniques. We will then review studies of unconstrained mental activity in symptomatic patients, which reveal the pattern of cerebral activity associated with the expression of schizophrenic symptoms. Following this, we will review neuropsychological challenge studies that examine cerebral activity during the performance of externally specified tasks. Finally, we will review the evidence regarding the effects of pharmacological agents on patterns of cerebral activity, emphasizing the light shed by functional imaging studies on the mechanism of antipsychotic drug action.

Imaging techniques

When neurons become active, there is local vasodilation producing an increase in regional cerebral blood flow (rCBF). This can be quantified by measuring the accumulation of a radioactive tracer that is distributed in proportion to local blood flow. In the case of PET, the most commonly used tracer is water labelled with the oxygen isotope ^{15}O, which has a half-life of approximately two minutes. In the case of SPET, the usual tracer is exametazime (also known as HMPAO) labelled with the metastable technetium isotope, ^{99m}Tc, which has a half-life of 6 hours. The much shorter half-life of the PET tracer allows the collection of multiple images, separated by approximately 10-minute intervals, within a single session. The relatively low radiation exposure per scan makes it possible to obtain at least 12 PET rCBF images per subject without exceeding allowed radiation exposure limits. Thus it is feasible to study the relationship between symptoms and cerebral activity in a single subject. In contrast, with SPET, if more than one image is to be collected in a day, the long half-life of the tracer makes it necessary to subtract residual radioactivity from any previous scan. The high radiation exposure per scan imposes a limit of two or three scans per individual per year.

Functional MRI is based on the fact that the increase in perfusion associated with neural activity exceeds that required to meet increased demand for oxygen, so that local concentration of deoxyhaemoglobin falls. Deoxyhaemoglobin is paramagnetic and creates local inhomogeneity in an applied magnetic field. Protons in the water in brain tissue rotate about an applied magnetic field. In MRI, radio frequency pulses are employed to synchronize the phase of the rotation of protons, and the subsequent decay of this synchronization is measured. Magnetic field inhomogeneity increases the rate of desynchronization of the proton rotation. Thus, when local neural activity increases, deoxyhaemoglobin concentration falls and the magnetic field homogeneity decreases; the phase coherence of rotating protons is lost more slowly, and there is an increase in the amount of residual magnetization detectable at a specified time after the radio frequency pulse. This is known as the Blood Oxygen Level Dependent (BOLD) effect. MRI images that reflect the local rate of loss of phase coherence of rotating protons (T2* weighted images) thus provide a measure of local neural activity .

Using fast MRI techniques, it is possible to obtain an image of the entire brain in a few seconds. Because there is no exposure to ionizing radiation, and it is not necessary to wait between scans for the clearance of an exogenous tracer, it is feasible to obtain hundreds of images of brain activity in a single subject in a single scanning session. However, the signal-to-noise ratio for each individual image is poor, and it is usual to average over several images in each brain state of interest. Slight movements of the subject can induce artefacts, and it is necessary to take great care to re-align images if reliable images are to be obtained.

Cerebral activity associated with expression of symptoms

It is probable that each specific schizophrenic symptom is associated with its own particular pattern of cerebral activity. However, the observation that certain types of symptoms tend to co-exist within an individual implies that particular patterns of abnormal psychological and cerebral activity are common to specific groups of symptoms. There are at least five major groups of symptoms that occur commonly in schizophrenia: reality distortion, disorganization, psychomotor poverty, psychomotor excitation and depression (Liddle, 1995). Three of these groups of symptoms, reality distortion, disorganization and psychomotor poverty are especially characteristic of schizophrenia, and we will therefore focus on the findings with regard to these three groups. Because interpretation of the data must take careful account of the study design, we will begin with a discussion of some design issues.

STUDY DESIGN

In view of the evanescent and idiosyncratic nature of human cerebral activity, a multiplicity of factors can contribute to variance in images of cerebral function. If the pattern of cerebral activity associated with symptoms is to be identified clearly, it is essential that investigations be designed so that the major source of variance between images is variance in symptoms. The interpretation of observed differences between images must take account of issues such as whether these differences might reflect the predisposition to suffer those symptoms or the actual experience of the relevant symptoms.

Three principal types of study design have been employed to determine the relationships between schizophrenic symptoms and patterns of cerebral activity: (i) determination of correlations between symptoms and rCBF across patients; (ii) comparison of rCBF in the presence and absence of symptoms within patients; (iii) determination of correlations between symptoms and rCBF within patients.

Correlations between symptoms and rCBF across patients

This strategy, which was introduced by Liddle *et al.* (1992), is the preferred strategy for determining the relationship between chronic symptoms and cerebral activity. In particular, it is the only strategy suitable for determining the pattern of cerebral activity associated with persistent negative symptoms. During stable phases of the illness, the three groups of characteristic schizophrenic symptoms are usually orthogonal, while symptoms of excitation and depression have a low prevalence, so the correlation between rCBF and any one of the three groups of characteristic symptoms is unlikely to be confounded by systematic differences between subjects in symptoms from a different group. This study design would be expected to reveal the pattern of cerebral activity associated not only with the experience of symptoms belonging to a given group, but also with the propensity to experience the relevant type of symptom. To minimize the potentially confounding influence of unavoidable medication in studies of patients during the stable phase of illness, all patients should receive medication of a single class, at a broadly similar dose.

The cross-sectional correlation design has also been applied to determine the correlation between rCBF and symptom profile in acutely ill patients (e.g. Ebmeier *et al.*, 1993). While it is possible to avoid the potential confounding effects of medication in acute patients, it is less easy to avoid confounding effects of other types of symptoms, because the different symptom groups might not be orthogonal in such patients.

Within-subject rCBF in the presence or absence of symptoms

In this type of study, patients are scanned during the presence of the symptom of interest, and again after resolution of that symptom. This study design is best exemplified by the SPET study of rCBF patterns associated with hallucinations by McGuire *et al.* (1993). As in cross-sectional correlational studies, those employing this design would be anticipated to reveal rCBF patterns associated with the propensity to suffer the symptom of interest in addition to cerebral activity associated with the occurrence of that symptom. The strength of this study design is the fact that comparisons within subjects are not prone to influence by irrelevant differences between subjects. The difficulty is that clinical features other than the symptom of interest might also change between the first and second scan. If systematic changes in any other symptoms occurs, the variance in rCBF accounted for by variance in these symptoms must be allowed for by analysis of covariance. There is also the possibility for confounding differences between the first and second scans due to inevitable differences in duration of medication.

Determination of correlations within patients

In this type of study, multiple scans are performed in each subject during a relatively brief period of time during which individual symptoms might fluctuate in intensity, but the overall clinical status of the patients would not be expected to change. Variation between scans in the severity or frequency of the symptom of interest is recorded and correlated with variation in rCBF. This type of design is only feasible for measuring cerebral activity associated with symptoms such as hallucinations that are transient in nature. It would be expected to reveal the pattern of rCBF associated with the actual experience of the symptom, rather than that associated with the propensity to suffer the symptom.

This type of study is exemplified by the PET study of rCBF associated with hallucinations performed by Silbersweig *et al.* (1995). They recruited a group of patients who exhibited frequent hallucinations and performed up to 20 PET scans in each individual, using the slow bolus water infusion technique. In this technique, water labelled with ^{15}O is injected over a period of 30 seconds. The accumulation of radioactivity at any brain site reflects local cerebral activity over the interval of approximately 30 seconds, during which the labelled water reaches the brain. Subjects were instructed to press a button to indicate the experience of hallucinations occurring during the scan. The images were analysed to determine those pixels in which variance in rCBF between scans (within each subject) was correlated with number of hallucinations occurring during the period in which labelled water was accumulating. Employing such a design, it is not possible to distinguish the pattern of rCBF associated with the symptom of interest from that associated with concomitant mental activity, such as the recognition and psychological response to the symptom, or the activity involved in reporting the experience of the symptom.

REALITY DISTORTION

The tendency for the severity of delusions and hallucinations to co-vary, both between subjects, and within a subject over time, indicates that these two types of clinical features share aspects of their underlying pathophysiology. It is likely that they have in common an abnormality of the mechanism for evaluating reality, and hence it is appropriate to employ the name reality distortion for this group of symptoms.

In their cross-sectional PET study of 30 schizophrenic patients with persistent, stable symptoms, Liddle *et al.* (1992) found that severity of reality distortion was positively correlated with rCBF in left medial temporal lobe, including the parahippocampal gyrus, left ventral striatum and left inferolateral prefrontal cortex (*see* Fig. 7.1). There were negative correlations between reality distortion and rCBF in the posterior cingulate cortex, and in left lateral temporoparietal cortex. Thus, the evidence suggests that a distributed array of cerebral sites is involved in reality distortion.

Subsequently, in their PET study of the correlations between occurrence of auditory hallucinations within individual schizophrenic patients, based on up to 30 scans per subject, Silbersweig *et al.* (1995) found that the occurrence of auditory hallucinations was associated with increased rCBF in medial temporal lobe (hippocampus and parahippocampal gyrus), ventral striatum, thalamus and orbital frontal cortex. While Silbersweig *et al.* confirmed the overactivity in medial temporal lobe and ventral striatum reported by Liddle *et al.* (1992), they did not find any areas of negative correlation between hallucinations and rCBF. The study design employed by Silbersweig would be expected to identify cerebral activity associated with the experience of symptoms, but not the propensity to suffer those symptoms. It is possible that in general, areas of underactivity are indicative of propensity to suffer symptoms, whereas the actual occurrence itself is associated with increase in cerebral activity.

SPET studies of rCBF associated with symptoms of reality distortion have reported abnormalities of temporal rCBF, but the direction of the reported change has been inconsistent. In a cross-sectional SPET study of 20 acutely ill unmedicated patients, Ebmeier *et al.* (1993) replicated Liddle's finding of a negative correlation between reality distortion and rCBF in lateral temporal lobe, but they did not find evidence of positive correlation with rCBF in medial temporal lobe. In contrast, in a longitudinal within-subject study, Suzuki *et al.* (1993) found occurrence of hallucinations to be associated with increased superior temporal rCBF. These observations are partially consistent with the hypothesis that temporal underactivity is associated with propensity to suffer hallucinations, while the actual occurrence of hallucinations is associated with temporal overactivity. However, it should be noted that Suzuki *et al.* (1993) observed overactivity in superior temporal lobe, not in medial temporal structures such as parahippocampal gyrus or hippocampus. SPET is relatively less sensitive than PET to areas deep in the brain.

The hypothesis that the propensity to suffer hallucinations is associated with lateral temporal underactivity while the occurrence of hallucinations is associated with medial temporal overactivity is supported by two studies by McGuire and colleagues (1993,1995). In a study employing SPET to measure rCBF in a cohort of 12 schizophrenic patients while they were experiencing auditory hallucinations, and again, a mean of 19 weeks later when the hallucinations had resolved, McGuire *et al.* (1993) found that rCBF was significantly greater during the experience of hallucinations in left inferolateral frontal cortex (Broca's area). There was also higher blood flow in

decreases   **increases**

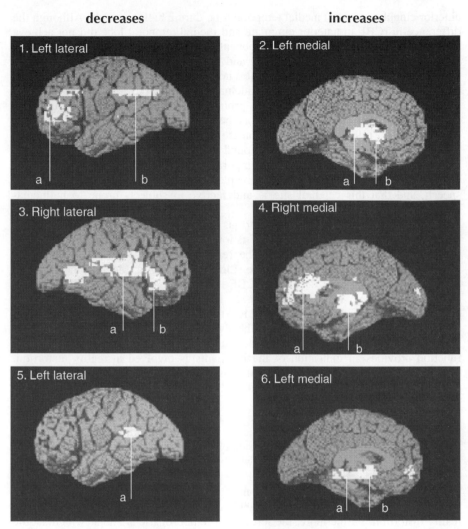

Fig. 7.1 Patterns of rCBF associated with schizophrenic symptoms (Liddle *et al.*, 1992). The areas of significant correlation between rCBF and severity of each of three syndromes of characteristic syndromes are shown rendered onto the cortical surface. rCBF was measured using PET. 1. Negative correlations of psychomotor poverty with rCBF in left lateral prefrontal cortex (a) and inferior parietal lobule (b). 2. Positive correlations of psychomotor poverty with rCBF in corpus striatum and thalamus. 3. Negative correlations of disorganization with rCBF in right ventro-lateral prefrontal cortex (a) and insula, rendered onto the overlying temporal cortex (b). 4. Positive correlations of disorganization with rCBF in right medial frontal cortex and thalamus (a). 5. Negative correlations of reality distortion with rCBF in left superior temporal gyrus (a). 6. Positive correlations of reality distortion with rCBF in left parahippocampal gyrus (a) and ventral striatum (b). This figure also appears in colour between pages 150 and 151.

anterior cingulate and left medial temporal lobe during hallucinations. Although the difference in rCBF in anterior cingulate and medial temporal lobe did not achieve statistical significance, principle component analysis demonstrated that rCBF in Broca's area, left medial temporal lobe and left cingulate gyrus loaded on a single component, implying that they constitute a network of cerebral areas in which correlated changes occur during auditory hallucinations.

In a subsequent study of six patients prone to persistent auditory hallucinations, six patients without a history of auditory hallucinations, and six healthy controls, McGuire *et al.* (1995) used PET to measure rCBF while the subjects imagined words spoken in an alien voice. They found that the hallucinators produced significantly less activation of left lateral temporal lobe. They interpreted their finding as evidence that left lateral temporal lobe plays a part in monitoring self-generated speech, and that this cerebral site is underactive in subjects prone to hallucinations.

Despite some discrepancies, these various studies of rCBF associated with either reality distortion (delusions and hallucinations), or with hallucinations alone, have produced some consistent findings. The replicated findings include evidence of increased rCBF in medial temporal lobe (Liddle *et al.*, 1992; McGuire *et al.*, 1993; Silbersweig *et al.*, 1995); decreased rCBF in lateral temporal lobe (Liddle *et al.*, 1992; Ebmeier *et al.*, 1993; McGuire *et al.*, 1995); increased rCBF in left inferolateral frontal cortex (Liddle *et al.*, 1992, McGuire *et al.*, 1993); and increased rCBF in ventral striatum (Liddle *et al.*, 1992; Silbersweig *et al.*, 1995).

Consideration of the roles that the identified cerebral areas play in normal brain function provides an indication of the mechanisms involved in reality distortion. The observed overactivity of left lateral frontal cortex might reflect the production of the verbal content of delusions and hallucinations, since this cerebral area is specialized for the generation of speech. Overactivity in the left medial temporal lobe possibly reflects aberrant function of a cerebral site that plays a role in the monitoring of self-generated mental activity. This possibility is supported by a PET study by Frith *et al.* (1992) of the cerebral activity associated with the learning of a novel eye movement task, which was designed so as to place heavy demands on the need to monitor self-generated actions. They found that the healthy individuals produced activation of left parahippocampal gyrus at a site within the area where Liddle *et al.* (1992) found increased rCBF associated with reality distortion. Furthermore, the left lateral temporoparietal site at which Liddle *et al.* (1992) had observed a negative correlation between rCBF and severity of reality distortion, is near to the site in left superior temporal gyrus at which McGuire *et al.* (1995) found involvement in monitoring self-generated speech. Thus, the available evidence indicates that both the medial and lateral temporal sites implicated in reality distortion might reflect involvement of the circuitry for monitoring self-generated mental activity.

The evidence for an association between reality distortion and increased rCBF in ventral striatum (Liddle *et al.*, 1992; Silbersweig *et al.*, 1995) might be of particular relevance to pharmacological treatment, in view of the evidence that ventral striatum is the site of action common to typical and atypical antipsychotic drugs (Robertson and Fibiger, 1992).

DISORGANIZATION

Formal thought disorder, inappropriate affect and bizarre behaviour form a group of related symptoms that appear to reflect disorganization of mental activity. Neuropsychological studies indicate that the disorganization is associated with impaired ability to suppress inappropriate responses. For example, severity of disorganization is correlated with impaired performance in the Stroop task, in which the subject is presented with colour names printed in ink of a colour that is incongruent with the colour name, and is required to name the ink colour (Liddle and Morris, 1991).

In their PET study of schizophrenic patients with persistent stable symptoms, Liddle *et al.* (1992) found that disorganization was associated with increased rCBF in anterior cingulate, and with decreased rCBF in the right ventral frontal cortex and contiguous insula, and in the parietal lobe bilaterally (*see* Fig. 7.1). The finding of an association between disorganization and increased rCBF in anterior cingulate was confirmed by Ebmeier *et al.* (1993) in their study of acute, unmedicated patients, and by Yuasa *et al.* (1995). In a study employing PET to measure regional cerebral metabolic rate for glucose, Kaplan *et al.* (1993) found a negative correlation between disorganization and parietal metabolism, consistent with the negative correlation between disorganization and parietal rCBF observed by Liddle *et al.* (1992), but they did not find a correlation between disorganization and metabolism in the anterior cingulate.

The involvement of parietal cortex and anterior cingulate in disorganization is consistent with the role of a distributed network embracing both of these cerebral areas in selective attention. In particular, the site of increased rCBF in anterior cingulate cortex associated with disorganization coincides with the site that Pardo *et al.* (1990) demonstrated to be maximally activated in healthy individuals during the Stroop task, consistent with the observation of an association between severity of disorganization and impaired performance in the Stroop task (Liddle and Morris, 1991). It should be noted that disorganization appears to be associated with pathological overactivity rather than underactivity at this site. In monkeys, lesions of ventral frontal cortex are associated with impaired ability to suppress inappropriate responses. This suggests the hypothesis that as a consequence of impaired ventral prefrontal cortex, patients with marked disorganization are subject to continual intrusion of inappropriate mental activity in conscious processing, and hence are continually subjected to the challenge of a Stroop-like experience, resulting in overactivity in anterior cingulate cortex.

PSYCHOMOTOR POVERTY

The core negative symptoms, flat affect, poverty of speech and decreased spontaneous movement, that make up the psychomotor poverty syndrome, appear to reflect a difficulty in initiating mental or motor activity. Liddle and Morris (1991) found that psychomotor poverty is associated with decreased or slowed output in tasks, such as word generation, that demand self-generated mental activity. Virtually all functional imaging studies that have examined the pattern of cerebral activity associated with psychomotor poverty symptoms have reported an association with underactivity of frontal cortex. In the first study of rCBF in schizophrenia, Ingvar and Franzen (1974) found hypofrontality in a group of patients who exhibited social withdrawal and motor underactivity. Liddle *et al.* (1992) found that severity of psychomotor poverty was correlated negatively with rCBF in lateral and medial prefrontal cortex, and in left parietal cortex, at a site which has strong reciprocal connections with lateral prefrontal cortex (*see* Fig 7.1). However, in addition to these areas of underactivity, Liddle *et al.* (1992) also found that psychomotor poverty was associated with increased rCBF in the corpus striatum bilaterally. This suggests that rather than being a reflection of fixed loss of cortical function, psychomotor poverty entails a dynamic imbalance between activity at different sites in the cortico-subcortical loops that connect frontal cortex, striatum and thalamus. Consistent with the observation that psychomotor poverty is associated with diminished output in word generation tasks, the site of negative correlation between psychomotor poverty and left lateral prefrontal rCBF coincided with the site which Frith *et al.* (1991) found to be maximally activated in healthy subjects during the generation of words.

Ebmeier *et al.* (1993) found a strong negative correlation between rCBF and left lateral frontal rCBF in their SPET study of acute unmedicated schizophrenic subjects, demonstrating that this negative correlation is not confined merely to patients with persistent stable symptoms. However, it is of interest to note that as a group, the patients studied by Ebmeier *et al.* (1993) exhibited increased frontal rCBF compared with healthy controls. This finding indicates that some other clinical feature of acute psychosis causes an increase in frontal rCBF. It is likely that psychomotor excitation, which would be anticipated in a group of acute, unmedicated patients, is associated with overactivity of frontal cortex, though this hypothesis has not been tested directly.

Differences in detail between different studies indicate that different aspects of psychomotor poverty might be preferentially associated with underactivity of different frontal areas. For example, in a study using PET to measure glucose metabolism, Wolkin *et al.* (1992) found that blunted affect was associated with decreased frontal activity only in the right prefrontal cortex. In contrast, Dolan *et al.* (1993) found that poverty of speech is associated with left prefrontal underactivity (in schizophrenia and also in depression).

Neuropsychological challenge

WISCONSIN CARD SORTING TEST (WCST)

This task, which demands a flexible approach to problem solving, entails several aspects of mental processing that place demands upon the frontal lobes, including working memory and ability to change mental set. The finding of diminished frontal activation in schizophrenic patients during performance of the WCST, originally reported by Weinberger *et al.* (1986), has been replicated on numerous occasions, both by Weinberger's own colleagues (e.g. Weinberger *et al.*, 1988; Berman *et al.*, 1992), and by others (Rubin *et al.*, 1991; Catafau *et al.*, 1994). In a study of monozygotic twins, Berman *et al.* (1992) demonstrated that in all twins pairs discordant for schizophrenia, the affected twin exhibited less activation of prefrontal cortex during the WCST than the healthy co-twin, even when both twins exhibited activation within the normal range. This suggests that a degree of diminution of ability to activate prefrontal cortex might be a characteristic of virtually all patients with schizophrenia. Furthermore, it indicates that diminished ability to activate prefrontal cortex is determined at least in part by non-genetic factors.

The degree of diminution of activation of prefrontal cortex is correlated with reduced hippocampal volume (Weinberger *et al.*, 1992). It is also associated with reduced dopaminergic activity as indicated by levels of the dopamine metabolite, homovanillic acid, in the cerebrospinal fluid (Weinberger *et al.*, 1988), and can be at least partially alleviated by the dopamine agonist, amphetamine (Daniel *et al,* 1991).

While there is an overall consensus that schizophrenic patients have a reduced ability to activate prefrontal cortex during the WCST, there are differences in detail of the findings from different studies demonstrating that the essential problem in schizophrenia is not merely a diminished ability to activate prefrontal cortex. For example, Catafau *et al.* (1994) found that the schizophrenic subjects had increased frontal rCBF in the resting state, but there was no significant difference between patients and controls during WCST performance. There are two possible interpretations: (i) The patients were engaged in generation of excessive spontaneous mental activity in both rest and test conditions and did not allocate frontal processing resources to the WCST; (ii) the subjects re-allocated frontal resources from excessive spontaneous generation of mental activity during the rest condition to WCST performance during the test condition, with no net increase in activity. The findings of Catafau *et al.* (1994) suggest that the essential problem is a difficulty in appropriate allocation of frontal processing resources, rather than inability to activate frontal lobe.

WORD GENERATION

Schizophrenic patients tend to perform poorly in word generation tasks in which the subject is instructed to produce words within a given semantic category (e.g. names of animals) or orthographic category (beginning with a specified letter). In healthy controls, both semantic and orthographic word generation tasks are associated with activation of frontal cortex (Frith *et al.*, 1991). While the area of maximal increase in rCBF is usually the left lateral frontal cortex other areas such as medial frontal cortex and thalamus also exhibit an increase in rCBF, while decreases occur in superior temporal gyrus.

Warkentin *et al.* (1989) reported that schizophrenic patients failed to produce the normal activation of prefrontal cortex during word generation. However, patients tended to generate fewer words than healthy control subjects. The question of whether or not patients exhibit a similar level of prefrontal activation as healthy controls when both groups generate words at the same rate was addressed by Frith *et al.* (1995) using a paced word generation task. The subjects were cued to generate words beginning with a specified letter at the rate of one every five seconds. Even patients with marked poverty of speech were able to generate words at that rate. Blood flow during word generation was compared with a reference condition in which subjects merely repeated words. Frith and colleagues found that the magnitude of the prefrontal activation was similar in patients and in healthy controls. However, unlike healthy controls, the patients did not exhibit a decrease in activity in the superior temporal gyrus. Thus, the findings of Frith *et al.* (1995) suggest that provided the patients are normally engaged in the task, the left lateral prefrontal cortex is activated to a normal degree, but the relationship between activity in frontal and temporal cortex is abnormal. The role of the interaction between frontal cortex and superior temporal gyrus during word generation is uncertain. One possibility is that corollary discharge from frontal cortex acts to suppress activity in auditory processing areas during self-generated speech, to minimize interference. A failure of this mechanism in schizophrenic patients might reflect a failure to recognize the origin of self -generated verbal material.

In a re-analysis of these data that examined more extensive areas of the brain, Liddle *et al.* (1997) found abnormalities of rCBF during word generation in diverse cerebral areas, including thalamus, bilateral temporal lobes, bilateral inferior parietal lobule and medial parietal cortex (*see* Fig 7.2). Liddle *et al.* (1997) also examined the patterns of covariance over six scans (within each subject) between rCBF in left lateral frontal cortex and rCBF in all other cerebral grey matter pixels. Consistent with the patterns of activity illustrated in Fig. 7.2, they found that the pattern of covariance differed from that in healthy controls not only for the relationship between left frontal cortex and left lateral temporal lobe, but also for the relationship between frontal cortex and thalamus, and between frontal cortex and medial posterior cortex, including posterior cingulate and precuneus. Patients differed from healthy controls in so far as patients showed a positive covariance between frontal cortex and left lateral temporal cortex, while the corresponding covariance was negative in healthy controls. In both patients and controls the covariance between left lateral frontal cortex and posterior cingulate gyrus and precuneus was negative, but significantly more negative in patients than in controls. In contrast, the covariance between left lateral frontal cortex and thalamus was positive in both patients and controls, but significantly less so in the patients.

Overall, the findings of Frith *et al.* (1995) and Liddle *et al.* (1997) indicate that the essential functional abnormality in schizophrenic patients during word generation is not decreased magnitude of activation in frontal cortex, but an abnormal relationship between activity in the frontal cortex and activity in other cerebral sites that are engaged during word generation. This might be described as an abnormalitiy of functional connectivity.

Yurgelun-Todd *et al.* (1995) used fMRI to examine frontal and temporal cerebral activity in schizophrenic patients and healthy controls during word generation. Rate of word generation was not paced, though in fact the patients produced as many words as the healthy subjects. Unfortunately, in the healthy subjects the signal in frontal cortex did not return to baseline during the periods of rest that alternated with periods of activity, making the interpretation of the findings ambiguous. In comparison with the initial baseline, the healthy subjects exhibited a greater frontal activation than controls. However, when active periods were compared to the rest conditions, patients and controls exhibited an equal degree of activation. In the superior temporal gyrus, shifting baseline was not a problem. Patients exhibited increased

Healthy subjects

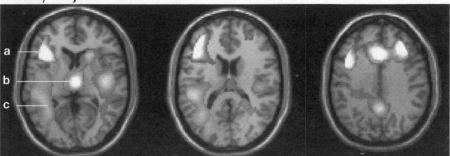

Range of z scores −4.7 < 2z <5.4

Schizophrenic subjects

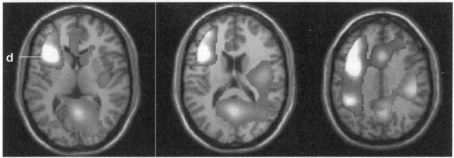

Range of z scores −6.2 < 2z <6.9

Change in healthy subjects *minus* change in schizophrenic subjects

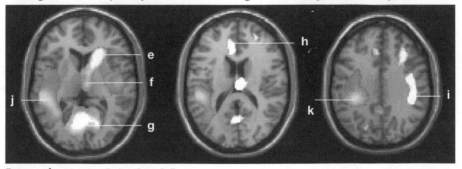

Range of z scores −5.4 < 2z <3.5

Fig. 7.2 Significant changes in rCBF measured with PET during paced word generation in healthy subjects and in schizophrenia (Liddle *et al.*, 1997). Increases relative to word repetition are shown in red-yellow hues and decreases in blue, in slices at 6 mm (left), 16 mm and 24 mm above the inter-commissural plane. In all the clusters of voxels shown in colour, the change is statistically significant at level *P*<0.05 after correcting for multiple comparisons. In healthy subjects, rCBF increases in left lateral frontal cortex (a) and thalamus (b), while it decreases in temporal cortex bilaterally (c). Schizophrenic subjects exhibit a normal increase in left lateral frontal cortex (d), but there are abnormalities in many other areas. Relative to healthy subjects, schizophrenic subjects exhibit significantly less increase in rCBF in right striatum (e), right thalamus (f), lingual gyrus (g), anterior cingulate (h) and right inferior parietal lobule (i), and significantly greater increase in temporal lobe bilaterally (j) and left inferior parietal lobule (k). This figure also appears in colour between pages 150 and 151.

activity during word generation while controls exhibited decreased activation, in accord with the findings of Frith *et al.* (1995).

Curtis *et al.* (1997) employed fMRI to compare schizophrenic patients with controls with respect to the activity during paced word generation relative to that during word repetition. The design of the word generation task was very similar to that employed by Frith *et al.* (1995), except that the subjects were not asked to say the words aloud. Both patients and healthy controls produced activation of left lateral frontal cortex, but the magnitude of this activation was less in patients than in controls. There were no significant changes in superior temporal gyrus in either patients or controls, consistent with the hypothesis that changes in this area only occur when subjects articulate self -generated speech aloud. In the precuneus, Curtis *et al.* (1997) found that the patients produced a significantly greater suppression of activity than controls, in accord with the findings of Liddle *et al.* (1997).

Overall, the question of the relative magnitude of frontal activation in patients and controls during word generation remains unanswered. However, there is consensus between the various studies that schizophrenic patients differ from healthy controls in the functional connectivity between frontal cortex and other cerebral areas, including superior temporal gyrus and precuneus.

SACCADIC EYE MOVEMENTS

A variety of eye movement abnormalities have been reported in schizophrenia. Of particular importance are the impairments in volitional saccadic movements made in the presence of distraction, as these movements are controlled by frontal circuits. Both Nakashima *et al.* (1994) and Crawford *et al.* (1996) have reported abnormalities of frontal rCBF during volitional saccade tasks, in which the subject was presented with a stimulus in one visual hemifield, and instructed to make a saccadic movement directed into the opposite hemifield. The two studies employed somewhat different tasks, and there are important differences in the details of their findings.

Nakashima *et al.* (1994) found that healthy controls exhibited a significant increase in rCBF of frontal eye fields in the volitional saccade task relative to the resting condition, while the schizophrenic subjects did not. However, schizophrenic subjects had greater rCBF in the frontal eye field at rest than the controls and did not differ significantly from the controls during the eye movement tasks. Thus, it is possible that these findings indicate that patients are subject to a greater need to suppress distraction even in the resting state, rather than having a reduced ability to activate frontal eye fields when required. Crawford *et al.* (1996) found that schizophrenic patients selected on the basis of poor antisaccade performance, exhibited lower rCBF in the anterior cingulate gyrus during an antisaccade task compared with healthy controls. No comparison with a reference condition such as rest, was performed, so it is not possible to determine whether or not the difference in rCBF was due to lower baseline activity in this patient group, or to a lesser degree of activation.

Overall, these two studies add to the evidence indicating abnormal frontal lobe function in schizophrenia. The findings of Nakashima *et al.* (1994) suggest aberrant allocation of processing resources rather than an intrinsic lack of ability to activate prefrontal cortex.

PLANNING

Andreasen _et al._ (1992) measured rCBF during the performance of the Tower of London test, a task that entails rearranging towers of coloured building blocks, so as to match a target arrangement within a specified number of moves. Advanced planning of moves is essential if the goal is to be achieved. They found that schizophrenic patients produced less activation of medial prefrontal cortex than healthy control subjects. Furthermore, the degree of diminution of prefrontal activation was significantly correlated with severity of negative symptoms.

FINGER–THUMB OPPOSITION

Elementary motor functions are relatively intact in schizophrenia, though there can be subtle impairments of relatively simple motor tasks, leading to poor co-ordination and clumsiness. Studies using the xenon inhalation method to measure cortical rCBF (Guenther _et al, 1991_) and using PET (Guenther _et al.,_ 1994), reported abnormal function of primary sensori-motor cortex during finger–thumb opposition, in schizophrenia. Guenther _et al._ (1991) found bilateral overactivation in the precentral gyrus in patients with positive symptoms, but decreased activation in patients with negative symptoms. Guenther _et al._ (1994) found that schizophrenic patients exhibited less activation of contralateral sensori-motor cortex than healthy controls. However, the schizophrenic patients exhibited aberrant activity in a variety of other cortical areas, consistent with the hypothesis that functional connectivity between cerebral areas is impaired in schizophrenia.

Three fMRI studies have reported abnormal lateralization of activation during finger–thumb opposition. Schroder _et al._ (1995) found that compared with healthy controls, the schizophrenic patients exhibited reduced activation of both sensori-motor cortex and supplementary motor cortex, together with evidence of reversal laterality of activation. Braus _et al._ (1997) confirmed the finding of reversed laterality of the activation, though in contrast to the findings of Schroder _et al._ (1995) they found that schizophrenic subjects produced significant activation in a larger number of pixels than healthy controls. Weinberger _et al._ (1996) found that the magnitude the contralateral sensori-motor activation was normal, but they too found a relative excess of ipsilateral activity.

Similar to studies of word generation, studies of cerebral activity during finger–thumb opposition in schizophrenia have yielded inconsistent findings regarding the magnitude of the activation at the primary site engaged in the task, namely of contralateral sensori-motor cortex, but all reveal a pattern of aberrant activity in other cerebral areas, especially ipsilateral cortex. These studies provide further support for the hypothesis that the essential functional abnormality in schizophrenia is a disorder of functional connectivity.

MEMORY

Memory impairments are a feature of schizophrenia. Some investigators (e.g. Saykin _et al.,_ 1991) have interpreted this as evidence of temporal lobe dysfunction because of the well established role of medial temporal lobe structures in episodic memory. However , PET studies of healthy individuals have demonstrated that other cerebral areas, including frontal cortex, medial parietal areas and cerebellum play an important role in memory tasks. In particular, many studies have shown that the left frontal lobe plays a cardinal role in encoding memories (irrespective of modality) while the right frontal lobe plays a cardinal role in recall (Tulving *et al.*, 1994). PET offers the possibility of determining whether or not the memory deficits in schizophrenia reflect a specific temporal lobe abnormality.

Busatto *et al.* (1994) measured rCBF during the performance of a verbal memory task in schizophrenic patients and healthy controls. In the healthy controls, there was a significant increase in rCBF in left medial temporal, left inferior frontal and anterior cingulate cortices, and right cerebellum during performance of the memory task. Despite significantly poorer performance, the degree of medial temporal activation measured in the schizophrenic patients was not significantly different from that found in the control group. The authors concluded that memory deficits in schizophrenia do not necessarily imply failure to activate the left medial temporal lobe.

In a PET study of verbal recall, Andreasen *et al.* (1996) reported that healthy controls activated a distributed circuit embracing frontal lobes, thalamus and cerebellum, while schizophrenic patients showed a lesser degree of activation in all of these regions, despite the fact that the patients achieved a similar level of performance to the controls. In a PET study of a graded word learning, Fletcher *et al.* (1998) found that healthy subjects exhibited increasing activity of left lateral frontal cortex as task demands increased, while in schizophrenic subjects initial increases in frontal lobe activity fell away with increasing memory load. They interpreted this as evidence that attenuation of left lateral frontal activation reflects diminished performance. Furthermore, they reported that the schizophrenic subjects failed to exhibit task-related decreases in the left superior temporal gyrus that occurred in healthy subjects, implying aberrant co-ordination of activity in frontal and temporal cortex.

Working memory, which is the ability to maintain information 'on-line' while it is needed for mental processing, is another aspect of memory that is impaired in schizophrenia. fMRI studies by Weinberger *et al.* (1996) and by Mellers *et al.* (1997) demonstrated that schizophrenic patients tend to exhibit an attenuated increase in frontal activity during the 'N-back' working memory paradigm, compared with healthy subjects. More recently, Liddle *et al.* (1999) demonstrated that schizophrenic subjects exhibit not only attenuated frontal activity, but also a failure to produce the concomitant bilateral decrease in activity in anterior temporal lobe that occurs in healthy subjects. Thus, during this task, as during word generation (Fig. 7.2) and verbal learning (Fletcher *et al.*, 1998), schizophrenic patients exhibit evidence of aberrant co-ordination between frontal and temporal lobes.

Overall, the evidence from functional imaging studies indicates that abnormalities of several aspects of memory, including both word learning, word recall, and also working memory, observed in schizophrenia, do not reflect under-activity of temporal lobes, but rather, abnormal function of distributed neural systems that embrace frontal and temporal cortex, thalamus, and cerebellum.

Pharmacological studies

Functional imaging techniques can be used to measure the effects of pharmacological agents on patterns of cerebral activity. Many psychoactive drugs act on monoaminergic neurotransmitters, which generally exert a modulatory role. That is, their effects depend on concurrent brain activity. Therefore, it is likely that the most informative study designs will be those that examine the effect of a pharmacological agent on the pattern of cerebral activity associated with a particular mental state. Few studies have done this in a systematic manner.

Although the resting state is a poorly controlled condition, studies of the effects of drugs on resting state blood flow or metabolism might be expected to show those effects that are common to various self-generated mental activities. The studies of sustained treatment with typical antipsychotic drugs on resting rCBF or metabolism in schizophrenic subjects consistently report an increase in basal ganglia flow or metabolism (Wolkin *et al.* 1985; DeLisi *et al.*, 1985; Cohen *et al.*, 1987; Buchsbaum *et al.*, 1987; Szechtman *et al.*, 1988; Wik *et al.*, 1989; Bartlett *et al.*, 1991; Buchsbaum *et al.*, 1992). Approximately half of these studies (DeLisi *et al.*, 1985; Cohen *et al.*, 1987; Bartlett *et al.*, 1991) also report a decrease in frontal lobe activity.

The extent to which these changes reflect therapeutic effects remains uncertain. In particular, it is possible that increased basal ganglia metabolism is related to extrapyramidal side-effects, while decreased frontal metabolism might be related, at least in part, to neuroleptic induced akinesia. In principle, this issue might be addressed by studying the effects of atypical antipsychotics, which cause fewer extrapyramidal side-effects and less akinesia. There have been a few small studies of the effects of treatment with atypical antispychotics. The first such study, by Berman *et al.* (1996), found that the atypical antipsychotic, risperdone, produced a reduction in frontal rCBF. A more recent study (Ngan *et al.*, 1998; Lane *et al.*, 1998) of the effect of the risperidone on regional metabolism, reveals that no evidence of increased basal ganglion metabolism, but did confirm that antipsychotic treatment is associated with decreased frontal lobe metabolism, and also with decreased metabolism in the left temporal lobe (*see* Fig. 7.3). Consistent with predictions based on the observed patterns of aberrant rCBF associated with disorganization and with reality distortion (Liddle *et al.*, 1992 *see also* Fig. 7.1), the reduction in medial frontal metabolism was associated with reduction in medial frontal activity, while the decrease in temporal metabolism was correlated with the reduction in severity of reality distortion.

Studies of the psychoto-mimetic glutamatergic antagonist, ketamine, provide indirect evidence about the cerebral sites likely to be involved in the mechanism of antipsychotic action. Ketamine produces schizophrenia-like symptoms in healthy individuals and transient exacerbations of psychosis in schizophrenic patients. Lahti *et al.* (1997) demonstrated that ketamine increased rCBF in anterior cingulate and contiguous medial frontal cortex, while decreasing rCBF in cerebellum, in schizophrenic patients and in healthy controls. Furthermore, changes in positive symptoms induced by ketamine correlated with rCBF changes in left medial temporal lobe and left ventral striatum, consistent with the findings by Liddle *et al.* (1992) and

Healthy subjects, 2 mg

Schizophrenic subjects, 2 mg

Schizophrenic subjects, 6 weeks

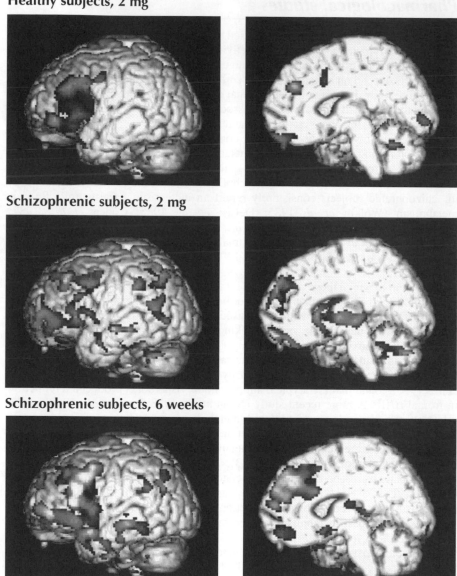

Fig. 7.3   Decreases in regional metabolism measured using PET in healthy subjects 90 min after 2 mg of risperidone; decreases in medication-free first episode schizophrenic patients 90 min after 2 mg of risperidone, and in the same patients after 6 weeks treatment with risperidone, rendered onto the left lateral cerebral (left) and right medial cortex (Ngan ct al., 1998; Lane et al., 1998). This figure also appears in colour between pages 150 and 151.

Silbersweig *et al.* (1995) that increased rCBF at these two sites is associated with reality distortion symptoms.

The combination of pharmacological challenge with neuropsychological challenge offers the possibility of determining the effects of drugs on the patterns of cerebral activity associated with the cognitive deficits of schizophrenia. The first such study (Daniel *et al.*, 1991) demonstrated that acute challenge with the indirect dopaminergic agonist amphetamine produces a modest alleviation of the impairment of frontal activation during the Wisconsin Card Sorting Test. More recently, Dolan *et al.* (1995) reported that apomorphine produces an enhanced activation of anterior cingulate cortex during word generation, in medication-naïve schizophrenic patients by comparison with healthy controls, though the interpretation of the findings is made complex because of variation in baseline activity. Thus, these two studies indicate that enhancement of dopaminergic neurotransmission has the potential to provide at least a modest beneficial effect on frontal lobe function in schizophrenia.

Conclusion

Functional imaging studies have revealed abnormalities of the function of diverse cortical and subcortical cerebral areas in schizophrenia. The studies of the relationships between symptoms and cerebral activity indicate that symptom expression is associated with aberrant activity in widespread areas of multimodal association cortex that play a major role in the selection, initiation and monitoring of self-generated mental activity.

Measurement of rCBF during a variety of different tasks provides further evidence of widespread functional impairment. In particular, many studies have demonstrated abnormal cerebral activity during tasks in which prefrontal cortex plays a cardinal role. Despite the differences in details between the findings of various studies, there is compelling evidence that prefrontal cortex itself is less active in schizophrenic patients than in healthy subjects, during some of these tasks. However, there does not appear to be a pervasive loss of ability to activate frontal cortex under all circumstances. Some of the evidence indicates abnormal allocation of processing resources.

The question of whether or not the widespread abnormalities of function reflect primary malfunction at one or more discrete sites remains an issue of major importance. Studies of word generation, verbal learning, working memory, and of finger–thumb opposition suggest that the essential functional abnormality in schizophrenia is not so much a fixed loss of function at any specific site, but rather a malfunction of the co-ordination of activity between different sites.

References

Andreasen, N.C., Rezai K., Alliger, R. *et al.* (1992) Hypofrontality in neuroleptic-naïve patients and in patients with chronic schizophrenia. Assessment with Xenon 133 single photon emission computed tomography and the Tower of London. *Arch Gen Psychiatry*, **49**, 943–58.
Andreasen, N.C., O'Leary D.S., Cizadlo, T. *et al.* (1996) Schizophrenia and cognitive dysme-

tria: a PET study of dysfunctional prefrontal-thalamic-cerebellar circuitry. *Proc Natl Acad Sci, USA*, **93**, 9985–90.

Bartlett, E.J., Wolkin, A, Brodie, J.D. *et al.* (1991) Importance of pharmacologic control in PET studies: effects of thiothixine and haloperidol on cerebral glucose utilization in chronic schizophrenia, *Psychiat Res*, **40**, 115–24.

Berman, I., Merson, A., Sison, C. *et al.* (1996) Regional cerebral blood flow changes associated with risperidone treatment in elderly schizophrenia patients: a pilot study. *Psychopharmacol Bull*, **32**, 95–100.

Berman, K.F., Torrey, E.F., Daniel, D.G., *et al.* (1992) Regional cerebral blood flow in monozygotic twins discordant and concordant for schizophrenia. *Arch Gen Psychiatry*, **49**, 927–35

Braus, D.F., Sartorius, A., Ende, G. *et al.* (1997) Schizophrenia as a misconnection syndrome: a fMRI study. *Neuroimage*, **5**, S293.

Buchsbaum, M.S., Wu, J.C., DeLisi, L.E. *et al.* (1987) Positron emission tomography studies of basal ganglia and somatosensory cortex neuroleptic drug effects. *Biol Psychiatry*, **22**, 479–94.

Buchsbaum, M.S., Potkin, S.G., Siegel, B.V. *et al.* (1992) Striatal metabolic rate and clinical response to neuroleptics in schizophrenia. *Arch Gen Psychiatry*, **49**, 966–74.

Busatto, G.F., Costa, D.C., Ell, P.J. *et al.* (1994) Regional cerebral blood flow (rCBF) in schizophrenia during verbal memory activation: a ^{99m}Tc-HMPAO single photon emission tomography (SPET) study. *Psychol Medicine*, **24**, 463–72.

Catafau, A., Parellada, E., Lomena, F. *et al.* (1994) Prefrontal and temporal blood flow in schizophrenia: resting and activation changes during Wisconsin Card Sorting Test by randomised ^{99m}Tc-HMPAO-SPECT. *J Nucl Med*, **35**(6), 935–41

Cohen, R.M., Semple, W.E., Gross, M. *et al.* (1987) Dysfunction in a prefrontal substrate of sustained attention in schizophrenia. *Life Sci*, **20**, 2031–9.

Crawford, T.J. Puri, B.K. Nijran, K.S. *et al.* (1996) Abnormal saccadic distractibility in patients with schizophrenia: a ^{99m}Tc-HMPAO SPET study. *Psychol Med*, **26**, 265–77.

Curtis, V.A., Bullmore, E.T., Brammer, H.J. *et al.* (1997) Attended frontal activation during a verbal fluency task in patients with schizophrenia. *Am J Psychiatry*, **155**, 1056–63.

Daniel, D.G., Weinberger, D.R., Jones, D.W. *et al.* (1991) The effect of amphetamine on regional cerebral blood flow during cognitive activation in schizophrenia. *J Neurosci*, **11**, 1907–17.

DeLisi, L.E., Holcomb, H.H., Cohen, R.M. *et al.* (1985) Positron emission tomography in schizophrenic patients with and without neuroleptic medication. *J Cerebral Blood Flow Metab*, **5**, 201–6.

Dolan, R.J., Bench, C.J., Liddle, P.F. *et al.* (1993) Dorsolateral prefrontal cortex dysfunction in the major psychoses; symptom or disease specificity? *J Neurol Neurosurg Psychiatry*, **56**, 1290–4.

Dolan, R.J., Fletcher, P., Frith, C. *et al.* (1995) Dopaminergic modulation of a functional deficit in anterior cingulate cortex in schizophrenia. *Nature*, **378**, 180–2.

Early, T.S., Reiman, E.R. and Raichle, M.E. (1987) Left globus pallidus abnormality in never-medicated patients with schizophrenia. *Proc Natl Acad Sci, USA*, **84**, 561–3.

Ebmeier, K.P., Blackwood, D.H.R., Murray, C. *et al.* (1993) Single photon emission tomography with ^{99m}Tc-exametazime in unmedicated schizophrenic patients. *Biol Psychiatry*, **33**, 487–95.

Fletcher, P.C., McKenna, P.J., Frith, C.D. *et al.* (1998) Brain activations in schizophrenia during a graded memory task studied with functional neuroimaging. *Arch Gen Psychiatry*, **55**, 1001–8.

Frith, C.D., Friston, K.J., Liddle, P.F. *et al.* (1991) Willed action and the prefrontal cortex in man: a study with PET. *Proc Roy Soc Lond B*, **244**, 241–246.

Frith, C.D., Friston, K.J., Liddle, P.F. *et al.* (1992) PET imaging and cognition in schizophrenia. *J Roy Soc Med*, **85**, 222–4.

Frith, C.D., Friston, K.J., Herold, S. *et al.* (1995) Regional brain activity in chronic schizophrenic patients during the performance of a verbal fluency task. *Br J Psychiatry*, **176**, 343–9.

Guenther, W., Petsch, R., Steinberg, R. *et al.* (1991) Brain dysfunction during motor activation and corpus callosum alterations in schizophrenia measured by cerebral blood flow and magnetic resonance imaging. *Biol Psychiatry*, **29**, 553–5.

Guenther, W., Brodiem J.D., Bartlet, E.J. *et al.* (1994) Diminished cerebral metabolic response to motor stimulation in schizophrenics: a PET study. *Euro Arch Psychiat Clin Neurosci*, **244**, 115–25.

Ingvar, D.H. and Franzen, G. (1974) Abnormalities of cerebral blood flow distribution in patients with chronic schizophrenia. *Acta Psychiat Scand*, **50**, 425–62.

Kaplan, R.D., Szechtman, H., Franco, S. *et al.* (1993) Three clinical syndromes of schizophrenia in untreated subjects: relation to brain glucose activity measured by positron emission tomography (PET). *Schizophr Res*, **11**, 47–54.

Lahti, A.C., Holcomb, H.H., Weiler, M.A. *et al.* (1997) Regional correlations between ketamine-induced actions on psychosis and regional cerebral blood flow (rCBF). *Schizophr Res*, **24**, 167–8.

Lane, C.J., Ngan, E.T.C. and Liddle, P.F. (1998) Effects of risperidone on cerebral activity and positive symptoms in first-episode schizophrenic subjects. *Neuroimage*, **7**, 236.

Liddle, P.F. (1995) Inner connections within the domain of dementia praecox: the role of supervisory mental processes in schizophrenia. *Eur Arch Psychiat Clin Neurosci*, **245**, 210–5.

Liddle, P.F. and Morris, D.L. (1991) Schizophrenic syndromes and frontal lobe performance, *Br J Psychiatry*, **158**, 340–5.

Liddle, P.F., Friston, K.J., Frith, C.D. *et al.* (1992) Patterns of cerebral blood flow in schizophrenia. *Br J Psychiatry*, **160**, 179–86.

Liddle, P.F., Mendrek, A., Smith, A.M. and Kiehl, K.A. (1999) An FMRI study of fronto-temporal coordination during working memory in schizophrenia. *Schizophr Res*, **36**, 225.

Liddle, P.F., Passmore, M., Friston, K.J. *et al.* (1997) Functional connectivity during word generation in schizophrenia. *Schizophr Res*, **23**, 168.

McGuire, P.K., Shah, G.M.S., Murray, R.M. (1993) Increased blood flow in Broca's area during auditory hallucinations in schizophrenia. *Lancet*, **342**, 703–6.

McGuire, P.K., Silbersweig, D.A., Wright, I. *et al.* (1995) Abnormal monitoring of inner speech: a physiological basis for auditory hallucinations. *Lancet*, **346**, 596–600.

Mellers, J.D.C., Wykes, T., Bullmore, E. *et al.* (1997) An fMRI study of verbal working memory in schizophrenia. *Schizophr Res*, **24**, 169–70.

Nakashima, Y., Momose, T., Sano, I. *et al.* (1994) Cortical control of saccade in normal and schizophrenic subjects: a PET study using a task-evoked rCBF paradigm. *Schizophr Res*, **12**, 259–64.

Ngan, E.T.C., Lane, C.T. and Liddle, P.F. (1998) Immediate and long term effects of risperidone on cerebral metabolism in schizophrenia. *Schizophr Res*, **29**, 173.

Pardo, J.V., Pardo, P.J., Janer, K.W. *et al.* (1990) The anterior cingulate mediates processing selection in the Stroop attentional conflict paradigm. *Proc Natl Acad Sci, USA*, **87**, 256–9.

Robertson, G.S. and Fibiger, H.C. (1992) Neuroleptics increase *c-fos* expression in the forebrain: contrasting effects of clozapine and haloperidol. *Neuroscience*, **46**, 315–28.

Rubin, P., Holm, S., Friberg, L. *et al.* (1991) Altered modulation of prefrontal and subcortical brain activity in newly diagnosed schizophrenia and schizophreniform disorder. *Arch Gen Psychiatry*, **48**, 987–95

Saykin, J.A., Gur, R.C., Gur, R.E. *et al.* (1991) Neuropsychological function in schizophrenia: selective impairment in memory and learning. *Arch Gen Psychiatry*, **48**, 618–24.

Schroder, J., Wenz, F., Schad, L.R. *et al.* (1995) Sensorimotor cortex and supplementary motor area changes in schizophrenia. A study with functional magnetic resonance imaging. *Br J Psychiatry*, **176**, 197–201.

Silbersweig, D.A., Stern, E., Frith, C.D. *et al.* (1995) A functional neuroanatomy of hallucinations in schizophrenia. *Nature*, **378**, 176–9.

Suzuki, M., Yuasa, S., Mintabi, Y. *et al.* (1993) Left superior temporal blood flow increases in schizophrenic and schizophreniform patients with auditory hallucinations. *Eur Arch Psychiat Clin Neurosci*, **242**, 257–61.

Szechtman, H., Nahmias, C., Garnett, E.S. *et al.* (1988) Effects of neuroleptics on altered cerebral glucose metabolism in schizophrenia. *Arch Gen Psychiatry*, **45**, 523–32.

Tulving, E., Kapur, S., Craik, F.I.M. *et al.* (1994) Hemispheric encoding/retreival asymmetry in episodic memory: positron emission tomography findings. *Proc Natl Acad Sci, USA*, **91**, 2016–20.

Warkentin, S., Nilsson, A., Risberg, J. and Karlson, S. (1989) Absence of frontal lobe activation in schizophrenia. *J Cerebral Blood Flow Metab*, **9** (Suppl.1), S354.

Weinberger, D.R., Berman, K.F. and Zec, R.F. (1986) Physiologic dysfunction of dorsolateral prefrontal cortex in schizophrenia. I. Regional cerebral blood flow evidence. *Arch Gen Psychiatry*, **43**, 114–24.

Weinberger, D.R., Berman, K.F. and Illowsky, B.P. (1988) Physiological dysfunction of the dorsolateral prefrontal cortex in schizophrenia. III. A new cohort and evidence for a monoaminergic mechanism. *Arch Gen Psychiatry*, **45**, 609–15.

Weinberger, D.R., Berman, K.F., Suddath, R. *et al.* (1992) Evidence of dysfunction of a prefrontal–limbic network in schizophrenia: a magnetic reasonance imaging and regional cerebral blood flow study of discordant monozygotic twins. *Am J Psychiatry*, **149**, 890–7.

Weinberger, D.R., Mattay, V., Callicot, J. *et al.* (1996) fMRI applications in schizophrenia research. *Neuroimage*, **4**, S118–S126.

Wik, G., Weisel, F-A., Sjogren, I. *et al.* (1989) Effects of sulpiride and chlorpromazine on regional cerebral glucose metabolism in schizophrenic patients as determined by positron emission tomography. *Psychopharmacol*, **97**, 309–18.

Wolkin, A., Jaeger, J., Brodie, J.D. *et al.* (1985) Persistence of cerebral metabolic abnormalities in chronic schizophrenia as determined by positron emission tomography. *Am J Psychiatry*, **142**, 564–71.

Wolkin, A., Sanfilipo, M., Wolf, A.P. *et al.* (1992) Negative symptoms and hypofrontality in chronic schizophrenia. *Arch Gen Psychiatry*, **49**, 959–65.

Yuasa, S., Kurachi, M., Suzuki, M. *et al.* (1995) Clinical symptoms and regional cerebral blood flow in schizophrenia. *Eur Arch Psychiat Clin Neurosci*, **246**, 7–12.

Yurgelun-Todd, D.A., Waternaux, C.M., Cohen, B.M. *et al.* (1995) Functional magnetic resonance imaging of schizophrenic patients and comparison subjects during word production. *Am J Psychiatry*, **153**, 200–5.

CHAPTER 8

Neurochemical imaging in schizophrenia

GÖRAN C. SEDVALL, LARS FARDE AND STEFAN PAULI

Introduction

Over the past 40 years a number of research findings have implicated important roles of central neurochemical signalling mechanisms in the pathophysiology of schizophrenia. The involvement of several neurotransmitter mechanisms has been suggested on the basis of pharmacological and biochemical evidence and also from post-mortem human brain studies. Special focus has been upon the role of neurotransmitters such as dopamine, noradrenaline, serotonin, glutamate and GABA. Several neuropeptides such as cholecystokinin, neurotensin and opiates have also been implicated. Recently a role for nitrous oxide (NO), the recently discovered neuromodulator, has also been suggested (Sedvall and Farde, 1995). Although some experimental proof has been put forward for each one of these hypotheses, there is still great controversy in the field, and most proposals have not been consistently replicated. This holds true for in-vitro studies on post-mortem brain material from schizophrenic patients as well as for studies in living patients.

During the past two decades a number of in-vivo brain imaging modalities have been developed, some of which are useful for neurochemical clinical studies. Among those, magnetic resonance spectroscopy (MRS), positron emission tomography (PET) and single photon emission computed tomography (SPECT), allow the recording of neurochemical variables in the living human brain.

MRS is useful for the measurement of biochemicals in the millimolar concentration range. Only a few biochemical entities can be recorded by this method and the resolution of currently used methods is low. PET and SPECT, on the other hand, are based upon the radiotracer approach, and allow measurement in the nanomolar range. Such a high sensitivity is a prerequisite to record aspects of neurochemical signalling mechanisms related to the neurotransmitters, receptors and transporters implicated in the pathophysiology of schizophrenia, and in the mechanisms of action of antipsychotic drugs.

In the present chapter the application of PET and SPECT in clinical studies with schizophrenic patients will be reviewed. Although such studies were initiated more than 15 years ago, because of the rapid development of technical aspects of these imaging techniques, as well as appropriate radiotracers, these methods will continue to yield increasingly important and penetrating information in the field of schizophrenia research for many years to come. Therefore, this chapter will begin with a brief description of the current technical methods.

Techniques of PET and SPECT

Both PET and SPECT are indirect brain imaging techniques that are dependent upon the use of a radiotracer molecule administered intravenously (Fig. 8.1). The rational n for using a radiotracer molecule is that the radiotracer follows and reflects a predicted role in participating in a physiological biochemical reaction or binds reversibly or irreversibly to a specific protein, a principle used to study its characteristics. The choice of radiotracer is primarily dependent upon the specific neurochemical aspect to be examined. Thus, radiolabelled 2-deoxyglucose can be used for examining regional glucose metabolism in the brain (Sokoloff *et al.*, 1977). Radiolabelled deprenyl, a monoamine oxidase inhibitor can be used to label monoamine oxidase. Radiolabelled neuroleptic-like compounds have been extensively applied to visualize binding sites for specific sub-types of dopamine and serotonin receptors in the brain (Wagner *et al.*, 1983; Farde *et al.*, 1986; Sedvall *et al.*, 1986a, 1986b).

In positron emission tomography (PET) short-lived positron emitting isotopes are used. Such isotopes, which occur naturally only in minute quantities, can be produced efficiently by nuclear reactions in a cyclotron. Carbon-11 [^{11}C], fluorine-18 [^{18}F] and oxygen-15 [^{15}O] have half-lives between 2–120 minutes and demand the availability of a cyclotron and a radiochemistry laboratory on site in order to produce the isotope and to introduce it rapidly and efficiently into the radiotracer molecule to be applied (Fig. 8.1). The selection of positron emitting isotopes for radiolabelling has important advantages. They can be produced in sufficiently high quantities and specific activities required to achieve an appropriate radioactivity signal for the measurement. The short physical half-life also guarantees that the time of radioactivity exposure will be short. Moreover, for the purpose of radioactivity quantification, the

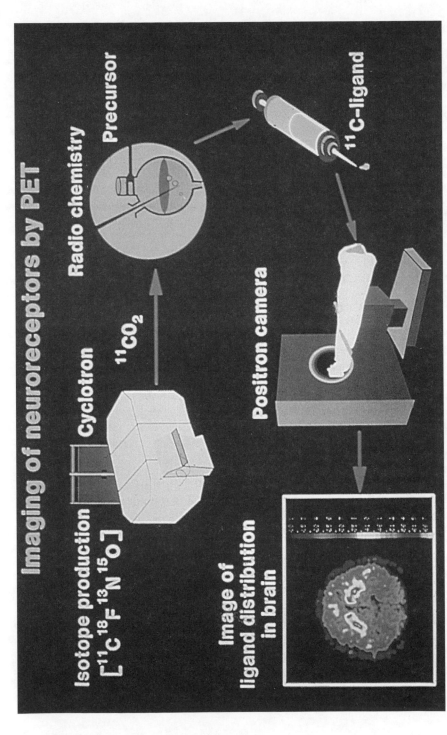

Fig. 8.1 Principles of PET and SPECT imaging of neuroreceptors.

physical character of positron disintegration is advantageous. When such isotopes disintegrate a positron is released. A positron can be regarded as antimatter and corresponds to a positively charged electron. After travelling for about two millimetres the positron will collide with an electron in the tissue. Their annihilation produces two antiparallel gamma rays. These gamma rays can travel through biological tissue without significant absorption and can be recorded by scintillation detectors. These are placed externally in relation to the brain location of the radiotracer that has reached the brain after being administered intravenously. By placing rings with a large number of small scintillation detectors around the head and using the technique of coincidence coupling of diametrically placed detectors antiparallel gamma rays produced by positron annihilation can be efficiently distinguished from the random noise of background gamma radiation. The technically most elaborate PET cameras produced today contain up to 20 rings, each one containing several hundred scintillation detectors. By coincidence coupling of diametrically placed scintillation detectors in each ring, and also between the rings, three-dimensional acquisition of the source of gamma rays (i.e. the positron and the radiotracer molecule) can be localized and displaced as two- or three-dimensional images of radiotracer distribution in the brain, by using the signals from the scintillation detectors and elaborate algorithms and computer facilities (Pauli and Sedvall, 1997). The distance travelled by the positron before annihilation with an electron is the resolution limiting factor in PET technology. In practice, resolution higher than about three millimetres cannot be obtained.

In single photon emission (computed) tomography (SPECT or SPET) gamma emitting isotopes instead of positron emitters are used to label the radiotracer. Thus [^{99m}Tc]HMPAO has been used extensively for measurement of regional blood flow in the brain. Iodine-123 [^{123}I] is a widely used gamma emitter with a longer half-life that can be applied for neurochemical brain imaging. [^{123}I]-BZM, a neuroleptic-like benzamide, was developed by Kung *et al.* (1990) to label D2 dopamine receptors. [^{123}I]-iodomazenil, a benzodiazepine receptor antagonist, has been used to visualize benzodiazepine receptor binding in the brain. In SPECT the distinction of specific gamma radiation from the radiotracer in relation to background gamma radiation is technically more difficult than with PET since only one gamma ray is released upon the disintegration of gamma-emitting isotopes as compared to two antiparallel ones for positron emitters. Also, quantification and resolution are not as efficient as in PET technology. On the other hand, the technical demands of SPECT cameras are less advanced than for PET, and therefore less expensive. Over the past few years the technical specifications of SPECT cameras have increased significantly, currently giving a resolution of the order of about five millimetres with a high sensitivity. Since gamma emitters as [^{123}I] have a fairly long half-life (10 days) the availability of an on-site cyclotron is not required. Therefore a SPECT operation unit will be less expensive in this regard also as compared to a corresponding PET facility. Thus, a radiochemical laboratory facility required for running a PET system is not an absolute requirement for a SPECT operation.

Radiotracer development

Besides the high technical requirements of a PET or a SPECT camera, the availability or need to develop appropriate radiotracer molecules is a second indispensable demand. PET and SPECT radiotracers when introduced intravenously are assumed to map and reflect exclusively the neurochemical component or pathway aimed for in the specific measurement. The selection of an appropriate radioligand for a specific neurochemical pathway is a demanding procedure that also has to take into account the need to develop an efficient organic radiochemical labelling procedure, and to clarify the kinetics and metabolism of the tracer (Halldin *et al.*, 1995). When a radiotracer has been prepared to high specific activity and purity, certain criteria have to be fulfilled in order for it to be appropriate for clinical experimental use. Some criteria formulated for ideal PET or SPECT tracers are listed in Table 8.1.

When pharmacokinetic and metabolic data for the radiotracer have been obtained in animals and in humans it may be possible to design radiotracer kinetic models that in mathematical form describe the kinetics of the radiotracer in different brain compartments, and which allow the quantification of significant neurochemical variables reflected by the assumed kinetics of the radioligand (Blomquist *et al.*, 1990). In this way, a sophisticated data analysis can be performed supplying data of clinical interest both in quantitative and in relative terms.

Fig. 8.2 shows the structural formulas and PET images of five radioligands binding with high selectivity to one of five distinct neuroreceptors in the human brain.

Table 8.1. Selection criteria for radioligands for human PET or SPECT studies

- Nanomolar binding affinity for receptors, transporters or other specific proteins in vitro
- High selectivity of binding in vitro
- Low non-specific binding
- Reversible binding
- Low competition by endogenous ligands
- Stereoselectivity of binding
- Rapid chemical labelling procedure
- Solubility properties suitable for i.v. administration
- Rapid transfer over blood–brain barrier
- Uniform distribution to free brain compartments
- Slow biotransformation and low accumulation of labelled metabolites
- Low toxicity allowing the administration of sub-saturating doses

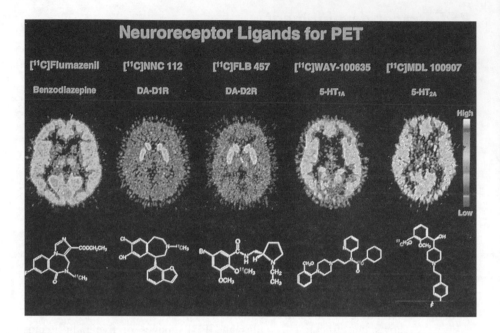

Radiotracer kinetics

After intravenous administration of a radiotracer the radioactivity is recorded in the brain regions over time with the human subject placed within a PET or SPECT camera system. For each radiotracer the kinetics of the radioactivity in the brain is assumed to reflect the kinetics of the radiotracer itself in the brain compartments. Since every radiotracer has its individual physicochemical properties, a specific radiotracer kinetic model has to be designed for each radiotracer in order to interpret how data on the radioactivity accumulation in the brain reflect the specific physiological or biochemical variable searched for, in order to obtain quantitative data concerning this variable. Some radiotracers have been selected because of their straightforward physicochemical characteristics, and simple models can be designed to obtain quantitative information from the radioactivity data. This holds true for the SPECT tracer [^{99m}Tc]HMPAO. This compound (hexamethyl propylene aminoxine) is a fat-soluble compound that easily passes the blood–brain barrier. The regional intensity of radioactivity uptake reflects the relative blood flow in the brain.

For the PET tracers [^{18}F]-2-deoxyglucose and [^{15}O] used to measure regional glucose metabolism and blood flow respectively in quantitative terms, more elaborate multicompartment kinetic models are used (Sokoloff *et al.*, 1977; Sheppard *et al.*, 1988).

For specific neurochemical imaging in schizophrenia, radiotracers labelling specific protein molecules in the brain are required. Since the radioactivity accumulation in the brain reflects concentrations of the radiotracer bound to the receptors as well as free radioligand concentration in the tissue and in blood, these radiotracers also require elaborate modelling with experimental analyses of the validity of these models. For neurochemical brain imaging a number of approaches have been used, most of them dealing with radioligand binding kinetics to D2 dopamine receptors (Huang *et al.*, 1986). The principle of radioligand binding to neuroreceptors in the brain is illustrated in Fig. 8.3. If the radioligand administered intravenously has a high specific activity, i.e. the proportion of labelled molecules is high in relation to the total mass of radioligand administered, only a small fraction of the receptors will be bound by the radioligand. With increasing dose of the radioligand, more and more receptors will be occupied until the receptor population is saturated. This is illustrated in Fig. 8.3 where the specific radioligand binding to a neuroreceptor population is illustrated. This figure also shows that the non-specific radioactivity uptake in the tissue is linearly related to the dose or concentration of the radioligand. At low doses (high specific activity) specific neuroreceptor binding will be high in proportion to non-specific binding. This gives the possibility to visualize radioligand binding to a specific neuroreceptor population in the brain during in-vivo conditions (Fig. 8.2). By systematically altering the specific activity or dose of the radioligand, quantitative data for the total number of receptors (B_{max}) and the binding affinity (K_d) can be obtained separately on the basis of certain assumptions (Farde *et al.*, 1986). This approach, based upon the assumption of a pseudoequilibrium in relation to a PET experiment, requires a series of PET experiments using different specific activities.

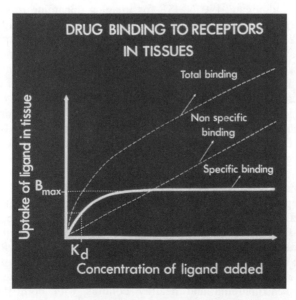

Fig. 8.3 Principles of radioligand binding

A simpler approach, that is usually applied in extensive clinical studies, uses only data from a single PET experiment using high specific radioactivity of the radioligand. Here the radioactivity uptake ratio for a brain region containing receptors in relation to a reference region with low receptor number is calculated. This ratio will reflect the total number of receptors in the region of interest, assuming constant receptor affinity during different experimental conditions as well as similar non-specific radioactivity accumulation in the reference region to the region of interest.

Another approach to obtain quantitative data from a PET experiment uses the data from the whole time course after a radioligand injection, and employs a multicompartment model to follow the radioactivity concentration in the different compartments including arterial blood. Such data give quantitative information on radioligand transport over the blood–brain barrier in addition to data on the specific receptor binding of the radioligand. For a detailed account of different kinetic approaches to examine neuroreceptors in vivo the reader is referred to Leenders *et al.* (1980).

Imaging of dopaminergic mechanisms

D2 DOPAMINE RECEPTORS

The potent effects of conventional antipsychotic drugs on D2 dopamine receptors has stimulated studies on such receptors in schizophrenia. Quite extensive PET and SPECT studies have been performed to examine whether the dense D2 dopamine receptor populations in the basal ganglia are altered in schizophrenic patients. Using their prototype radioligand [^{11}C]NMSP for imaging dopamine receptors, Wagner, Wong and their collaborators in initial experiments claimed a substantial elevation of D2 dopamine receptor densities in the brains of drug-naïve schizophrenic patients (Wong *et al.*, 1986). Using the selective D2 dopamine receptor radioligand [^{11}C]raclopride, Farde *et al.* (1987) employed a pseudoequilibrium model for quantifying the B_{max} and K_d in the basal ganglia of schizophrenic patients which failed to confirm an alteration of D2 dopamine receptor characteristics in the basal ganglia of drug-naïve schizophrenic patients. In fact, the Scatchard plots obtained from those experiments (Fig. 8.4) indicated similar B_{max} and K_d values for the basal ganglia in patients with schizophrenia as compared to healthy controls. These data also indicated that endogenous dopamine release in the two subject groups were similar, since there were no differences in radioligand binding at low doses of the radioligand. Subsequent similar studies by other groups also failed to show an elevation of D2 dopamine receptor densities in patients with schizophrenia (Hietala *et al.*, 1994). Also with SPECT and the radioligands [^{123}I]IBZM or [^{123}I]epidepride similar binding potential was found in the basal ganglia for healthy controls and schizophrenic patients (Pilowsky *et al.*, 1996; Tibbo *et al.*, 1997). Claims that [^{11}C]NMSP and [^{11}C]raclopride bind to different subsets of D2 dopamine receptors were refuted by Nordström *et al.* (1995). The latter authors found similar binding parameters in patients with schizophrenia and healthy controls with both [^{11}C]NMSP and [^{11}C]raclopride.

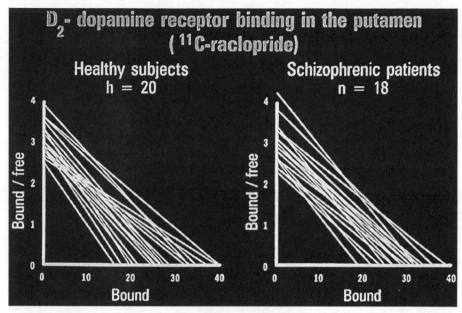

Fig. 8.4 D2 dopamine receptor binding in drug-naïve schizophrenic patients and healthy control subjects as measured by PET. The radioligand [^{11}C]raclopride was given in two specific activities. The graph demonstrates Scatchard plots. The intercept between the lines and the abscissa indicates the B_{max} values. The slope of the line represents the affinity of binding.

The fact that most studies have failed to demonstrate alterations of D2 dopamine receptor characteristics in the basal ganglia does not exclude the possibility that minor alterations may occur in parts of this brain region or that minor assymetries may occur (Pilowsky *et al.*, 1996). The studies performed so far also give no clues concerning the role of D2 dopamine receptors in extrastriatal regions of the brain. Recently, new high affinity radioligands have been developed giving the possibility also to image D2 dopamine receptors in extrastriatal brain regions. Thus, Farde *et al.* (1997) using [^{11}C]-FLB 457 obtained good signals for D2 dopamine receptor binding in some nuclei of the thalamus and in basal frontal and temporal brain regions of healthy control subjects. This is illustrated in Fig. 8.5 where D2 dopamine receptor binding is visualized in three dimensions in a healthy human subject. So far, systematic studies on possible alterations of these extrastriatal D2 dopamine receptor populations have not been performed in patients with schizophrenia.

D1 DOPAMINE RECEPTORS

The selective D1 dopamine receptor antagonist SCH-23390 was developed as the prototype PET radioligand for D1 dopamine receptors (Sedvall *et al.*, 1986b; Farde

D₁ and D₂ Dopamine Receptor Binding in the Human Brain

[¹¹C]NNC112   [¹¹C]FLB 457

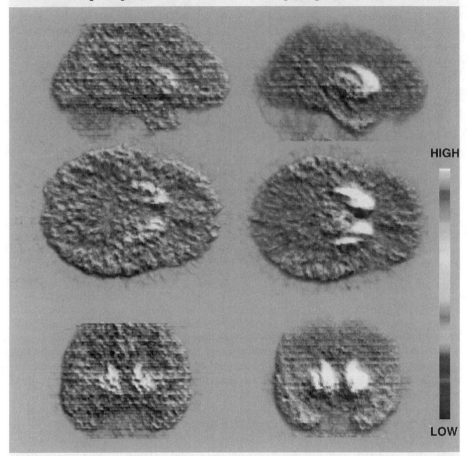

S. Pauli et al 1998

Fig. 8.5   Three-dimensional presentation of D1 (*left*) and D2 (*right*) dopamine receptor binding in the brain of two healthy human subjects. The radioligand used for D1 dopamine receptors was [¹¹C]NNC-112 and for D2 dopamine receptors [¹¹C]FLB-457. This figure also appears in colour between pages 150 and 151.

et al., 1989). This radioligand binds to D1 as well as D5 dopamine receptors. Since the D5 receptors are present only in very low densities, the radioactivity signal using [^{11}C]SCH-23390 should reflect predominantly D1 dopamine receptor binding. In the first preliminary studies with this radioligand no major alteration of D1 dopamine receptor binding could be obtained in the basal ganglia, nor in neocortical brain regions (L. Farde and G. Sedvall, unpublished data). Although, detailed analyses of these data indicated that reductions of D1 dopamine receptor binding might be present in subcompartments of the basal ganglia (Sedvall and Farde, 1995), subsequent studies disclosed large variability in the group of schizophrenic patients, which made interpretation of the results difficult. In subsequent studies Okubo *et al.* (1997) reported reduced binding potential for [^{11}C]SCH-23390 in the frontal cortex of drug-naïve schizophrenic patients but unchanged binding in the basal ganglia. The reduction of D1 dopamine receptor binding in the cortex was related to high scores for negative symptomatology. These data were of interest in relation to the negative therapeutic effect of the D1 dopamine receptor antagonist SCH-39166 in schizophrenic patients (Karlsson *et al.*, 1995a, 1995b).

[^{11}C]SCH-23390 has a short half-life with rapid metabolism and a relatively low ratio of specific to non-specific binding on the brain. Recently, [^{11}C]NNC-112 has been developed as a more optimal radioligand for D1 dopamine receptors (Halldin *et al.*, 1998, Fig. 8.5, *left*). [^{11}C]NNC-112 has the potential to explore striatal as well as extrastriatal D1 dopamine receptors in schizrenia during more optimal experimental conditions as with the previous radioligand. Such studies are currently in progress.

DOPAMINE TRANSPORTER

Cocaine and several of its analogues have high affinities for monoamine transporters. Fairly selective PET and SPECT radioligands for the dopamine transporter have been developed (Bergström *et al.*, 1995; Lundqvist *et al.*, 1997). [^{11}C]- or [^{18}F]-labelled β-CITFP and [^{123}I]-labelled β-CIT represent such radioligands. These radiotracers supply information concerning the dopamine transporter located at dendritic and terminal regions of brain dopamine neurons. With [^{11}C]-labelled β-CIT a good signal is obtained from the basal ganglia as well as several cortical regions and thalamic nuclei. This radiotracer and some of its recently developed analogues may be useful in examining densities of the dopamine transporters in these brain regions. However, so far, studies in schizophrenic patients have not been reported.

DOPAMINE RELEASE

[^{11}C]raclopride binds reversibly to D2 dopamine receptors. Animal and clinical experimentation indicates that endogenous concentrations of dopamine in the tissue compete with [^{11}C]raclopride for its binding sites in the brain. Thus, reserpine treatment, which causes a reduction of brain dopamine concentrations, has been shown to elevate [^{11}C]raclopride binding in the monkey brain. Amphetamine administration that releases dopamine into the synapse has been shown to reduce [^{11}C]raclopride binding in studies in monkeys as well as in human subjects. Similar results have been obtained with [^{123}I]-labelled BZM.

Laurelle *et al.* (1996) were the first in a clinical study to take advantage of the fact that radioligand binding to D2 dopamine receptors is affected by amphetamine treatment. These authors compared the effect of amphetamine administration on [^{123}I]BZM binding in groups of drug-free schizophrenic patients and healthy control subjects. As demonstrated in Fig. 8.6 amphetamine treatment resulted in a greater reduction of [^{123}I]BZM binding in patients with schizophrenia as compared to control subjects. These results are compatible with the view that amphetamine treatment causes a more marked dopamine release in schizophrenic patients as compared to healthy subjects. These results were replicated in a recent PET study where [^{11}C]raclopride was used as the radioligand (Breier *et al.*, 1997). Although obtained with an indirect pharmacological technique, these results indicated that schizophrenia may be related to a presynaptic alteration of dopaminergic synapses in the basal ganglia of schizophrenic patients.

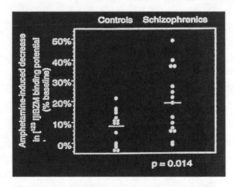

Fig. 8.6 Amphetamine induced reduction of radioligand binding in schizophrenic patients and control subjects (Laurelle *et al.*, 1996)

DOPAMINE SYNTHESIS

Tyrosine hydroxylation is the rate-limiting step in brain dopamine synthesis. Conversion of tyrosine into dopamine is too slow, however, to use radiolabelled tyrosine as a PET radiotracer for in-vivo studies of dopamine synthesis. However, radiolabelled DOPA or fluoro-DOPA, compounds that are converted by L-aromatic amino acid decarboxylase (AAD) to the corresponding amines have been used as radiotracers to study DOPA decarboxylation. AAD is a non-specific enzyme that occurs in high abundance in brain monoaminergic neurons. Using radiolabelled L-DOPA some, but not all investigators, found evidence for increased conversion of the radiotracer to dopamine in drug-free schizophrenic patients. Thus, Hietala *et al.*

(1994) using [^{18}F]DOPA found significantly higher radioactivity uptake in the basal ganglia in schizophrenic patients as compared to controls. Similar results were recently obtained by Lindström (personal communication) using [^{11}C]-labelled DOPA. The latter author also found increased uptake in frontal neocortical brain regions. These results are interesting since they point to the possibility of a presynaptic alteration in dopaminergic transmission in the brain of schizophrenic patients. Thus, these data appear to be consistent with the previously mentioned studies on amphetamine-induced dopamine release performed by Laurelle *et al.* (1996) and Breier *et al.* (1997).

Imaging of serotonergic mechanisms

The well-known hallucinogenic effects of LSD25 and other indolamines has stimulated interest in serotonergic mechanisms in schizophrenia. The potent effect of atypical antipsychotic drugs such as clozapine on serotonin 5HT2 receptors has placed further emphasis on the role of serotonin-mediated effects in the brain in schizophrenia. Among the extensive series of recently cloned sub-types of serotonin receptors most interest has been focused on serotonin 5HT2A and 5HT1A receptors. Several post-mortem studies have inferred the occurrence of alterations of these two receptor sub-types in post-mortem brain tissue from schizophrenic subjects (Bennett *et al.*, 1979; Arora and Meltzer, 1991; Hashimoto *et al.*, 1993; Dean and Hayes, 1996).

SEROTONIN 5HT2 RECEPTORS

The prototype neuroreceptor radioligand [^{11}C]NMSP has high affinity for 5HT2A and 5HT2C serotonin receptors. This radioligand gives a signal from neocortical 5HT2, receptors in human PET experiments. In their pioneering studies in drug naïve schizophrenic patients Wong *et al.* (1986) used this signal to record possible changes in brain 5HT2 receptors. Similar studies were performed by Nordström *et al.* (1995). None of these groups could demonstrate any marked alterations in 5HT2 receptor binding using this ligand. However, NMSP as a radioligand is far from ideal because of the fairly short time-window for radioactivity uptake in the neocortex and also the fact that no valid model was demonstrated using this ligand for 5HT2 receptor binding.

Recently the selective 5HT2A receptor ligand MDL-100907 was labelled with carbon-11 for PET experiments (Lundkvist *et al.*, 1996; Ito *et al.*, 1998). [^{11}C]MDL-100907 binding in the human brain discloses an excellent signal from a number of neocortical brain regions with practically no signal from the basal ganglia disclosing the low density of 5HT2A receptors in this region (Fig. 8.2). Pharmacological specificity studies in monkeys verify the high selectivity of [^{11}C]MDL-100907 for 5HT2A receptor binding (Ito *et al.*, 1998). [^{11}C]MDL-100907 also exhibits good kinetic properties and low metabolism, which makes this radioligand an excellent tool for in-vivo studies on 5HT2A receptors in schizophrenia. So far, no clinical comparison between schizophrenic patients and healthy controls using this radioligand has been reported.

SEROTONIN 5HT1A RECEPTORS

In-vitro studies indicate that 5HT1A receptors occur in high densities in a number of neocortical brain regions. Recent in-vitro studies indicate that densities of this receptor may be increased in several brain regions in schizophrenia. [^{11}C]-WAY-100635 was recently introduced as a suitable PET ligand for this receptor (Farde *et al.*, 1997). As shown in Fig. 8.2 [^{11}C]-WAY-100635 gives an excellent PET signal for neocortical brain regions and also a significantly higher uptake in the medial temporal cortex, where high densities of this receptor have been demonstrated. It is significant that using this radioligand a distinct signal can also be obtained from the serotonin pericarya located in the raphe nuclei of the brain stem. So far, no clinical studies using this radioligand in schizophrenia have been reported. Such studies should be pertinent to validate the recently presented post-mortem studies indicating that 5HT1A receptors are increased in the brain of schizophrenic patients (Dean and Hayes, 1996).

SEROTONIN TRANSPORTER

Although extensive experimental studies aimed at developing selective radioligands for PET studies of the serotonin transporter have been performed, so far only partially selective compounds are available, none of which has been systematically used for studies in schizophrenia.

Imaging of benzodiazepine receptors

The benzodiazepine flumazenil and its iodinated analogue iomazenil have been used in PET and SPECT studies on benzodiazepine receptors in the brain (Persson *et al.*, 1989). With regard to the recent interest in GABA-ergic mechanisms in schizophrenia it should be of interest to examine how the GABA$_A$ receptor-coupled benzodiazepine receptors are possibly changed in this disorder. Also in-vitro evidence indicates that reductions of benzodiazepine receptors may occur in some neocortical regions of brain in schizophrenia. The high densities of GABA$_A$ receptor-coupled benzodiazepine receptors in the human brain also make this receptor useful for examining gross changes of neocortical structures in schizophrenia. Since a number of studies indicate that a significant fraction of patients with schizophrenia exhibit such neocortical changes, brain imaging studies of the benzodiazepine receptor complex are well motivated. In a recent SPECT study Busatto *et al.* (1997) demonstrated reduced in-vivo benzodiazepine receptor binding using [^{123}I]-ionomazenil. The reduction of benzodiazepine receptor binding was correlated to severity of psychotic symptoms in schizophrenic patients.

Imaging of cholinergic mechanisms

In spite of extensive attempts to find suitable radioligands to label the subtypes of nicotinic and muscarinic cholinergic receptors during in-vivo conditions such attempts have, so far, not been highly successful. Nicotine itself shows binding kinetics that are extensively influenced by regional blood flow. For muscarinic receptors it has been very difficult to develop compounds with selectivity for the receptor subtypes. Some radioligands have been developed that exhibit partial separation between binding to M1 and M2 muscarinic receptors. However, none of these compounds has, so far, been used to explore receptor binding in schizophrenia.

Effect of antipsychotic drugs

In order to explore the mechanism of action for antipsychotic drugs in schizophrenia and to localize the effects of these drugs PET and SPECT have been extensively applied. PET and SPECT tracers such as [^{18}F]-2-deoxyglucose and [^{15}O], reflecting brain energy metabolism and blood flow, have generally demonstrated *small or no effect* of antipsychotic drug treatment in schizophrenia. Conventional antipsychotic drugs such as haloperidol have demonstrated a slight elevation of glucose level and metabolism in the basal ganglia in some studies (Buchsbaum and Hazlett, 1998; Andreasen *et al.*, 1997). However, these results have not been consistently replicated in all studies.

Radioligand binding studies, on the other hand, using selective radioligands for D2 dopamine receptors and 5HT2A receptors have demonstrated marked and highly consistent effects of different chemical classes of antipsychotic drugs on brain D2 dopamine and 5HT2 serotonin receptors (Sedvall *et al.*, 1986a; Nyberg *et al.*, 1993, 1997; Nordström *et al.*, 1993; Farde *et al.*, 1994; Kapur *et al.*, 1996). Thus, clinical doses of conventional antipsychotic drugs produced a marked blockade of radioligand binding, indicating competition at the receptor sites by the conventional drug treatment. PET and SPECT data presented, so far, are consistent in demonstrating relationships between high D2 dopamine receptor occupancy in the basal ganglia and the occurrence of extrapyramidal side-effects in drug-treated patients (Farde *et al.*, 1989; Nordström *et al.*, 1993; Scherer *et al.*, 1994; Goyer *et al.*, 1996).

It is also consistent that the atypical antipsychotic drug clozapine discloses a significantly lower D2 dopamine receptor occupancy than the conventional drugs (Farde *et al.*, 1992; Schlösser *et al.*, 1997). The recently developed new atypical antipsychotics risperidone, olanzapine, sertindole and ziprasidone appear to occupy a dose-dependent intermediate position between clozapine and the conventional drugs (Bench *et al.*, 1996; Fischman *et al.*, 1996; Klemm *et al.*, 1996; Seibyl *et al.*, 1996; Nyberg *et al.*, 1997; Schlösser *et al.*, 1997; Farde *et al.*, 1997). Current PET studies indicate that there are thresholds for D2 dopamine receptor occupancy and the clinical manifestation of antipsychotic drug action (Fig. 8.7). Thus, extrapyramidal side-effect frequency is significantly increased at occupancy levels above 80 per cent for D2 dopamine receptors (Farde *et al.*, 1992). The therapeutic antipsychotic actions seem to be induced at lower occupancy levels than 80 per cent. Here positive and negative symptoms may also exhibit different occupancy thresholds. Thus, significant therapeutic effects on positive symptoms were induced at occupancy levels above 50 per cent in a controlled study by Nordström *et al.* (1993). Martinot *et al.* (1994) reported therepeutic effects on negative symptoms already at low occupancy levels below 30 per cent using the selective D2 antagonist amisulpride. Further

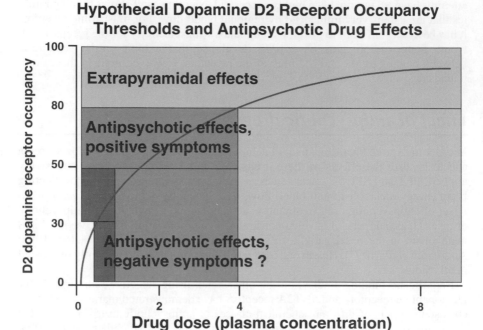

Fig. 8.7   Relationships between central D2 dopamine receptor occupancy and dose or plasma concentration of antipsychotic drugs. Note different occupancy windows for extrapyramidal effects and the effects on psychotic symptom profiles

controlled studies with different doses of conventional and unconventional compounds are required in order to explore and validate the suggested relationships between clinical therapeutic effects of antipsychotic drugs and dopamine D2 receptor occupancy as disclosed by PET and SPECT (Fig. 8.7). It should also be kept in mind that the occupancy levels demonstrated by in-vivo imaging studies do not disclose to what extent the occupancy induced by the drugs on the receptors reflect exclusively antagonistic binding to the receptor or whether partial agonistic effects may also be induced.

Using [¹¹C]NMSP and [¹¹C]MDL-100907 as radioligands it has also been disclosed that some of the conventional and practically all of the new atypical antipsychotic drugs also have marked effects on brain 5HT2 receptors (Fig. 8.8). Thus, clozapine, risperidone, olanzapine, seroquel, sertindole and ziprasidone all exhibit a marked occupancy of neocortical 5HT2 receptors when administered in clinical doses (Nyberg *et al.*, 1993; Farde *et al.*, 1994; Fishman *et al.*, 1996; Nordström *et al.*, 1998). Although, it has been claimed that this high occupancy level results in lower frequency of extrapyramidal side-effects of those drugs, it is still too early to draw firm conclusions concerning the clinical implications of high 5HT2 occupancy and antipsychotic drug action. New selective compounds have to be developed to answer this question.

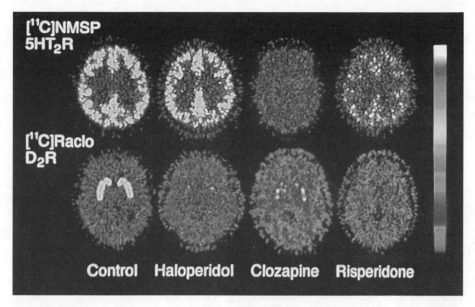

Fig. 8.8 PET visualization of serotonin 5HT2 (top panels) and D2 dopamine (lower panels) receptor binding in a healthy man (control) and three schizophrenic patients treated with haloperidol, clozapine, and risperidone. [¹¹C]NMSP and [¹¹C]raclopride were used as radioligands visualizing 5HT2 binding in the neocortex (upper panels) and D2 binding in the striatum (lower panels). Note striking reduction of 5HT2 binding after clozapine and risperidone treatment but not haloperidol. Note also reduction of D2 receptor binding which is striking after haloperidol and risperidone but less after clozapine. (Courtesy of Dr Svante Nyberg and Dr Anna-Lena Nordström). This figure also appears in colour between pages 150 and 151.

The selective D1 dopamine antagonist [¹¹C]SCH-23390 could be used to demonstrate that clozapine and thioxantine derivatives induce a significant but low degree of occupancy of D1 dopamine receptors (Farde *et al.*, 1992). It could also be demonstrated that the selective and potent D1 antagonist SCH-39166 could induce a high degree (>70 per cent) of D1 dopamine receptor occupancy when administered in high doses in clinical studies (Karlsson *et al.*, 1995a). Since this compound did not exhibit significant therapeutic effects in schizophrenia it could be concluded that selective occupancy of D1 dopamine receptors was not related to an antipsychotic drug action (Karlsson *et al.*, 1995b).

The neurochemical brain imaging studies performed so far, indicate specific patterns of relationship between drug effects on different neuroreceptors in the brain and the manifestation of therapeutic effects in schizophrenia and the occurrence of extrapyramidal side-effects. These relationships are schematically illustrated in Table 8.2.

Table 8.2. Monoamine receptor occupancy – antipsychotic action

Drug	D1	D2	D3	D4	5HT2	Antipsychotic action
Haloperidol	–	++	++	+(+)	–	yes
Clozapine	+	+	+	+(+)	++	yes
Amisulpride	–	++	++	–	–	yes
SCH-39166	++	–	–	–	(+)	no
L-745870	–	–	–	+(+)	–	no?
MDL 100907	–	–	–	–	++	?

– indicates no occupancy; + indicates significant occupancy.

Concluding remarks

Neurochemical brain imaging in schizophrenia is a young research field with an expanding number of studies over the past 10 years. During this period a rapid development of experimental tools has led to higher standards with regard to selectivity of radiotracers, sensitivity and resolution of the technical methodology.

The following conclusions can be drawn regarding possible neurochemical alterations in schizophrenia on the basis of studies performed so far. Although consistent evidence for general alterations of D2 dopamine receptors has not been obtained for the basal ganglia, new tracers allow the exploration of extrastriatal dopamine D2 receptors that may be involved in the pathophysiology of schizophrenia. PET studies using amphetamine challenge of D2 receptor binding and also studies with labelled DOPA analogues indicate that presynaptic alterations may occur in dopaminergic synapses in schizophrenic patients. Such changes may be present in the basal ganglia as well as in neocortical brain regions. The observations performed indicate that schizophrenic patients might have an altered release mechanism for dopamine related to hyperfunction at dopaminergic synapses.

Possible alterations of D1 dopamine receptors have to be further explored in more extensive studies. This also holds true for the preliminary studies on brain benzodiazepine receptors. Systematic studies on sub-types of serotonin receptors are now feasible, since suitable radioligands have recently been developed.

Neurochemical imaging in schizophrenia has been most rewarding in the field of clinical pharmacology of antipsychotic drugs. Here distinct and marked effects on D2 dopamine and 5HT2 receptors have been disclosed by PET and SPECT imaging. These studies have demonstrated significant differences between the action profiles of chemically different classes of antipsychotic drugs and have also pointed to significant relationships between receptor effects and some of the clinical manifestations of these drugs. In this way the neurochemical imaging methods have been shown to be powerful tools to explore relationships between molecular events in the living human brain and their relationship to clinical manifestations in schizophrenia.

Acknowledgement

Original work described in this paper was supported by the following grants: NIMH (44814-9A), Swedish Medical Research Council (03560) and the Wallenberg Foundation.

References

Andreasen, N. C., O'Leary, D. S., Flaum, M., Nopoulos, P., Watkins, G. L., Boles Ponto, L. L. and Hichwa, R. D. (1997) Hypofrontality in schizophrenia: distributed dysfunctional circuits in neuroleptic-naive patients. *Lancet*, **349**, 1730–4.

Arora, R. C. and Meltzer, H. Y. (1991) Serotonin2 (5-HT2) receptor binding in the frontal cortex of schizophrenic patients. *J Neural Transm Gen Sect*, **85**, 19–29.

Bench, C. J., Lammertsma, A. A., Grasby, P. M., Dolan, R. J., Warrington, S. J., Boyce, M., Gunn, K. P., Brannick, L. Y. and Frackowiak, R. S. (1996) The time course of binding to striatal dopamine D2 receptors by the neuroleptic ziprasidone (CP-88, 059-01) determined by position emission tomography. *Psychopharmacology*, **124**(1–2), 141–7.

Bennett, J. P., Jr, Enna, S. J., Bylund, D. B., Gillin, J. C., Wyatt, R. J. and Snyder, S. H. (1979) Neurotransmitter receptors in frontal cortex of schizophrenics. *Arch Gen Psychiatry*, **36**, 927–34.

Bergström, K. A. (1995) *Radiosynthesis, Pharmacokinetics and Evaluation of [123I]-2β-Carbomethoxy-3β- (4-iodophenyl)tropane as a Single Photon Emission Tomography Tracer of Dopamine and Serotonin Transporters in the Living Human Brain*. Kuopio.

Blomqvist, G., Stone-Elander, S., Halldin, C., Långström, B. and Wiesel, F. A. (1990) Positron emission tomographic mesurements of cerebral glucose utilization using (1-^{11}C)-D-glucose. *J Cereb Blood Flow Metab*, **10**, 467–483.

Breier, A., Su, T. P., Saunders, R., Carson, R. E., Kolachana, B. S., de Bartolomeis, A., Weinberger, D. R., Weisenfeld, N., Malhotra, A. K., Eckelman, W. C. and Pickar, D. (1997) Schizophrenia is associated with elevated amphetamine-induced synaptic dopamine concentrations: evidence from a novel positron emission tomography method. *Proceedings of the National Academy of Sciences of the United States of America*, **94**(6), 2569–74.

Buchsbaum, M. S. and Hazlett, E. A. (1998) Positron emission tomography studies of abnormal glucose metabolism in schizophrenia. *Schizophr Bull*, **24**, 343–64.

Busatto, G. F., Pilowsky, L. S., Costa, D. C., Ell, P. J., David, A. S., Lucey, I. V. and Kerwin, R. W. (1997) Correlation between reduced in vivo benzodiazepine receptor binding and severity of psychotic symptoms in schizophrenia [published erratum appears in *Am J Psychiatry* 1997 May 154(5): 722] (see comments) *Am J Psychiatry*, **154**(1), 56–63.

Dean, B. and Hayes, W. (1996) Decreased frontal cortical serotonin2A receptors in schizophrenia. *Schizophr Res*, **21**, 133–9.

Farde, L., Ginovart, N., Ito, H., Lundkvist, C., Pike, V. W., McCarron, J. A. and Halldin, C. (1997) PET-characterization of [carbonyl-11C]WAY-100635 binding to 5-HT1A receptors in the primate brain. *Psychopharmacology*, **133**, 196–202.

Farde, L., Mack, R. J., Nyberg, S. and Halldin, C. (1997) D2 occupancy, extrapyramidal side effects and antipsychotic drug treatment: a pilot study with sertindole in healthy subjects. *Int Clin Psychopharmacol*, **12** Suppl 1: S3–7.

Farde, L., Nordstrom, A. L., Nyberg, S., Halldin, C. and Sedvall, G. (1994) D1, D2 and 5HT2 receptor occupancy in clozapine-treated patients. *J Clin Psychiatry*, **55** Suppl B: 67–9.

Farde, L. Wiesel, F.-A., Hall, H., Halldin, C., Stone-Elander, S. and Sedvall, G. (1987) No D$_2$ receptor increase in PET study of schizophrenia. *Arch Gen Psychiatry* 44: 671–2.

Farde L., Wiesel, F.-A., Nordström, A.-L., Sedvall, G. (1989) D1 and D2 dopamine receptor occupancy during treatment with conventional and atypical neuroleptics. *Psychopharmacology*, **99**, S28–S31.

Farde, L., Hall, H., Ehrin, E. and Sedvall, G. (1986) Quantitative analysis of D2 dopamine receptor binding in the living human brain by PET. *Science*, **231**, 258–61.

Fischman, A. J., Bonab, A. A., Babich, J. W., Alpert, N. M., Rauch, S. L., Elmaleh, D. R., Shoup, T. M., Williams, S. A. and Rubin, R. H. (1996) Positron emission tomographic analysis of central 5-hydroxytryptamine2 receptor occupancy in healthy volunteers treated with the novel antipsychotic agent, ziprasidone. *J Pharmacol Exp Ther* **279**(2), 939–47.

Goyer, P. F., Berridge, M. S., Morris, E. D., Semple, W. E., Compton-Toth, B. A., Schulz, S. C., Wong, D. F., Miraldi, F. and Meltzer, H. Y. (1996) A PET measurement of neuroreceptor occupancy by typical and atypical neuroleptics. *J Nuclear Med*, **37**(7), 1122–7.

Halldin, C., Foged, C., Karlsson, P. *et al.* (1988) [¹¹c]NNC112: A radioligand for PET examination of striatal and neocortical D¹-dopamine receptors. *J Nucl Med*, **39**, 2061–8.

Halldin, C., Swahn, C. -G., Farde, L. and Sedvall, G. (1995) Radioligand disposition and metabolism – key information in early drug development. In: Comer D, ed. *PET for drug development and evaluation*. The Netherlands: Kluwer Academic Publishing, 55–65.

Hashimoto, T., Kitamura, N., Kajimoto, Y., Shirai, Y., Shirakawa, O., Mita, T., Nishino, N. and Tanaka, C. (1993) Differential changes in serotonin 5-HT1A and 5-HT2 receptor binding in patients with chronic schizophrenia. *Psychopharmacology*, **112**, S35–S39.

Heinz, A., Knable, M. B. and Weinberger, D. R. (1996) Dopamine D2 receptor imaging and neuroleptic drug response. *J Clin Psychiatry*, **57** Suppl 1§1: 84–8, discussion 89–93.

Hietala, J., Syvalahti, E., Vuorio, K., Rakkolainen, V., Bergman, J., Haaparanta, M., Solin, O., Kuoppamaki, M., Kirvela, O., Ruotsalainen, U., *et al.* (1995) Presynaptic dopamine function in striatum of neuroleptic-naive schizophrenic patients. *Lancet*, **346**, 1130–1.

Hietala, J., Syvalahti, E., Vuorio, K., Nagren, K., Lehikoinen, P., Ruotsalainen, U., Rakkolainen, V., Lehtinen, V. and Wegelius, U. (1994) Striatal D2 dopamine receptor characteristics in neuroleptic-naive schizophrenic patients studied with positron emission tomography [Journal Article] *Arch Gen Psychiatry*, **51**(2), 116–23.

Huang, S. C., Barrio, J. R. and Phelps, M. E. (1986) Neuroreceptor assay with positron emission tomography: Equilibrium versus dynamic approaches. *J Cereb Blood Flow Metab*, **6**, 515–21.

Ito, H., Nyberg, S., Halldin, C., Lundkvist, C. and Farde, L. (1998) PET imaging of central 5-HT2A receptors with carbon-11-MDL. *J Nucl Med*, **39**, 208–14.

Kapur, S., Remington, G., Jones, C., Wilson, A., DaSilva, J., Houle, S. and Zipursky, R. (1996) High levels of dopamine D2 receptor occupancy with low-dose haloperidol treatment: a PET study *Am J Psychiatry*, **153**(7), 948–50.

Karlsson, P., Sedvall, G., Halldin, C., Swahn, C.-G. and Farde, L. (1995a) Evaluation of SCH 39166 as PET ligand for central D1-dopamine receptor binding and occupancy in man. *Psychopharmacology*, **121**, 300–8.

Karlsson, P., Smith, L., Farde, L., Härnryd, C., Sedvall, G. and Wiesel, F.-A. (1995b) Lack of apparent antipsychotic effect of the D1-dopamine receptor antagonist SCH39166 in acutely ill schizophrenic patients. *Psychopharmacology*, **121**, 309–16.

Klemm, E., Grunwald, F., Kasper, S., Menzel, C., Broich, K., Danos, P., Reichmann, K., Krappel, C., Rieker, O., Briele, B., Hotze, A. L., Moller, H. J. and Biersak, H. J. (1996) IBZM SPECT for imaging of striatal D2 dopamine receptors in 56 schizophrenic patients taking various neuroleptics. *Am J Psychiatry*, **153**(2), 183–90.

Kung, H. F., Alavi, A., Chang, W., Kung, M. P., Keyes, J. W. Jr, Velchik, M. *et al.* (1990) In vivo SPECT imaging of CNS D-2 dopamine receptors: initial studies with iodine-123-IBZM in humans. *J Nucl Med*, **31**(5), 573–9.

Laurelle, M., Abi-Dargham, A., van Dyck, C. H., Gil, R., D'Souza, C. D., Erdos, J., McCance, E., Rosenblatt, W., Fingado, C., Zoghbi, S. S., Baldwin, R. M., Seibyl, J. P., Krystal, J. H.,

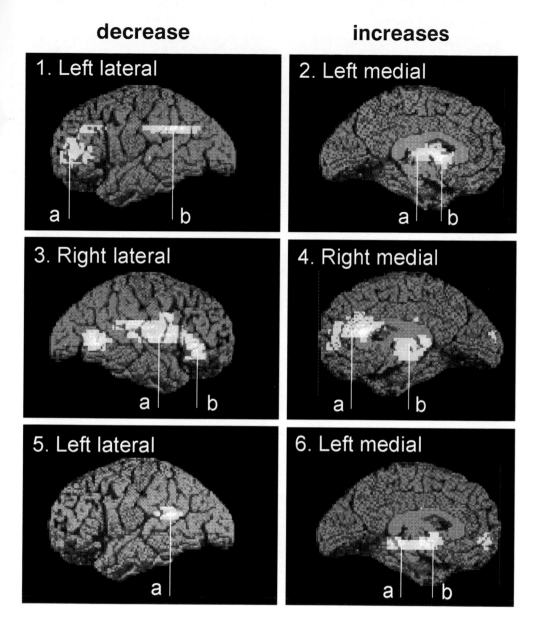

decrease **increases**

1. Left lateral   2. Left medial

a   b   a   b

3. Right lateral   4. Right medial

a   b   a   b

5. Left lateral   6. Left medial

a   a   b

Plate 1 Patterns of rCBF associated with schizophrenic symptoms (Liddle *et al.*, 1992). The areas of significant correlation between rCBF and severity of each of three syndromes of characteristic syndromes are shown rendered onto the cortical surface. rCBF was measured using PET. 1. Negative correlations of psychomotor poverty with rCBF in left lateral prefrontal cortex (a) and inferior parietal lobule (b). 2. Positive correlations of psychomotor poverty with rCBF in corpus striatum and thalamus. 3. Negative correlations of disorganization with rCBF in right ventro-lateral prefrontal cortex (a) and insula, rendered onto the overlying temporal cortex (b). 4. Positive correlations of disorganization with rCBF in right medial frontal cortex and thalamus (a). 5. Negative correlations of reality distortion with rCBF in left superior temporal gyrus (a). 6. Positive correlations of reality distortion with rCBF in left parahippocampal gyrus (a) and ventral striatum (b)

Healthy subjects

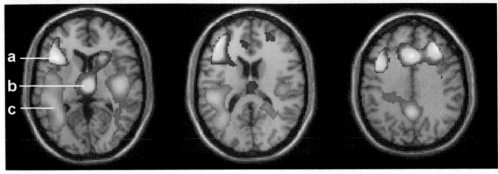

Range of z scores -4.7<2z<5.4

Schizophrenic subjects

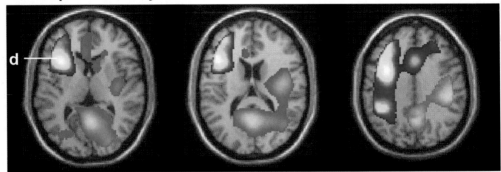

Range of z scores -6.2<2z<6.9

Change in healthy subjects *minus* change in schizophrenic subjects

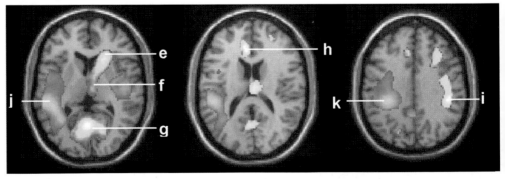

Range of z scores -5.4<2z<3.5

Plate 2 Significant changes in rCBF measured with PET during paced word generation in healthy subjects and in schizophrenia (Liddle *et al.*, 1997). Increases relative to word repetition are shown in red-yellow hues and decreases in blue, in slices at 6mm (left), 16 mm and 24 mm above the inter-commissural plane. In all the clusters of voxels shown in colour, the change is statistically significant at level *P*<0.05 after correctiong for multiple comparisons. In healthy subjects, rCBF increases in left lateral frontal cortex (a)and thalamus (b); while it decreases in temporal cortex bilaterally (c). Schizophrenic subjects exhibit a normal increase in left lateral frontal cortex (d), but there are abnormalities in many other areas. Relative to healthy subjects, schizophrenic subjects exhibit significantly less increase in rCBF in right striatum (e), right thalamus (f), lingual gyrus (g), anterior cingulate (h) and right inferior parietal lobule (i), and significantly greater increase in temporal lobe bilaterally (j) and left inferior parietal lobule (k).

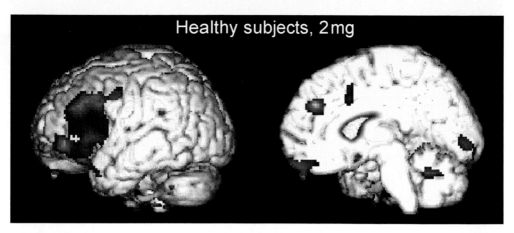

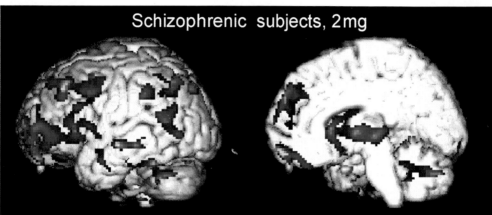

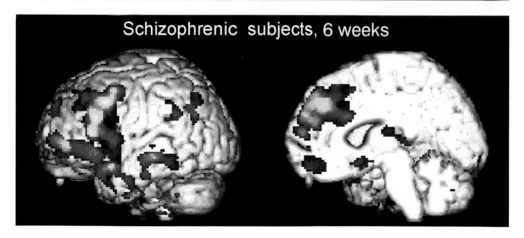

Plate 3 Decreases in regional metabolism measured using PET in healthy subjects 90 minutes after 2 mg of risperidone; decreases in medication-free first episode schizophrenic patients 90 minutes after 2 mg of risperidone, and in the same patients after 6 weeks treatment with risperidone, rendered onto the left lateral cerebral (left) and right medial cortex (Ngan *et al.*, 1998, Lane *et al.*, 1998).

D₁ and D₂ Dopamine Receptor Binding in the Human Brain

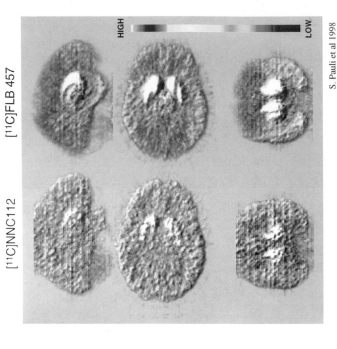

[¹¹C]NNC112   [¹¹C]FLB 457

HIGH
LOW

S. Pauli et al 1998

Plate 6 Three-dimensional presentation of D1 (left) and D2 (right) dopamine receptor binding in the brain of two healthy human subjects. The radioligand used for D1 dopamine receptors was [¹¹C]NNC-112 and for D2 dopamine receptors [¹¹C]FLB-457.

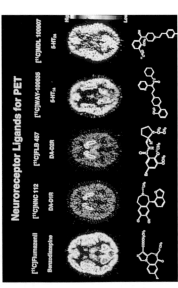

Plate 4 PET image from human subjects showing radioactivity distribution after administration of selective radioligands: benzodiazepine receptors, D1 dopamine receptors, 5HT1A receptors, D2 dopamine receptors, 5HT1A receptors, and 5HT2A receptors.

Plate 5 PET visualization of serotonin 5HT2 (top panels) and D2 dopamine (lower panels) receptor binding in a healthy man and three schizophrenic patients treated with haloperidol, clozapine, and risperidone. [¹¹C]NMSP and [¹¹C]raclopide were used as radioligands visualizing 5HT2 binding in the neocortex (upper panels) and D2 binding in the striatum (lower panels). Note striking reduction of 5HT2 binding after clozapine and risperidine treatment but not haloperidol. Note also reduction of D2 receptor binding which is striking after haloperidol and risperidone but less after clozapine. (Courtesy of Dr Svante Nyberg and Dr Anna-Lena Nordström.)

Charney, D. S. and Innis, R. B. (1996) Single photon emission computerized tomography imaging of amphetamine-induced dopamine release in drug-free schizophrenic subjects. *Proc Natl Acad Sci USA*, **93**, 9235–9240.

Leenders, K. L., Gibbs, J. M., Frackowiak, R. S. J., Lammertsma, A. A. and Jones, T. (1980) Positron emission tomography of the brain: New possibilities for the investigation of human cerebral pathophysiology. *Prog Neurobiol*, **23**, 1–38.

Lundkvist, C., Halldin, C., Ginovart, N., Nyberg, S., Swahn, C.-G., Carr, A. A., Brunner, P. and Farde, L. (1996) [11C]MDL 100907, a radioligand for selective imaging of 5-HT2A receptors with positron emission tomography. *Life Sci*, **58**(10), PL 187–92.

Lundkvist, C., Halldin, C., Ginovart, N., Swahn, C.-G. and Farde, L. (1997) [18F]β-CIT-FP is superior to [11C]β-CIT-FP for quantitation of the dopamine transporter. *Nuclear Med Biol*, **24**, 621–7.

Martinot, J. L., Paillere-Martinot, M. L., Loc'h, C., Lecrubier, Y., Dao-Casterllana, M. H., Aubin, F., Allilaire, J. F., Mazoyer, B., Mazière, B. and Syrota, A. (1994) Central D2 receptors and negative symptoms of schizophrenia. *Br J Psychiatry*, **164**(1), 27–34.

Martinot, J. L., Paillere-Martinot, M. L., Poirier, M. F., Dao-Castellana, M. H., Loc'h, C. and Mazière, B. (1996) *In vivo* characteristics of dopamine D2 receptor occupancy by amisulpride in schizophrenia. *Psychopharmacology*, **124**(1–2), 154–8.

Nordström, A.-L., Farde, L. and Halldin, C. (1993) High 5-HT$_2$ receptor occupancy in clozapine treated patients demonstrated by PET. *Psychopharmacology*, **110**, 365–7.

Nordström, A.-L., Farde, L., Eriksson, L. and Halldin, C. (1995) No elevated D2 dopamine receptors in neuroleptic-naive schizophrenic patients revealed by positron emission tomography and [11C]N-methylspiperone. *Psychiatry Research: Neuroimaging*, **61**, 67–83.

Nordström, A.-L., Nyberg, S., Olsson, H. and Farde, L. (1998) PET-finding of a high striatal D2 receptor occupancy in olanzapine treated patients. *Arch Gen Psychiat*, **55**, 283–4.

Nyberg, S., Farde, L., Eriksson, L., Halldin, C. and Eriksson, B. (1993). 5-HT$_2$ and D$_2$ dopamine receptor occupancy in the living human brain: a PET study with risperidone. *Psychopharmacology*, **110**, 265–72.

Nyberg, S., Farde L. and Halldin C. (1997) A PET study of 5HT2 and D2 dopamine receptor occupancy induced by olazapine in healthy subjects. *Neuropsychopharmacology*, **16**(1), 1–7.

Okubo, Y., Suhara, T., Suzuki, K., Kobayashi, K., Inoue, O., Terasaki, O., Someya, Y., Sassa, T., Sudo, Y., Matsushima, E., Iyo M., Tateno, Y. and Toru, M. (1997) Decreased prefrontal dopamine D1 receptors in schizophrenia revealed by PET *Nature*, **385**(6617), 634–6.

Pauli, S. and Sedvall, G. (1997) Three dimensional visualization and quantification of the benzodiazepine receptor population within a living human brain using PET and MRI. *Eur Arch Psychiat Clin Neurosci*, **247**, 61–70.

Persson, A., Pauli, S., Halldin, C., Stone-Elander, S., Farde, L., Sjögren, L. and Sedvall, G. (1989) Saturation analysis of specific 11C Ro 15-1788 binding to the human neocortex using positron emission tomography. *Hum Psychopharmacol*, **4**, 21–31.

Pilowsky, L. S., Costa, D. C., Ell, P. J., Verhoeff, N. P., Murray, R. M. and Kerwin, R. W. (1996) D2 dopamine receptor binding in the basal ganglia of antipsychotic-free schizophrenic patients. An 123I-IBZM single photon emission computerised tomography study *Br J Psychiatry*, **164**(1), 16–26.

Scherer, J., Tatsch, K., Schwarz, J., Oertel, W. H., Konjarczyk, M. and Albus, M. (1994) D2 dopamine receptor occupancy differs between patients with and without extrapyramidal side effects. *Acta Psychiatr Scand*, **90**(4), 266–8.

Schlosser, R., Schlegel, S., Hiemke, C. *et al.* (1997) [^{123}I]IBZM SPECT in patients treated with typical and atypical neuroleptics: relationship to drug plasma levels and extrapyramidal side effects. *Psychiatr Res*, **75**, 103–14.

Schroder, J., Bubeck, B., Demisch, S. and Sauer, H. (1997) Benzodiazepine receptor distribution and diazepam binding in schizophrenia: an exploratory study. *Psychiatry Res*, **68**(2–3), 125–31.

Sedvall, G., Farde, L. A., Persson, A. and Wiesel, F. A. (1986a) Imaging of neurotransmitter receptors in the living human brain. *Arch. Gen. Psychiat*, **43**, 995–1005.

Sedvall, G., Farde, L., Stone-Elander, S. and Halldin, C. (1986b) Dopamine D_1 receptor binding in the living human brain. In Breese G. R., Creese I. (eds), *Neurobiology of Central D_1 dopamine Receptors*. New York: Plenum, 119–124.

Sedvall, G. and Farde, L. (1995) Chemical brain anatomy in schizophrenia. *Lancet*, **346**, 743–749.

Seibyl, J. P., Zea-Ponze, Y., Brenner, L., Baldwin, R. M., Krystal, J. H., Offord, S. J., Mochoviak, S., Charney, D. S., Hoffer, P. B. and Innis, R. B. (1996) Continuous intravenous infusion of iodine 123 IBZM for SPECT determination of human brain dopamine receptor occupancy by antipsychotic agent RWJ-37796. *J Nucl Med*, **37**(1), 11–15.

Sheppard, G., Manchanda, R., Gruzelier, J., Hirsch, S. R., Wise, R., Frackowiak, F. and Jones, T. (1988) O^{15}-positron emission tomographic scanning in predominantly never-treated acute schizophrenic patients. *Lancet*, **2**, 1448–1452.

Sokoloff, L., Reivich, M., Kennedy, C., DesRosiers, M. H., Patlak, C. S., Pettigrew, M. D., Sakurada, I. and Shinohara, M. (1977) The deoxyglucose method for the measurement of local cerebral glucose utilization: Theory, procedure and normal values in the conscious and anesthetized albino rat. *J Neurochem*, **28**, 897–916.

Tibbo, P., Silverstone, P. H., McEwan, A. J., Scott, J., Joshua, A. and Golberg, K. (1997) A single photon emission computed tomography scan study of striatal dopamine D2 receptor binding with 123I-epidepride in patients with schizophrenia and controls. *J Psychiatry Neurosci*, **22**(1), 39–45.

Wagner, H. N., Burns, H. D., Dannals, R. F., Wong, D. F., Langstrom, B., Duelfer, T., Frost, J. J., Raert, H. T., Links, J. M., Rosenblom, S. B., Lukas, S. E., Kramer, A. V. and Kuhar, M. J. (1983) Imaging dopamine receptors in the human brain by positron tomography. *Science*, **221**, 1264–66.

Wong, D. F., Wagner, H. N., Tune, L. E., Dannals, R. F., Pearlson, G. D., Links, J. M., Tamminga, C. A., Broussolle, E. P., Ravert, A. I., Wilson, A. A., Toung, J. K. T., Malat, J., Williams, J. A., Otuama, L. A., Snyder, S. H., Kuhar, M. J. and Gjedde, A. (1986) Positron emission tomography reveals elevated D_2 dopamine receptors in drug-naive schophrenics. *Science*, **234**, 1558–63.

CHAPTER 9

The neuropsychology of schizophrenia

ANN M. MORTIMER

Introduction

This review sets out the nature of cognitive impairment in schizophrenia, and its importance particularly with respect to pharmacological remediation. There follows an outline of the function of brain systems susceptible to neuroleptics, and a summary of studies on cognitive change produced by both conventional and atypical drugs. Interest in neuropsychological abnormalities in schizophrenia has two origins (McKenna, 1994): poor performance by patients on a wide range of standard psychometric tests; and the possibility that specific cognitive abnormalities may underlie particular symptom classes.

What are the neuropsychological deficits in schizophrenia?

GENERAL COGNITION

One review of 94 studies of schizophrenic patients' performance on neuropsychological tests concluded that acute, mixed and chronic patients were increasingly difficult to distinguish from patients with organic brain disease (Heaton *et al.*, 1978). Subsequent studies have confirmed that schizophrenia is characterized by a compromise of intellectual function, ranging from a fall in IQ, through decline in a wide range of tests (Kolb and Whishaw, 1983; Nelson *et al.*, 1990; Frith *et al.*, 1991) to frank dementia (Owens and Johnstone, 1980; Liddle and Crow, 1984; Davidson and Haroutunian, 1996). Evidence of independent dementia pathology in schizophrenic post-mortem brain samples is, however, conspicuous by its absence (Purohit *et al.*, 1993; Humphries *et al.*, 1996). Therefore the assumption that intellectual deterioration in schizophrenia is related to fixed structural abnormalities cannot yet be supported: some other process must be responsible, perhaps a neurochemical derangement susceptible to pharmacological intervention. This issue is of obvious interest in the context of neuroleptic treatment.

DISPROPORTIONATE DEFICITS IN SCHIZOPHRENIA

One of the few studies to compare schizophrenics with patients suffering from affective psychosis (Goldberg *et al.*, 1993a) concluded that patients with schizophrenia consistently performed at lower levels on tests of psychomotor speed, attention, memory and problem solving despite controlling for the effects of a fall in IQ in the schizophrenic group. Disproportionate deficits, which stand out as significantly compromised even in the presence of intact general cognition, have provoked a great deal of interest given their potential to identify candidate areas for schizophrenia pathophysiology.

MEMORY

Episodic and semantic memory are disproportionately impaired in schizophrenia (Shallice *et al.*, 1991; Tamlyn *et al.*, 1992; Duffy and O'Carroll, 1994; McKay *et al.*, 1996) with preservation of implicit memory and procedural learning (Goldberg *et al.*, 1993d; Clare *et al.*, 1993), a pattern which corresponds to the classic amnesic syndrome. The question of working memory deficits in schizophrenia is a vexed one. There is no evidence that 'slave systems' are impaired in the absence of general cognitive deficit, nor that the 'central executive' is impaired disproportionately, nor that 'central executive' function corresponds to other aspects of executive function (Rubinsztein *et al.*,1997). However, studies of executive function are frequently called upon when arguments for working memory dysfunction in schizophrenia are presented (e.g. Goldberg and Weinberger, 1995).

EXECUTIVE FUNCTION

Poor performance on tests of executive ('frontal') function has been found repeatedly (Goldberg et al.,1987; Morice, 1990; Liddle and Morris, 1991). Single case neuropsychological studies demonstrate the ubiquity of degrees of frontal impairment, and their disproportionate occurrence in schizophrenia even when there is no significant general cognitive dysfunction (Shallice et al., 1991). However, executive function is not as well characterized as memory in terms of doubly dissociable components: much remains to be done to tease out which aspects are relevant to schizophrenia and the brain systems which subserve them. A recent study demonstrated that executive dysfunction could not be ascribed to memory impairment, or vice versa: the two dysfunctions were doubly dissociable (Evans et al., 1997).

Influence of symptoms and institutional care on cognitive deficit

Are symptoms responsible for some compromise of cognitive performance? Many patients in both acute relapse and chronic severe states are completely untestable: furthermore, in older patients the effects of 'institutionalization' have been implicated. However, several lines of evidence refute these propositions. Cross-sectional studies find equivalent levels of impairment in different groups of co-operative schizophrenic patients despite wide ranges of age and illness duration (Goldberg et al., 1993c; Heaton et al., 1994; Hyde et al., 1994). Substantial levels of cognitive impairment can be found at illness onset (Bilder et al., 1992b; Hoff et al., 1992) including in drug-naïve patients (Saykin et al., 1994). Comparable levels of deficit have been reported in both first-episode and chronic patients (Hoff et al., 1992) while in the most severely affected, often the older group who became ill before neuroleptics were available, there is evidence of slow progressive cognitive decline (Davidson and Haroutunian, 1996). Finally, although overall symptom severity may be a strong concomitant of neuropsychological deficit (Bornstein et al., 1990) studies which investigated cognition longitudinally from relapse have demonstrated both positive (Sweeney et al., 1991) and negative (Goldberg et al., 1993b; Cantor-Graae et al., 1995) findings despite ubiquitous symptomatic recovery. One study which explored the influence of symptoms on cognition (Goldberg et al., 1993a) found that symptoms only accounted for 5% of the variance in schizophrenia, as opposed to 30% of the variance in affective disorder.

Cognitive abnormalities: relationship to symptom classes?

A 'levels of explanation' model of schizophrenia (Frith et al., 1991b; Mortimer, 1994) suggests that symptoms or symptom classes can be the result of specific neuropsychological deficits, which in turn are the result of particular pathophysiological phenomena in the brain. However, the demonstration of specific cognitive abnormalities with a causal role in symptom origin has generally been less than successful. One promising candidate, a deficit in selective attention, afforded much theoretical explanatory power for several symptom classes: repeated attempts to observe it in patients have been fruitless overall (McKenna, 1994). It has been pointed out (Cutting, 1985) that attention is not usually a problem in schizophrenia patients anyway, at least compared to manic patients. A reasoning bias towards 'jumping to conclusions' has been hypothesized to underlie delusions, and indeed schizophrenic patients do demonstrate such a bias compared to controls (Garety, 1991) but unfortunately it is not specific to deluded patients, nor does it bear any relationship to the severity of deludedness (Mortimer *et al.*, 1997).

A relatively rare class of delusion, alienation (passivity) of thought and action, has been linked to a disorder of self-monitoring observed during a visual motor task (Frith and Done, 1989; Mlakar *et al.*, 1994). Although this adduces support for a general self-monitoring deficit hypothesized to explain a wide range of symptoms classes (Frith, 1992) much more work is needed to test this theory on a broader range of more frequent symptoms.

Formal thought disorder has been replicably and specifically related to 'overinclusiveness' (Payne, 1993) but this concept remains undefined in cognitive psychological terms. A perusal of the tasks used to rate overinclusiveness shows that the verbal ones could be subsumed under the auspices of tests of semantic memory, while the non-verbal tests appear to tap executive function. There is a large body of evidence implicating semantic memory disorder in schizophrenia (Clare *et al.*, 1993; McKay *et al.*, 1996) some of it demonstrating a specific relationship with thought disorder (Mortimer *et al.*, 1995). Executive dysfunction on the other hand can be convincingly argued as the substrate for thought disorder (McGrath, 1991) but some studies do not find the two to be related (Clark and O'Carroll, 1997; Mortimer *et al.*, 1997).

Although it may seem likely on common sense grounds that the cognitive impairments picked up on routine testing may approximate to those responsible for symptoms, there is no reason *a priori* why this should be the case: such narrow specific deficits, if they exist at all, may merely form a subset or be quite unrelated. This, plus the natural tendency to use standard tests which were never designed with the objective of potential symptom correlation in mind, may be one reason why studies to date in this area have been generally disappointing. Many of these tests are poorly defined if at all in cognitive neuropsychological terms (intelligence tests being a prime example) and very few are based on animal work, or originate from anatomical or physiological studies. Most rely on a combination of mental functions. However, designing tasks which appear conceptually likely to reflect symptom classes may be no more than an exercise in inviting the patient to produce symptoms, and then quantitating these with numbers. The alternative, using a parallel task (for instance a non-verbal task against symptoms which are usually couched in verbal terms) may not only lack face validity as a predictor but may fail to tap the hypothesized cognitive function at fault. On the other hand, the 'levels of explanation' model of schizophrenia may simply be inaccurate.

Course of cognitive decline

Like everything else that has been investigated in schizophrenia, the course of cognitive decline appears to be extremely variable. Several studies have produced inconsistent results, the main argument being between schizophrenia as a static encephalopathy with most of the damage done in the first five years after onset (Heaton and Drexler, 1987), versus schizophrenia as a very slow and poorly understood degenerative or progressive process with gradual cognitive decline over many years (Miller, 1989). Some authorities describe a series of stages (Goldberg and Gold, 1995) beginning with poor premorbid function in childhood (Offord and Cross, 1971; Walker and Lewine, 1990) followed by further decline around onset and first episode (Goldberg *et al.*, 1988; Bilder *et al.*, 1992; Hutton *et al.*, 1997). Deterioration continues for a limited period beyond first episode (Lubin *et al.*, 1962), then the impairment stabilizes (Smith, 1960; Klonoff *et al.*, 1970; Chaikelson and Schwartzman, 1983). Two studies of age-stratified groups have verified this static phase (Goldstein and Zubin, 1990; Hyde *et al.*, 1994), apparent cognitive decline being attributable solely to the effects of ageing.

Conflicting studies have failed to replicate an abrupt decline in the wake of the first episode (Nopoulos *et al.*, 1994). Further decline has been demonstrated in elderly patients (Waddington *et al.*, 1995; Harvey *et al.*, 1997). A most interesting recent finding (Scully *et al.*, 1997) concerns elderly patients who became ill before the neuroleptic era. Duration of initially untreated psychosis was a strong predictor of current negative symptoms and general cognitive impairment; duration of treated psychosis was not related to any variable, even though on average it was twice as long. Executive function was severely impaired and unrelated to untreated psychosis: this may indicate that executive function is a very early, deeply ingrained phenomenon in schizophrenia. Finally, new research (Johnstone *et al.*, 1999) suggests that structurally the brains of learning disabled individuals with comorbid schizophrenia resemble (on MRI scan) those of schizophrenics: the conclusion was drawn that the learning disability was secondary to a schizophrenia process of very early onset, characterized by severe cognitive deficit.

Variability in the course of cognitive impairment perhaps represents nothing more than a function of neuroleptic treatment, in terms of historical availability, compliance and response, coupled with the usual considerations of illness severity and chronicity. It is, however, noteworthy that 11% of patients are neuropsychologically normal, yet have the same degree of positive symptoms as impaired patients (Palmer *et al.*, 1997).

Cognition and neuroleptics

The cognitive effects of neuroleptic drugs are important for both theoretical models of schizophrenia, and for patient outcome.

MODELS OF SCHIZOPHRENIA

The 'levels of explanation' model of schizophrenia (see above) is supported by studies relating alienation to self-monitoring (Frith and Done, 1989; Mlakar *et al.*, 1994).

Similarly, performance on executive tasks reflects failure to activate the prefrontal cortex (Weinberger *et al.*, 1986; Lewis *et al.*, 1992; Andreasen *et al.*, 1992). Therefore, manipulation of cognitive performance by drugs should reflect prior changes in brain physiology, and should bring about relevant symptomatic adjustments as a consequence.

An alternative model of schizophrenia (Carpenter *et al.*, 1989) sees cognitive impairment (here defined as attentional deficit and formal thought disorder) as a 'domain' of schizophrenia pathology, other 'domains' being other groups of symptoms, social and neurological abnormalities etc. Although there is quite a good argument for relating thought disorder to executive dysfunction (McGrath, 1991) there is an inherent problem in mixing up symptoms rated impressionistically with neuropsychological deficit measured psychometrically, within a cognitive domain. An implication of this model is that symptoms and cognition may not be causally related to each other either way, although of course they may co-exist or be related to prior variables associated with both: they are independent variables.

A third model (Van Praag *et al.*, 1990) relates 'dimensions' of behavioural psychopathology – inertia/action, aggression/anxiety and anhedonia/hedonia – to altered neurophysiology of the transmitter systems utilizing dopamine, serotonin and noradrenaline respectively. Since neuroleptics block receptors for these amines to varying degrees this model would predict fundamental effects of neuroleptics on specific behaviours that may enable cognitive change as a result.

COGNITION AND PATIENT OUTCOME

An increasing body of research indicates that cognitive deficits are substantial correlates of psychiatric disability (Kolb and Whishaw, 1983; Evans *et al.*, 1997) and psychosocial status (Kolakowska *et al.*, 1985; Perlick *et al.*, 1992; Goldberg and Gold, 1995). Indeed, a recent review (Green, 1996) found that verbal memory and certain aspects of executive performance – the Wisconsin Card Sorting Test (Breier *et al.*, 1991) and the Continuous Performance Task – were replicably associated with community functioning, social problem solving and skill acquisition. By contrast, psychotic symptoms were not correlated with functional outcome (Jonsson and Nyman, 1991; Green, 1996).

Because memory and executive functions are disproportionately compromised in schizophrenia, remediation of these deficits has the potential to overcome rate-limiting steps in rehabilitation and thus to improve outcome. Given the enormous costs of treatment and support for these patients, it is clear that any drug which remediates cognitive deficit – a 'smart drug' for schizophrenia – would have major advantages.

Why should neuroleptics modify cognition?

All neuroleptics come into the general category of cerebral depressant drugs which can impair performance on a wide variety of neuropsychological tests when given in acute doses. However, any theoretical account of their expected cognitive properties must rest upon bringing together what is known about their neurotransmitter receptor blocking attributes, coupled with available knowledge on the function of these neurotransmitter systems in both normal and pathological situations. The latter aspect has recently been reviewed (Robbins and Everitt, 1995).

Relevant neurotransmitter systems are monoaminergic (noradrenaline, dopamine), indoleaminergic (serotonin) and cholinergic (acetylcholine). All are components of the ascending reticular activating system, whose function is arousal. Arousal overall is the sum of interplay between these systems: each has its own tonic pattern of firing, and characteristic phasic responses to various environmental stimuli such as reinforcers and noxious events. The effect of increased firing of noradrenergic, cholinergic and possibly dopaminergic neurons is to sensitize cortical regions to sensory stimuli, i.e. increase signal-to-noise, increasing arousal. By contrast serotonin blunts evoked responses, a 'de-arousing' effect. Animal behavioural work suggests that the noradrenergic system is essential for controlled, rather than automatic, responses to stimuli. Rats whose noradrenergic systems have been chemically destroyed are impaired on a continuous performance task when they are distracted by bursts of noise or irregular stimulus presentation, which arouse them beyond normal test conditions. In humans, the noradrenergic system can be downgraded by clonidine, which impairs performance on both a continuous performance task and an executive task (Tower of London). This system seems to have a protective function of maintaining discriminability in stressful circumstances, sustaining alertness to the most salient stimuli.

The dopaminergic system appears to activate behaviour in response to cues that signal the availability of incentives or reinforcers. In humans, low doses of amphetamine cause impulsive responding to an attentional task, and dopamine depletion increases latency of responding, but neither affects accuracy of response. Behaviour activated by the dopamine system includes basic functions such as eating and drinking as well as newly learned responses. The mechanism seems to be the bringing about of a state of 'motor readiness' or response preparation, so that cues are acted upon quickly. In addition, work with Parkinsonian patients whose L-DOPA is withdrawn suggests that the dopaminergic system is involved in more complicated cognitive functions such as the planning and organizing of sequences of behaviour: the modulation of an 'executive network'.

Serotonin downregulation has been shown to improve memory, while upregulation can impair it. Massive serotonin depletion in animals leads to over-arousal in terms of behavioural disinhibition, manifested as impulsive responding on an attentional task.

The cholinergic system has a general arousing effect, enhancing stimulus processing in many cortical areas serving numerous cognitive functions. Depletion in experimental animals disrupts continuous performance task ability in the easiest paradigm. In humans, Alzheimer's disease, in which all cognitive functions are impaired, is characterized by marked widespread deficiencies in cholinergic function.

Several points are suggested by these data. Neuroleptics have the potential to modify cognition; its nature will depend on the pattern of receptor blockade produced; relatively pure blockers of one system may generate more predictable effects than 'dirty' drugs such as chlorpromazine. However, different tasks may well require different levels of arousal for optimum performance according to which functions are under scrutiny. Alteration of cognitive performance in patients, in whom there is reason to suspect intrinsic neurotransmitter derangement, may differ from that seen in controls. In conclusion, cognitive effects in patients will be very difficult to predict; it is hardly surprising that studies of neuroleptics and cognition have for the most part been empirical rather than theoretically driven.

In healthy volunteers, sedating neuroleptics such as thioridazine impair performance on tests of attention more than less sedating drugs such as haloperidol and remoxipride (Hindmarch and Tiplady, 1994). Impairment is particularly marked in time-limited tasks (Broadbent, 1984). Extrapyramidal side-effects (EPS) are especially relevant to motor paradigms. The anticholinergic effects of drugs added to control Parkinsonian side-effects, and similar properties intrinsic to some neuroleptics, have amnestic results in healthy volunteers (Plisken *et al.*, 1987; King, 1990). One study (Saletu *et al.*, 1987) found that the atypical neuroleptic clozapine, which has pronounced antimuscarinic activity, produced memory deficits in volunteers: their EEG became similar to that produced by anticholinergic antidepressant medication.

It has been suggested that dopaminergic and cholinergic agonists should be investigated as possible specific remedies for cognitive impairment (Davidson and Keefe, 1995), although this would risk antagonism of the antipsychotic effects of neuroleptics, and worsening of Parkinsonism.

Do conventional neuroleptics change cognitive performance?

GENERAL COGNITION

The efficacy of neuroleptics in controlling psychotic symptoms is such that neuroleptic treatment has become mandatory for schizophrenia. Perhaps the necessity for lifelong therapy, cerebral depressant effects and concerns about long-term side-effects, have combined to generate much work on the cognitive ramifications of neuroleptic treatment. EPS will inextricably confound therapeutic benefits to the mental component of motor tasks, but the literature contains many studies utilizing such tasks (*see* Medalia *et al.*, 1988). However, several recent, comprehensive and thorough reviews have all concluded that the chronic effects of conventional neuroleptics on a variety of cognitive functions in schizophrenic patients are small (Heaton and Crowley, 1981; Medalia *et al.*, 1988; Spohn and Strauss, 1989; Cassens *et al.*, 1990). One study (Seidman *et al.*, 1993), in which dose was reduced by 80–90% in chronic stable patients, found no deleterious or favourable effects on cognition or symptoms after 6 weeks.

It has been pointed out (Goldberg and Weinberger, 1996) that the majority of studies of the Continuous Performance Task indicate an advantage for medicated patients over those unmedicated or on placebo. However, this task has not been characterized in cognitive neuropsychological terms (for instance, does 'attention' comprise working memory, executive function, motor speed, some of each or something completely different?) and experimental paradigms have varied considerably between these studies. Therefore, the meaning of these results is unclear and there is little information on if or how improvements translate to symptomatic or functional improvement.

MEMORY

It is plausible that anticholinergic drugs and low potency neuroleptics with similar effects contribute to the failure of typical neuroleptics to improve memory performance in schizophrenia (Hagger *et al.*, 1993). However, one study (Tamlyn *et al.*, 1992) was unable to demonstrate any influence of anticholinergics on memory. There are no studies of typical or atypical neuroleptics and narrowly defined working memory, i.e., slave systems +/– central executive.

One study (Plisken *et al.*, 1987) suggested improvement in a measure of semantic memory thought to be sensitive to frontal dysfunction, on haloperidol: this improvement was lost when treatment was stopped, and regained when treatment was reinstituted.

EXECUTIVE FUNCTION

Executive function similarly seems impervious to typical neuroleptics. Tests examined include the Wisconsin Card Sorting Test (Cleghorn *et al.*, 1990; King and Henry, 1992; Seidman *et al.*, 1993), the Stroop Test (Medalia *et al.*, 1988), the Digit Symbol Test (Medalia *et al.*, 1988; Cassens *et al.*, 1990) and verbal fluency (Cleghorn *et al.*, 1990; Seidman *et al.*, 1993). Verbal fluency is distinguished by two further studies, one showing improvement on neuroleptics compared with placebo (Verdoux *et al.*, 1995) and the other showing deterioration (Bilder *et al.*, 1992a). Some improvement has been found on the Continuous Performance Task, which arguably includes some aspects of executive function (Spohn and Strauss, 1989; Pigache, 1993). Some very old work on maze tests, which require intact frontal function according to neurosurgical data (Riddle and Roberts, 1978), suggests deterioration on neuroleptic treatment independent of motor effects (Medalia *et al.*, 1988). A recent hypothesis (Goldberg, 1995) proposes that neuroleptics interfere with dopaminergic innervation from mesocortical systems to the frontal lobes, and that this compromises executive performance. This would predict that lower potency drugs may spare frontal function. However, there is no evidence for this: perhaps a 'floor' effect occurs, whereby executive performance is so compromised by integral frontal dysfunction that high potency drugs have little to take from it.

Possibility of practice effects in schizophrenia

There is a dearth of literature on practice effects in schizophrenia, possibly because so few instances of improvement have been reported. One study (Hagger *et al.*, 1993) tested 9 stable treatment resistant patients taking clozapine on 9 executive and memory measures, repeating the tests 3 weeks later; no evidence of practice effects was found. Another small study (Serper *et al.*, 1990) succeeded in normalizing dual task performance in a schizophrenic patients on medication, but not unmedicated patients, relative to healthy volunteers (group $ns = 4$) following intensive daily practice over 4 weeks. The task was a 'consistent-mapping procedure' i.e. capable of becoming 'automated' with such practice. Medication consisted of haloperidol plus an anticholinergic.

The point is made that this finding is unlikely to be generalizable to more complex tasks, including those encountered by patients in everyday life which it is not feasible to practise so intensively. However, where complex tasks cannot only be practised regularly but also broken down into components that can be automated, there may be some benefit of medication.

Atypical neuroleptics and cognitive performance

Atypical neuroleptics are defined as effective antipsychotics that do not cause catalepsy in rats (Kerwin, 1994). Several new atypical neuroleptics are now available, or about to become so. They aim to combine the same, or improved, antipsychotic efficacy as conventional neuroleptics with a milder side-effect profile, particularly for EPS. Pharmacologically, they fall into two categories: firstly those which preferentially block dopamine (D2) receptors or D2 and serotonin (5HT2) receptors, and secondly those which block multiple receptors without strong affinity for D2 (Gerlach and Peacock, 1995). The first group includes risperidone, ziprasidone and amisulpiride. Risperidone at recommended doses has few EPS (placebo level at 6 mg daily) and may be advantageous in the treatment of negative symptoms (Marder and Meibach, 1994). Amisulpiride has affinity for D2 and D3 receptors only: D3 affinity may confer a degree of limbic selectivity, resulting in placebo level EPS at low doses with a dose-related increase at higher doses. Efficacy for negative and depressive symptoms may be greater than for conventional drugs (*see* Mortimer, 1998). Ziprasidone is still undergoing clinical trials: it appears as effective as conventional treatments, and causes less EPS (Daniel *et al.*, 1997).

The second group of atypicals includes olanzapine, seroquel (quetiapine), zotepine and clozapine. Olanzapine (which is structurally very similar to clozapine) was launched in 1996, seroquel in 1998 and zotepine in 1999. Olanzapine induces EPS at placebo rates (Beasley *et al.*, 1996a, 1996b; Anonymous, 1997): antipsychotic efficacy is superior to conventional neuroleptics for negative symptoms (Beasley *et al.*, 1996b). Seroquel appears equivalent in efficacy to conventional antipsychotics (Rak and Arvanitis, 1997), EPS incidence being the same as placebo (Borison *et al.*, 1996; Goldstein and Arvanitis, 1997). Zotepine may cause less EPS than conventional neuroleptics, and has equivalent efficacy for positive symptoms (Raniwalla *et al.*, 1996) with possibly better efficacy for negative symptoms (Barnas *et al.*, 1992). Finally, clozapine is the original exemplar of atypical neuroleptics: evidence for its superior antipsychotic efficacy is not easy to refute (Mortimer, 1994a) and EPS are conspicuous by their absence.

The novel mechanisms of action of atypical neuroleptics may afford them the potential to have favourable effects on cognition. Despite the difficulties in predicting the results of their actions (particularly when multiple receptors are affected) it could be argued on purely 'common sense' grounds that a greater improvement in symptoms (particularly negative) could improve cognitive performance. From an amine perspective, drugs which block serotonin receptors may have the potential to improve memory, while poor dopamine blockers (of which clozapine is the most notable) may improve executive function.

Cognitive studies of atypical neuroleptics apart from clozapine are few in number, reflecting both the recent introduction of these drugs and the even more recent awareness of the importance of cognition in outcome. Many remain in abstract form: nearly all are relatively atheoretical in terms of any sophisticated appraisal of neuropsychological deficits in schizophrenia, and have been hampered by other methodological factors. These include the following:

- Small patient numbers
- Short (weeks) therapeutic trials
- Normal control group
- No control group
- Control group has single comparison drug in fixed dose
- Baseline data from acute phase of illness
- Baseline data from drug free patients
- Groups not adequately matched at baseline
- Polypharmacy
- No focus on cognitive functions known to be impaired in schizophrenia

This has led one influential reviewer (Lader, 1994) to conclude that the question of cognitive improvements resulting from clozapine treatment remains to be answered. However, a summary of studies of cognition in relation to clozapine, and newer atypicals, follows below.

CLOZAPINE

Classen and Laux (1988) were unable to establish differences in motor function, reaction time, tests of verbal/spatial ability and Stroop (executive) test scores, between parallel groups of patients on normal therapeutic doses of haloperidol, flupenthixol or clozapine. Numbers were small (total $n = 50$), patients were 'acute inpatients' matched on age and sex only; there was no baseline assessment, patients being tested once after just one week's treatment.

Meltzer (1992) studied 25 treatment-resistant patients who were tested on attention, working memory, executive function and semantic memory. Both measures of semantic memory had improved at 6 months, and these improvements were independent of changes in psychopathology. There was no comparison group. Goldberg *et al.* (1993b) studied 15 assorted psychotic patients up to 15 months after beginning clozapine treatment and found no change in a number of memory and executive tests, with deterioration in visual memory (attributed to clozapine's anticholinergic effects). The problems of small numbers and adjunctive medications were obvious drawbacks, but the long follow-up, within-subjects design and finding of a 40% decline in symptoms scores add some weight to these results. Hagger *et al.* (1993) studied 36 treatment-resistant patients for 6 months. There were significant improvements from baseline in semantic memory and attention. However, baseline data were obtained from patients in near drug-free states, and the confounding effects of high symptom scores on baseline performance could not be excluded. Other tests of memory and executive function were unchanged. Improvements in Brief Psychiatric Rating Scale were positive and overall scores were significant, but very small (3.5 and 2.3 points respectively). There was no comparison group.

Hoff *et al.* (1993), in a study of 17 patients after 12 weeks of clozapine treatment, confirmed Goldberg's finding of a decrement in visual memory. However, there were improvements in concentration, speed and spatial functions despite little symptomatic improvement. An apparent follow-up on an expanded sample of 30 patients, now said to be treatment-resistant (Hoff *et al.*, 1996) confirmed poor symptomatic improvement unrelated to cognitive change. Neuropsychological tests showed a pattern of improvement and deterioration, which was interpreted as improvements in mental and motor speed and concentration at the expense of executive function and short term visual memory: however, this rests on assumptions about the 'executive' nature of some tests (for instance, verbal fluency, which many would class as an executive test, improved).

Buchanan *et al.* (1994) studied 38 treatment-resistant patients randomized to fixed dose haloperidol or clozapine. The groups were well matched at baseline, and were reassessed after 10 weeks: no measure distinguished the groups. 33 patients either continued or commenced clozapine after 10 weeks, and were evaluated a third time after 1 year. There were significant improvements in semantic memory, executive function and trends to improvement in long-term memory. Memory measures were significantly correlated with quality of life. There was no comparison group for this extension of the study. Cognitive changes were not related to symptoms or side-effects.

Lee *et al.* (1994) investigated 48 non-treatment-resistant patients randomly assigned to clozapine or conventional neuroleptics for 12 months, plus 36 treatment-resistant patients treated with clozapine for 12 months. Test results were reported mostly as *P* values between groups, or described qualitatively for treatment-resistant patients. Improvement in the latter was limited to responders (>20% reduction in BPRS score) on tests of verbal fluency (which became normal), memory and attention. In the non-treatment-resistant group, Wisconsin Card Sorting Test performance (executive), verbal fluency, memory and attention improved on clozapine, while only memory improved on typical neuroleptics. The findings were attributed to a possible normalization of dopaminergic function on clozapine. This study was somewhat hampered by the unusually sketchy exposition of results in quantitative terms, and the superficial description of patients and their medication: for instance it was stated that EPS and tardive dyskinesia (*sic*) did not differ between groups at any time points, which seems most unlikely. The extent of EPS was not made clear, and the typically treated group were given unquantified anticholinergic treatment as required.

Grawe and Levander (1995) evaluated smooth pursuit eye movements and neuropsychological performance on a wide range of tests, in 29 patients on clozapine or conventional treatment and 22 controls. No differences attributable to treatment type were found. This was a cross-sectional study published as an abstract with no data on possible confounds.

Dye and Mortimer (1997) studied 29 stable but severely ill chronic patients, of whom 16 were started on clozapine and 13 remained on treatment-as-usual. Subsequently 5 clozapine and 7 treatment-as-usual patients had been followed up for 2 years. This was a naturalistic study: patients were not randomized and the groups were not well matched for motor disorder at baseline. However, all other measures were comparable. For the clozapine patients, significant improvements on an ecologically sound test of long-term memory and three measures of executive function were demonstrated, but these improvements did not take place convincingly until after 12 months. There were strong trends towards improvement on clozapine in tests of general cognition (Mini-Mental State (MMS), Middlesex Elderly Assessment of Mental State, current IQ estimate) frontal tests (verbal fluency) semantic memory (Graded Naming Test) and long-term memory (Recognition Memory Test) on course to become significant when all patients had completed 2-year assessments. At 6 months there were major improvements in positive and negative symptoms, and very large improvements in social competence and behaviour problems. The authors concluded that there was no evidence for cognition as the primary substrate for the action of clozapine, but that disproportionately affected cognitive functions with the greatest room for improvement indeed improved substantially as part of a general process of recovery.

Grace *et al.* (1996) administered clozapine and an enhanced psychosocial treatment programme to 31 treatment-resistant inpatients over 3 years. An extensive cognitive battery (13 tests incuding IQ sub-tests, short- and long-term memory tests and executive tests) was given. Performance improved on all tests and was significant in 15 of 21 sub-tests: 19 patients were discharged from hospital, There was no relationship of symptomatic to cognitive improvement.

Schall *et al.* (1996) studied 20 patients 6 months after starting to administer clozapine. Several measures of executive function were improved (significance not given) while P3b amplitude (an event-related potential measure) increased, implying an improvement of task-relevant stimulus processing with clozapine therapy.

Purdon *et al.* (1996) reported (in abstract form) particular gains on tests tapping 'frontal and temporal lobe functions' in 12 treatment-resistant patients after 8 weeks on clozapine.

Potkin *et al.* (1997) studied 27 patients using a double blind crossover methodology (phases 5–6 weeks long) comparing clozapine with haloperidol. Clozapine significantly improved performance on Trails B and verbal fluency (executive tests) and long-term verbal memory, and 'tended to increase performance on most measures compared to haloperidol'. Cognitive improvement was not due to symptom amelioration.

Stone *et al.* (1997) studied 12 patients on conventional treatment, who were then drug free for 2–6 weeks before starting on clozapine. After 12 weeks on clozapine there were 'modest trends' to improvement from baseline impairment, particularly for verbal memory.

RISPERIDONE

McGurk *et al.* (1996) examined spatial working memory in 30 patients before and after 4 weeks on risperidone or haloperidol under blind conditions. There was a trend for better performance on risperidone.

Berman *et al.* (1995a) studied 20 elderly schizophrenic patients on very reasonable doses of risperidone or haloperidol under double blind conditions for 'at least weeks'. Adjunctive medication was allowed, but kept stable. Risperidone treatment brought about significant improvements in the Boston Naming Test (semantic memory) and the MMS (general cognition). No other tests, nor symptoms, improved overall: it is not clear if the MMS improvement was sufficient to be clinically significant. The same authors reported regional cerebral blood flow results in a sub-set of 6 patients whose MMS and positive symptoms had both improved (Berman *et al.*, 1995b). Reductions in frontal and temporal perfusion were correlated with less positive symptoms, but not improved MMS. This study tends to suggest a dissociation between physiological, neuropsychological and symptom changes, at least when they may be attributable to risperidone treatment, and thus casts no light on the mechanisms involved. A final paper by most of the authors (Berman *et al.*, 1996) reported upon 10 elderly patients who took risperidone up to 6 mg daily for up to 6 weeks under open conditions. MMS scores improved by a mean of 3 points, taking the group mean into the normal range for this test. Several other cognitive measures covering executive function and memory also improved significantly, with the exception of the Trails Test and verbal fluency.

Rossi *et al.* (1995) studied 28 patients suffering from preponderant negative symptoms who were treated with open risperidone in very modest doses for 4 weeks. Significant improvements in negative symptoms were correlated with improvements on the Wisconsin Card Sorting Test, a measure of executive function involving set shifting and maintenance.

Williams *et al.* (1995) studied 20 stable schizophrenic outpatients switched to risperidone 3 mg twice daily dosage for 13 weeks. There was 'marked clinical improvement' on two executive tasks (Trails and Block Design) and a digit span measure of working memory: no means or P values were given.

Gallhofer *et al.* (1996a) studied 6 groups of 10 subjects: unmedicated first episode patients; unmedicated chronic patients with acute exacerbation; medicated first episode patients on risperidone (7) or zotepine (3); medicated chronic patients with acute exacerbation on risperidone (3), zotepine (4) or clozapine (3); healthy age matched controls for the first episode groups; and healthy age-matched controls for the chronic groups. All patients were of the paranoid sub-type, and unmedicated first episode did not mean drug-naïve. (There is no information on the duration of neuroleptic treatment.) Tests of working memory and executive function were given. Both executive tests (maze tests and a joystick task of choice reaction time) could be anticipated to be confounded by motor side-effect considerations, which were not assessed in this study. On digit span, medicated patients did better than the unmedicated groups on the forward but not on backward spans. On choice reaction time, unmedicated chronic patients did much worse than any of the other groups, which were similar for all degrees of test difficulty. On maze tests, chronic medicated patients did better than chronic unmedicated on time to completion.

The implications of this study are severely limited by small numbers, no comparison with conventional treatment, uninvestigated potential motor confounds and heterogeneity of atypical drug treatment: the only conclusion that may tentatively be drawn is that it is better to be on an atypical neuroleptic than nothing, particularly for chronic patients.

Stip and Lussier (1996) studied 13 patients switched to risperidone after 6 weeks and after 6 months. All but one patient were on procyclidine and some on quite large doses of conventional neuroleptics initially: 4 were still on procyclidine 6 months later despite taking 6 mg or less of risperidone per day. A variety of neuro-psychological tasks were administered. There were no improvements in working or long-term memory, but significant improvements on a reaction time task of alertness.

Wirshing _et al._ (1996) studied 22 treatment-refractory patients randomized for 8 weeks to risperidone or haloperidol under blind conditions. There were trends to superior performance on spatial working memory and the Trails Test of frontal function. The same authors reported an expanded study (McGurk _et al._, 1996) on 41 randomized patients treated under double blind conditions. Once again there were trends to better performance on risperidone (at 4 weeks): baseline performance was correlated with 3 executive tests. Anticholinergic medication had a detrimental effect on spatial working memory, and it may be assumed that more haloperidol than risperidone patients were on such antidotes, although this is not stated. The authors concluded that acetyl cholinergic neurotransmission supports a variety of cognitive functions thought to be carried out by the prefrontal cortex.

A further study (Simms _et al._, 1996) utilizing a test related to prefrontal/temporal network function, the Controlled Word Association Test (COWA), compared 6 patients on risperidone with 15 patients on assorted conventional treatments and 19 controls matched for age and premorbid IQ estimate. This cross-sectional investigation demonstrated marked and significantly poorer COWA performance by patients on conventional treatment compared to patients on risperidone (who were worse than controls but not significantly so).

CLOZAPINE COMPARED WITH RISPERIDONE

Gallhofer _et al._ (1996b) used maze tests (despite the aforementioned motor confounds) to compare haloperidol or fluphenazine with risperidone and clozapine. There were 16 patients in each group, plus a fourth group of unmedicated patients. As might be expected, conventional neuroleptic treated patients were slower to complete the mazes than those treated with clozapine or risperidone or unmedicated patients. Velocity, i.e. speed of moving the computer mouse used to trace the route, was significantly faster for those treated with clozapine than those on conventional neuroleptics but velocity on risperidone treatment was not significantly faster. There was no difference in velocity between conventionally treated and unmedicated patients. Clozapine- and risperidone-treated patients maintained better motor co-ordination than conventional neuroleptic-treated patients: the unmedicated patients appeared to resemble the atypical treated groups. It is claimed that both atypical drugs 'preserved patients' cognitive abilities better than conventional neuroleptics' and that frontal function was particularly well spared. However, there was surprisingly no assessment of motor side-effects in any of the groups and it is not possible to rule out that the differences were simply a result of greater EPS in the conventional treated group.

Goldman _et al._ (1996) reported a double-blind trial of clozapine or haldol in

22 treatment refractory patients, focusing on memory. At 29 weeks there was no improvement on clozapine, as opposed to a trend with depot haloperidol, but the clozapine patients were functioning better at entry suggesting a ceiling effect.

Daniel *et al.* (1996) compared clozapine and risperidone in 20 patients utilizing a 6 week crossover design. No consistent or significant pattern of differences on a number of neuropsychological tests emerged. However, a previous abstract of apparently the same study (Daniel *et al.* 1995) linked patients' preference for risperidone over clozapine to their subjective self-reports of cognitive impairment and sedation on clozapine compared to risperidone.

Lindenmayer *et al.* (1997) compared 28 treatment-resistant patients on risperidone or clozapine in an open 12 week study. Neither drug improved attention, memory or executive function: the dose of risperidone was higher than that recommended by the manufacturers (mean 11.6 mg).

Taylor *et al.* (1995) compared 12 patients on clozapine with 13 on risperidone, just prior to discharge from hospital. There were no differences in executive function, or short- or long-term memory. The groups did not differ in age, chronicity, IQ or symptom severity, but the drawbacks of small numbers and cross-sectional design, plus the lack of information on length of treatment, do not fully support the conclusion that differential effects on cognition are subtle or non-existent.

OLANZAPINE

Although the effect of olanzapine on cognition has not been systematically investigated, there is a suggestion that it resembles clozapine, at least in that it attenuates the diminished prepulse inhibition of startle reflex which occurs in response to phencyclidine treatment in rats. Conventional neuroleptics have no effect on diminished prepulse inhibition in these circumstances. Phencyclidine is an NMDA (glutamate receptor) antagonist: the finding that disruption of glutamatergic transmission impinges on a rat version of cognition (Verma and Moghaddam, 1995) taken with the observation that schizophrenic patients display diminished prepulse inhibition of startle reflex spontaneously (Tollefson, 1996) suggest that some of the cognitive deficits in schizophrenia may be secondary to an impairment of glutamatergic neurotransmission. This hypothesis is supported by a post-mortem study of genetic expression of the NR1 subunit of the glutamate receptor: there were strong correlations between a deficit in expression and two measures of dementia, plus a strong correlation between a deficit in expression and estimated premorbid IQ (Humphries *et al.*, 1996).

In a study of 14 healthy elderly volunteers, Beuzen *et al.* (1997) compared olanzapine, haloperidol and placebo in a three-way crossover design in which participants received each drug for 4 days separated by 16 days drug-free between treatments in random order and under double blind conditions. Attention, motor control and memory tests were given. On day 1, both active drugs impaired all tests but this quickly normalized in olanzapine treated patients and by day 4 performance was no different on olanzapine from on placebo: halperidol performance remained impaired.

QUETIAPINE

Fleming *et al.* (1997) tested 18 stable schizophrenic patients on open quetiapine after 10 days, and observed significant improvements in several tests generally ascribed to the prefrontal cortex. Such a rapid effect invites further investigation under blind conditions with a comparator.

Conclusions

That schizophrenia is a disorder in which cognitive impairments occur is hardly surprising given the evidence (albeit circumstantial) for derangement of neurotransmitter systems responsible for differentiated components of arousal. However, cognition is not affected by conventional neuroleptic treatment. Clozapine is slightly different: because clozapine is distinguished by poor blockade of D2 receptors, it and similar drugs may have a 'cognitive sparing' effect. This would be particularly relevant to executive tasks that require self-generated action given the apparent role of dopamine in response readiness, motor preparation and control of an 'executive network'. The anticholinergic effects of clozapine suggest some adverse effects on memory, but its ability to block serotonin receptors would suggest memory enhancement. These hypotheses are partly supported by some studies: clozapine is the only neuroleptic that has replicably improved aspects of cognition in schizophrenia. Although risperidone looks promising, and olanzapine and quetiapine potentially very interesting, the methodology of almost all studies leaves a great deal to be desired. The majority of studies reporting negative findings were either cross-sectional or employed treatment intervals of only a few weeks; it seems as a general impression that the longer treatment is continued the more chance of demonstrating an advantage for atypical over conventional treatment. This is in stark contrast to the effects of neuroleptics on symptoms, where (once again with the exception of clozapine) improvement is usually complete after a few weeks' treatment.

Much work remains to be done if studies of the type carried out to date can be harnessed to assess the validity of competing models of schizophrenia: there is, however, little if any support for 'levels of explanation' so far. More crucially, there is a notable lack of application to real life in this research, despite the emerging importance of cognitive function in patient outcome. What the clinician needs to know is, will my patients be any better on an expensive new drug than on their current medication? 'Better' to the clinician, and perhaps to the patient and carer, means issues like independence, the ability to look after oneself, to survive in society, to communicate and to master the kinds of community skills which we all take for granted. Very few studies address these issues. The current state of knowledge leaves us nowhere near an appraisal of the cognitive changes brought about by atypical drugs or the impact of these changes on outcome. This issue is of considerable importance and urgency given the increasing preponderance of care in the community and the relatively high cost of atypical drugs. Neither is the mechanism of cognitive change clear: we do not know if cognition is spared by atypicals simply because of their milder EPS profile, or because of different effects on dopaminergic transmission in regions outwith the basal ganglia, or if they can improve cognition by independent means. From a practical point of view this may seem unimportant, but an understanding of the mechanism at a neurophysiological level may facilitate the development of treatment strategies which could possibly bring about enhanced cognition – truly 'smart drugs' for schizophrenia which could lead to more reliable, better outcomes for more patients.

As yet there is no culture of addressing cognitive impairment as a specific target for treatment in schizophrenia: this can easily be understood given that proper intellectual assessment is not a routine part of clinical practice. Deficits are overlooked in favour of symptomatology, which psychiatrists are trained to elicit, but which unlike cognition may change rapidly despite relatively minor effects on outcome.

There is a clear need for further psychologically sophisticated, hypothesis-driven studies of atypical neuroleptics and cognition. Such studies should include proper assessment of the impact of cognitive improvement on outcome, and ideally a neuroimaging component. The development and funding of such research should be a high priority for pharmaceutical companies, national grant awarding bodies and health service research and development initiatives in the future.

References

Anonymous (1997) Patients considered 'at risk' and who should not receive serdolect. Pamphlet issued by Lundbeck Limited. Milton Keynes: Lundbeck Limited.

Andreasen, N.C., Resai, K., Alliger, R. *et al.* (1992) Hypofrontality in neuroleptic naive patients and in patients with chronic schizophrenia. *Arch Gen Psychiatry,* **49**, 943–58.

Barnas, C., Stuppack, C.H., Miller, C. *et al.* (1992) Zotepine in the treatment of schizophrenic patients with prevailingly negative symptoms, a double blind trial vs. haloperidol. *Int Clin Psychopharmacol,* **7**, 3–27.

Beasley, C.M., Sanger, T. and Satterlee, W. (1996a) Olanzapine versus placebo: results of a double-blind fixed dose olanzapine trial. *Psychopharmacology,* **124**, 159–67.

Beasley, C.M., Tollefson, G. and Tran, P. (1996b) Olanzapine versus haloperidol and placebo: acute phase results of the North American double-blind olanzapine trial. *Neuropsychopharmacology,* **14**, 111–24.

Berman, I., Merson, A., Allan, E., Alexis, C. and Losonczy, M. (1995a) Effect of risperidone on cognitive performance in elderly schizophrenic patients: a double-blind comparison study with haloperidol. *Psychopharmacol Bull,* **31**, 552(Abstr).

Berman, I., Merson, A., Allan, E., Sison, C.E. and Losonczy, M. (1995b) Regional cerebral blood flow changes associated with risperidone treatment in elderly schizophrenic patients. *Psychopharmacol Bull,* **31**, 553(Abstr).

Berman, I., Merson, A., Rachov-Pavlov, J., Allan, E., Davidson, M. and Losonczy, M. (1996) Risperidone in elderly schizophrenic patients. *Am J Geriatr Psychiatry,* **4**, 173–9.

Beuzen, J.N., Wesnes, K. and Wood, A. (1997) The effect of olanzapine on cognition and psychomotor function in healthy elderly volunteers. Poster presented at closed symposium, Eli Lilly, Indianapolis, USA, April 1997.

Bilder, R.M., Lieberman, J.A., Kim, Y., Alvir, J. and Reiter, G. (1992a) Methylphenidate and neuroleptic effects on oral word production in schizophrenia. *Neuropsychiat Neuropsychol Behav Neurol,* **5**, 262–71.

Bilder, R.M., Lipshutz-Broch, L., Reiter, G., Geisler, S.H., Mayerhoff, D.I. and Lieberman, J.A. (1992b) Intellectual deficits in first-episode schizophrenia: evidence for progressive deterioration? *Schizophr Bull,* **18**, 437–48.

Borison, R.L., Arvanitis, L.A. and Miller, B.G. (1996) A comparison of five fixed doses of 'Seroquel' (ICI 204,636) with haloperidol and placebo in patients with schizophrenia. *Schizophrenia Res,* **18**, 132.

Bornstein, H.A., Nasrallah, H.A., Olson, S.C., Coffman, J.A., Torello, M. and Schwarzkopf, S.B. (1990) Neuropsychological deficit in schizophrenic subtypes: paranoid, nonparanoid and schizoaffective subgroups. *Psychiat Res,* **31**, 15–24.

Breier, A., Schreiber, J.L. and Dyer, J. (1991) National Institute of Mental Health longitudinal study of chronic schizophrenia. *Arch Gen Psychiatry,* **48**, 239–46.

Broadbent, D.E. (1984) Performance and its measurement. *Br J Clin Pharmacol,* **18**, 5S–9S.

Buchanan, R.W., Holstein, C. and Breier, A. (1994) The comparative efficacy and long-term effect of clozapine treatment on neuropsychological test performance. *Biol Psychiatry,* **36**, 717–25.

Cantor-Graae, E., Warkentin, S. and Nilsson, A. (1995) Neuropsychological assessment of schizophrenic patients during a psychotic episode: persistent cognitive deficit? *Acta Psychiat Scand,* **91**, 283–8.

Carpenter, W.T., Buchanan, J.R. and Buchanan, R.W. (1989) Domains of psychopathology relevant to the study of etiology and treatment in schizophrenia. In: S.C. Schulz and C.A. Tamminga (eds.) *Schizophrenia: scientific progress.* Oxford: Oxford University Press, 13–22.

Cassens, G., Inglis, A.K., Appelbaum, P.S. and Gotheil, T.G. (1990) Neuroleptics: effects on neuropsychological function in chronic schizophrenic patients. *Schizophr Bull,* **16**, 477–99.

Chaikelson, J.S. and Schwartzman, A.E. (1983) Cognitive changes with ageing in schizophrenia. *J Clin Psychol,* **39**, 25–30.

Clare, L., McKenna, P.J., Mortimer, A.M. and Baddeley, A.D. (1993) Memory in schizophrenia: what is impaired and what is preserved? *Neuropsychologia,* **31**, 1225–41.

Clark, O. and O'Carroll, R. (1997) An examination of the relationship between executive function and rehabilitation status in schizophrenia. *Neuropsychological Rehabilitation* (in press).

Classen, W. and Laux, G. (1988) Sensorimotor and cognitive performance of schizophrenic patients treated with haloperodol, flupenthixol, or clozapine. *Pharmacopsychiatry,* **21**, 295–7.

Cleghorn, J.M., Kaplan, R.D., Szechtman, B., Szetchman, H. and Brown, G.M. (1990) Neuroleptic drug effects on cognitive function in schizophrenia. *Schizophr Res,* **3**, 211–19.

Cutting, J. (1985) *The psychology of schizophrenia.* Edinburgh: Churchill Livingstone.

Daniel, D.G., Goldberg, T.E., Lubick, L.J., Weinberger, D.R., Kleinman, J.E., Pickar, D. and Williams, T.S. (1995) Self-reported cognitive impairment predicts patient preference between risperidone and clozapine. *Schizophr Res,* **15**, 147–8.(Abstr).

Daniel, D.G., Goldberg, T.E., Weinberger, D.R. *et al.* (1996) Different side effect profiles of risperidone and clozapine in 20 outpatients with schizophrenia or schizoaffective disorder: a pilot study. *Am J Psychiatry,* **153**, 417–19.

Daniel, D.G., Reeves, K. and Harrigan, E.P. (1997) The efficacy and safety of ziprasidone 80 mg/day and 160 mg/day in schizophrenia and schizoaffective disorder. *Schizophr Res,* **24**, 204(Abstr).

Davidson, M. and Haroutunian, V. (1996) Cognitive impairment in geriatric schizophrenic patients: clinical and postmortem characterization. In: F.E. Bloom and D.J. Kupfer, (eds.), *Psychopharmacology: the fourth generation of progress.* New York: Raven Press.

Davidson, M. and Keefe, R.S.E. (1995) Cognitive impairment as a target for pharmacological treatment in schizophrenia. *Schizophr Res,* **17**, 123–9.

Duffy, L. and O'Carroll, R. (1994) Memory impairment in schizophrenia – a comparison with that observed in the alcoholic Korsakoff syndrome. *Psychol Med,* **24**, 155–66.

Dye, S. and Mortimer, A.M. (1997) Remediation of neuropsychological impairments with clozapine. *Schizophr Res,* **24**, 187.

Evans, J.J., Chua, S.E., McKenna, P.J. and Wilson, B.A. (1997) Assessment of the dysexecutive syndrome in schizophrenia. *Psychol Med*, **27**, 635–46.

Fleming, K., Kalali, A., Yeh, C., Vargo, D.L., Thyrum, P.T. and Potkin, S.G. (1997) The neurocognitive effects of quetiapine ('seroquel', ICI 204,636). *Schizophr Res*, **24**, 197(Abstr).

Frith, C.D., Leary, J., Cahill, C. and Johnstone, E.C. (1991) Performance on psychological tests: demographic and clinical correlates of the results of these tests. *Br J Psychiatry*, **159**, 26–9.

Frith, C.D. (1992) *The cognitive neuropsychology of schizophrenia*. Hove, Sussex: Lawrence Erlbaum.

Frith, C.D. and Done, D.J. (1989) Experiences of alien control in schizophrenia reflect a disorder in the central monitoring of action. *Psychol Med*, **19**, 359–63.

Gallhofer, B., Bauer, U., Gruppe, H., Kreiger, S. and Lis, S. (1996a) First episode schizophrenia: the importance of compliance and preserving cognitive function. *J Prac Psychol Behav Health*, **2**, 16S-24S.

Gallhofer, B., Bauer, U., Lis, S., Kreiger, S. and Gruppe, H. (1996b) Cognitive dysfunction in schizophrenia: comparison of treatment with atypical antipsychotic agents and conventional neuroleptic drugs. *Eur Neuropsychopharmacol*, **6**, 13–20.

Garety, P. (1991) Reasoning and delusions. *Br J Psychiatry*, **159**, 14–18.

Gerlach, J. and Peacock, L. (1995) New antipsychotics: the present status. *Int Clin Psychopharmacol*, **10**, 39–48.

Goldberg, E. (1995) Akinesia, tardive dysmentia, and frontal lobe disorders in schizophrenia. *Schizophr Bul*, **11**, 255–63.

Goldberg, T.E., Weinberger, D.R., Berman, K.F., Plisken, N. and Podd, M.H. (1987) Further evidence for dementia of prefrontal type in schizophrenia? *Arch Gen Psychiatry*, **44**, 1008–14.

Goldberg, T.E., Karson, C.N. and Leleszi, P.J. (1988) Intellectual impairment in adolescent psychosis: a controlled psychometric study. *Schizophr Res*, **1**, 261–6.

Goldberg, T.E., Gold, J.M., Greenberg, R. *et al.* (1993a) Contrasts between patients with affective disorders and patients with schizophrenia on a neuropsychological test battery. *Am J Psychiatry*, **150**, 1355–62.

Goldberg, T.E., Greenberg, R.D. and Griffin, S.J. (1993b) The effect of clozapine on cognition and psychiatric symptoms in patients with schizophrenia. *Br J Psychiatry*, **162**, 43–8.

Goldberg, T.E., Hyde, T.M., Kleinman, J.E. and Weinberger, D.R. (1993c) Course of schizophrenia: neuropsychological evidence for a static encephalopathy. *Schizophr Bull*, **19**, 797–804.

Goldberg, T.E., Torrey, E.F., Gold, J.M., Ragland, J.D., Bigelow, L.D. and Weinberger, D.R. (1993d) Learning and memory in monozygotic twins discordant for schizophrenia. *Psychol Med*, **23**, 71–85.

Goldberg, T.E. and Gold, J.M. (1995) Neurocognitive deficits in schizophrenia. In: S.R. Hirsch and D.R. Weinberger (eds.) *Schizophrenia*. London: Blackwell Science.

Goldberg, T.E. and Weinberger, D.R. (1995) Thought disorder, working memory and attention: interrelationships and the effects of neuroleptic medications. *Int Clin Psychopharmacol*, **10**, 99–104.

Goldberg, T.E. and Weinberger, D.R. (1996) Effects of neuroleptic medications on the cognition of patients with schizophrenia: a review of recent studies. *J Clin Psychiatry*, **57** (Suppl. 9) 62–5.

Goldman, R.S., Bates, J.A., Bilder, R.M., Kane, J., Schooler, N. and Marder, S. (1996) The effects of clozapine and haldol on memory functioning in treatment refractory schizophrenics. *Schizophr Res*, **18** (Special Issue), 221 (Abstr).

Goldstein, G. and Zubin, J. (1990) Neuropsychological differences between young and old schizophrenics with and without associated neuropsychological dysfunction. *Schizophr Res*, **3**, 117–26.

Goldstein, J.M. and Arvanitis, L.A. (1997) 'Seroquel' (quetiapine) is not associated with dose-related extrapyramidal symptoms: overview of clinical results. *Schizophr Res,* **24**, 198(Abstr).

Grawe, R.W. and Levander, S. (1995) Smooth pursuit eye movements and neuropsychological impairments in schizophrenia. *Acta Psychiat Scand,* **92**, 108–14.

Grace, J., Bellus, S.R., Raulin, M.L. *et al.* (1996) Long-term impact of clozapine and psychosocial treatment on psychiatric symptoms and cognitive functioning. *Psychiat Services,* **47** (1), 41–5.

Green, M.F. (1996) What are the functional consequence of neurocognitive deficits in schizophrenia? *Am J Psychiatry,* **153**, 321–30.

Hagger, C., Buckley, P., Kenny, J.T., Friedman, L., Ubogy, D. and Meltzer, H.Y. (1993) Improvement in cognitive functions and psychiatric symptoms in treatment-refractory schizophrenic patients receiving clozapine. *Biol Psychiatry,* **34**, 702–12.

Harvey, P.D., Powchik, P., Mohs, R.C. and Davidson, M. (1997) Cognitive decline in geriatric schizophrenic patients. *Schizophr Res,* **24**, 107(Abstr).

Heaton, R.K., Baade, L.E. and Johnson, K.L. (1978) Neuropsychological test patterns associated with psychiatric disorders in adults. *Psycholog Bull,* **85**, 146–62.

Heaton, R.K., Paulsen, J.S. and McAdams, L.A. (1994) Neuropsychological deficits in schizophrenics. Relationship to age, chronicity and dementia. *Arch Gen Psychiatry,* **51**, 469–76.

Heaton, R.K. and Crowley, T.J. (1981) Effects of psychiatric disorders and their somatic treatments on neuropsychological test results. In: S.D. Filskov and T.J. Boll (eds.), *Handbook of clinical neuropsychology.* New York: John Wiley & Sons.

Heaton, R.K. and Drexler, M. (1987) Clinical neuropsychological findings in schizophrenia and ageing. In: N.E. Miller and G.D. Cohen, (eds.) *Schizophrenia and ageing.* New York: Guilford Press, 145–61.

Hindmarch, I. and Tiplady, B. (1994) A comparison of the psychometric effects of remoxipride with those of haloperidol, thioridazine and lorazepam in healthy volunteers. *Human Psychopharmacol,* **9**, 43–9.

Hoff, A.L., Riordan, H., O'Donnell, D.W., Morris, L. and De Lisi, L.E. (1992) Neuropsychological functioning of first-episode schizophreniform patients. *Am J Psychiatry,* **149**, 898–903.

Hoff, A.L., Faustman, W.O., Wieneke, M., Espinoza, S., Costa, M., Wolkowitz, O. and Csernansky, J.G. (1996) The effects of clozapine on symptom reduction, neurocognitive function, and clinical management in treatment-refractory state hospital schizophrenic patients. *Neuropsychopharmacology,* **15** (4), 361–69.

Hoff A.L., Wieneke M. and DeVilliers D. (1993) Effects of clozapine on cognitive function. *New Research Program and Abstracts of the 146th Annual Meeting of the American Psychaitric Association, May 25, 1993.* San Francisco, California: American Psychiatric Association. Abstract NR254, p. 124.

Humphries, C.R., Mortimer, A.M., Hirsch, S.R. and de Belleroche, J. (1996) N-methyl-D-aspartate receptor mRNA correlation with antemortem cognitive impairment in schizophrenia. *Neuroreport* **7**, 2051–5.

Hutton, S.B., Puri, B.K., Duncan, L., Robbins, T.W., Barnes, T.R.E. and Joyce, E.M. (1997) Memory and executive function in first-episode schizophrenia. *Schizophr Res,* **24**, 109 (Abst).

Hyde, T.M., Nawroz, S. and Goldberg, T.E. (1994) Is there cognitive decline in schizophrenia? A cross-sectional study. *Br J Psychiatry,* **164**, 494–500.

Johnstone, E.C., Best, J.J.K., Doody, G.A., Owens, D.G.C. and Sanderson, T. (1999) A controlled study of the neuroanatomy of comorbid schizophrenia and learning disbility. *Schizophr Res,* **36**, 201 (Abstr).

Jonsson, H. and Nyman, A.K. (1991) Predicting long-term outcome in schizophrenia. *Acta Psychiat Scand,* **83**, 342–6.

Kerwin, R.W. (1994) The new atypical antipsychotics. *Br J Psychiatry,* **164**, 141–8.

King, D.J. (1990) The effect of neuroleptics on cognitive and psychomotor function. *Br J Psychiatry,* **157**, 799–811.

King, D.J. and Henry, G. (1992) The effect of neuroleptics on cognitive and psychomotor function, a preliminary study in healthy volunteers. *Br J Psychiatry,* **160**, 647–53.

Klonoff, H., Fibiger, C.H. and Hutton, G.H. (1970) Neuropsychological patterns in chronic schizophrenia. *J Nervous Mental Dis,* **150**, 291–300.

Kolakowska, T., Williams, A.O. and Ardern, M. (1985) Schizophrenia with good and poor outcome. I: early clinical features, response to neuroleptics and signs of organic dysfunction. *Br J Psychiatry,* **146**, 229–46.

Kolb, B. and Whishaw, I.Q. (1983) Performance of schizophrenic patients on tests sensitive to right or left frontal, temporal or parietal function in neurological patients. *J Nervous Mental Dis,* **171**, 435–43.

Lader, M. (1994) Does clozaril improve the cognitive and psychomotor function of schizophrenic patients? *Clozaril Newslett,* **8**, 1–3.

Lee, M.A., Thompson, P.A. and Meltzer, H.Y. (1994) Effects of clozapine on cognitive function in schizophrenia. *J Clin Psychiatry,* **55**, 82–7.

Lewis, S.W., Ford, R.A., Syed, G.M., Reveley, A.M. and Toone, B.K. (1992) A controlled study of 99mTc-HMPAO single photon emission imaging in chronic schizophrenia. *Psychol Med,* **22**, 27–35.

Liddle, P.F. and Crow, T.J. (1984) Age disorientation in chronic schizophrenia is associated with global intellectual impairment. *Br J Psychiatry,* **144**, 193–9.

Liddle, P.F. and Morris, D.L. (1991) Schizophrenic syndromes and frontal lobe performance. *Br J Psychiatry,* **158**, 340–5.

Lindenmayer, J., Iskander, A., Park, M., Smith, R., Apergi, F. and Czobor, P. (1997) Psychological and neuropsychological profile of clozapine vs. risperidone in refractory schizophrenics. *Schizophr Res,* **24**, 195 (Abstr).

Lubin, A., Gieseking, C.F. and Williams, H.L. (1962) Direct measurement of cognitive deficit in schiozphrenia. *J Consult Psychology,* **26**, 139–43.

Marder, S.R. and Meibach, R.C. (1994) Risperidone in the treatment of schizophrenia. *Am J Psychiatry,* **151**, 825–35.

McGrath, J. (1991) Ordering thoughts on thought disorder. *Br J Psychiatry,* **158**, 307–16.

McGurk, S.R., Green, M.F., Wirshing, W.C., Ames, D., Marshall, B.D. and Marder, S.R. (1996) The effects of risperidone vs. haloperidol on spatial working memory in treatment-resistant schizophrenia. *Biol Psychiatry,* **39**, 571 (Abstr).

McGurk, S.R., Green, M.F., Wirshing, W.C., Ames, D., Marshall, B.D., Marder, S.R. Effects of risperidone on spatial working memory. Paper presented at the 148th Annual Meeting of the American Psychiatric Association, Miami, Florida USA, May 20–25, 1995.

McKay, A.P., McKenna, P.J., Bentham, P., Mortimer, A.M., Holbery, A. and Hodges, J.R. (1996) Semantic memory is impaired in schizophrenia. *Biol Psychiatry,* **39**, 929–37.

McKenna, P.J. (1994) The psychology and neuropsychology of schizophrenia. In: *Schizophrenia and related syndromes.* Oxford: Oxford Medical Publications, 164–95.

Medalia, A., Gold, J.M. and Merriam, A. (1988) The effects of neuroleptics on neuropsychological test results of schizophrenics. *Arch Clin Neuropsychol,* **3**, 249–71.

Meltzer, H.Y. (1992) Dimensions of outcome with clozapine. *Br J Psychiatry,* **160**, 46–53.

Miller, R. (1989) Schizophrenia as a progressive disorder: relations to EEG, CT, neuropathological and other evidence. *Prog Neurobiol,* **33**, 17–44.

Mlakar, J., Jensterle, J. and Frith, C.D. (1994) Central monitoring deficiency and schizophrenic symptoms. *Psychol Med,* **24**, 557–64.

Morice, R. (1990) Cognitive inflexibility and pre-frontal dysfunction in schizophrenia and mania. *Br J Psychiatry,* **157**, 50–4.

Mortimer, A.M. (1994a) Newer and older antipsychotics. A comparative review of appropriate use. *CNS Drugs,* 2, 381–96.

Mortimer, A.M. (1994b) Levels of explanation - symptoms, neuropsychological deficit and morphological abnormalities in schizophrenia. *Br J Psychiatry,* 24, 541–5.

Mortimer, A.M., Corridan, B.J., Rudge, S.D.E. *et al.* (1995) Thought, speech and language disorder and semantic memory in schizophrenia. In: A.C.P. Sims, (ed.) *Speech and language disorders in psychiatry.* London: Gaskell, 70–80.

Mortimer, A.M., Bentham, P., McKay, A.P. *et al.* (1997) Delusions in schizophrenia: a phenomenological and psychological exploration. *Cogn Neuropsychiatry,* 1, 289–303.

Mortimer A.M. (1998) Atypical antipsychotic drugs and their place in therapy. *Progr Neurol Psychiatry,* 2, 41–5.

Nelson, H.E., Pantelis, C., Carruthers, K., Speller, J., Baxendale, S. and Barnes, T.R.E. (1990) Cognitive functioning and symptomatology in chronic schizophrenia. *Psychol Med,* 20, 357–65.

Nopoulos, P., Flashman, L. and Flaum, M. (1994) Stability of cognitive functioning early in the course of schizophrenia. *Schizophr Res,* 14, 29–37.

Offord, D.R. and Cross, L.A. (1971) Adult schizophrenia with scholastic failure or low IQ in childhood: a preliminary report. *Arch Gen Psychiatry,* 24, 431–6.

Owens, D.G.C. and Johnstone, E.C. (1980) The disabilities of chronic schizophrenia: their nature and the factors contributing to their development. *Br J Psychiatry,* 136, 384–93.

Palmer, B.W., Heaton, R.K., Paulsen, J.S. *et al.* (1997) Is it possible to be schizophrenic yet neuropsychologically normal? *Neuropsychology,* 11, 437–46.

Payne, R.W. (1993) Cognitive abnormalities. In: H.J. Eysenck, (ed.) *Handbook of abnormal psychology.* London: Pitman, 420–83.

Perlick, D., Mattis, S. and Stastny, P. (1992) Neuropsychological discriminators of long-term inpatient or outpatient status in chronic schizophrenia. *J Neuropsychiat Clin Neurosci,* 4, 428–34.

Pigache, R.M. (1993) The clinical relevance of an auditory attention task (PAT) in a longitudinal study of chronic schizophrenia, with placebo substitution for chlopromazine. *Schizophr Res,* 10, 39–50.

Plisken, N., Raz, N., Raz, S. and Weinberger, D.R. (1987) Neuroleptic withdrawal and deterioration of verbal fluency in schizophrenia: a preliminary report. *J Clin Exp Neuropsychol,* 9, 62.

Potkin, S.G., Fleming, K., Telford, J., Costa, J., Gulasekaram, B. and Jin, Y. (1997) Clozapine enhances neurocognition and clinical symptoms more than standard neuroleptics. *Schizophr Res,* 24, 188 (Abstr).

Purdon, S.E., Jones, B., Labelle, A. and Boulay, L. (1996) Neuropsychological change to clozapine. *Schizophr Res,* 18 (Special Issue), 221 (Abstr).

Purohit, D.P., Davidson, M., Perl, D.P. *et al.* (1993) Severe cognitive impairment in elderly schizophrenic patients: a clinicopathological study. *Biol Psychiatry,* 33, 255–60.

Rak, I.W. and Arvanitis, L.A. (1997) Overall view of the efficacy of 'seroquel' (quetiapine). *Schizophr Res,* 24, 199 (Abstr).

Raniwalla, J., Tweed, J.A., Dollfus, S. and Petit, M. (1996) A comparison of an atypical (zotepine) and classical (haloperidol) antipsychotic in patients with acute exacerbation of schizophrenia. *Schizophr Res,* 18, 133.

Riddle, M. and Roberts, A.H. (1978) Psychosurgery and the Porteus Maze Tests. *Archives of Gen Psychiatry,* 35, 493–7.

Robbins, T.W. and Everitt, B.J. (1995) Arousal systems and attention. In: M. Gazzaniga, (ed.) *The cognitive neurosciences.* Cambridge, MA: MIT Press, 703–20.

Rossi, A., Mancini, F., Marola, V. *et al.* (1995) Risperidone, negative symptoms and cognitive deficit in schizophrenia: an open study. *Eur Neuropsychopharmacol,* 5, 351 (Abstr).

Rubensztein, J., McKenna, P.J. and Baddeley, A.D. (1997) Working memory is spared in schizophrenia. *Schizophr Res,* **24**, 136 (Abstr).

Saletu, B., Grunberger, J. and Linzmayer, L. (1987) Comparative placebo-controlled pharmacodynamic studies with zotepine and clozapine utilizing pharmaco-EEG and psychometry. *Pharmacopsychiatry,* **20**, 12–27.

Saykin, A.J., Shtasel, D.L., Gur, R.E. *et al.* (1994) Neuropsychological deficits in neuroleptic naive patients with first-episode schizophrenia. *Arch Gen Psychiatry,* **51**, 124–31.

Schall, U., Catts, S.V., Chaturvedi, S., Redenbach, J., Karayanidis, F. and Ward, P.B. (1996) The effect of clozapine therapy on psychometric and event-related potential (ERP) measures on cognitive dysfunction in schizophrenia. *Schizophr Res,* **15**, 164 (Abstr).

Scully, P.J., Coakley, G., Kinsella, A., Waddington, J.L. (1997) Negative symptom severity and general cognitive impairment increase with duration of initially untreated psychosis. *Schizophr Res,* **24**, 22 (Abstr).

Seidman, L.J., Pepple, J.R. and Faraone, S.V. (1993) Neuropsychological performance in chronic schizophrenia in response to neuroleptic dose reduction. *Biol Psychiatry,* **33**, 575–84.

Serper, M.R., Bergman, R.L. and Harvey, P.D. (1990) Medication may be required for the development of automatic information processing in schizophrenia. *Psychiat Res,* **32**, 281–8.

Shallice, T., Burgess, P. and Frith, C.D. (1991) Can the neuropsychological case study be applied to schizophrenia? *Psychol Med,* **21**, 661–73.

Simms, M.G.N., Patel, J.K., Dursun, S.M., Burke, J.G. and Reveley, M.A. (1996) The effects of risperidone and typical antipsychotic drug treatments on the functional state of the prefrontal-temporal-cortical network in schizophrenia. *J Psychopharmacology,* **10**, 4(Abstr).

Smith, A. (1960) Mental deterioration in chronic schizophrenia. *J Nervous Mental Dis,* **139**, 479–87.

Spohn, H.E. and Strauss, M.E. (1989) Relation of neuroleptic and anticholinergic medications to cognitive functions in schizophrenia. *J Abnormal Psychol,* **98**, 367–80.

Stip, E. and Lussier, I. (1996) The effect of risperidone on cognition in patients with schizophrenia. *Can J Psychiatry,* **41**, 35–40.

Stone, W.S., Seidman, L.J., Kalinowski, A. *et al.* (1997) Effects of clozapine on cognitive functions in treatment-refractory schizophrenia. *Schizophr Res,* **24**, 188–9 (Abstr).

Sweeney, J.A., Haas, G.L., Keilp, J.G. and Long, M. (1991) Evaluation of neuropsychological function after acute episodes of schizophrenia: one-year followup study. *Psychiatr Res,* **38**, 63–76.

Tamlyn, D., McKenna, P.J., Mortimer, A.M., Lund, C.E., Hammond, S. and Baddeley, A.D. (1992) Memory impairment in schizophrenia: its extent, affiliations and neuropsychological character. *Psychol Med,* **22**, 101–15.

Taylor, S.F., Goldman, R., Smet, I.C. and Tandon, R. (1995) Atypical neuroleptics and neuropsychological function in schizophrenia. *Biol Psychiatry,* **37**, 675 (Abstr).

Tollefson, G.D. (1996) Cognitive function in schizophrenic patients. *J Clin Psychiatry,* **57**, 31–9.

Van Praag, H.M., Asnis, G.M. and Kahn, R.S. (1990) Monoamines and abnormal behaviour. A multi-aminergic perspective. *Br J Psychiatry,* **157**, 723–34.

Verdoux, H., Magnin, E. and Bourgeois, M. (1995) Neuroleptic effects on neuropsychological test performance in schizophrenia. *Schizophr Res.* **14**, 133–9.

Verma, A. and Moghaddam, B. (1995) The role of excitatory amino acids in prefrontal cortex function as assessed by spatial delayed alternation performance in rats: modulation by dopamine. Presented at the 34th annual meeting of the American College of Neuropharmacology: December 1–15, 1995: San Juan, Puerto Rico.

Waddington, J.L., Youssef, H.A. and Scully, P.J. (1995) The evolution of negative symptoms and cognitive (executive) dysfunction over the course of illness in schizophrenia. Presented at the 34th annual meeting of the American College of Neuropsychopharmacology; December 11–15, 1995; San Juan, Puerto Rico.

Walker, E. and Lewine, R.J. (1990) Prediction of adult-onset schizophrenia from childhood home movies of the patients. *Am J Psychiatry,* **147**, 1052–6.

Weinberger, D.R., Berman, K.F. and Zec, R.F. (1986) Physiological dysfunction of dorsolateral prefrontal cortex in schizophrenia. *Arch Gen Psychiatry,* **43**, 114–24.

Williams, R., Dickson, R., Caliguiri, M., Mahoney, A., Dalby, J.T. and Yuen, O. (1995) Improvement in tardive dyskinesia, laterality of TD and cognition in schizophrenic patients changed from typical neuroleptics to risperidone. *Eur Neuropsychopharmacol,* **5**, 352 (Abstr).

Wirshing, W.C., Ames, D., Marder, S.R., Marshall, B.D., Green, M. and McGurk, S.R. (1996) Risperidone versus haloperidol in treatment resistant schizophrenia: preliminary results. *Schizophr Res,* **18**, 130 (Abstr).

CHAPTER 10

Movement disorders associated with antipsychotic drugs: clinical and biological implications

THOMAS R.E. BARNES AND SEAN A. SPENCE

Introduction

Pharmacological therapies have transformed the clinical management of schizophrenia, facilitating a full recovery in some and a return to community living for the majority of patients. Nevertheless, the therapeutic benefits of antipsychotic drugs are gained at the expense of a range of unwanted effects (Edwards and Barnes, 1993). Disturbances of movement are perhaps the most obvious, and have long been a defining feature of antipsychotic drug therapy. The term 'neurolepsis' was initially used to describe the behavioural syndrome induced in patients by the early neuroleptic agents (which would now be regarded as conventional antipsychotic drugs, in contrast to the newer, so-called atypical drugs). Such neurolepsis comprised psychomotor slowing, emotional flattening and affective indifference (Stahl, 1996). These effects may be mediated predominantly via the dopaminergic systems of the brain (see below).

The movement disorders associated with antipsychotic drugs can be classified into acute extrapyramidal side-effects and tardive syndromes. The acute extrapyramidal side-effects consist of three distinct syndromes: parkinsonism, akathisia and acute dystonia. The tardive syndromes are tardive dyskinesia, tardive dystonia and chronic akathisia, which are generally associated with prolonged use of antipsychotic medication. The acute extrapyramidal side-effects can have a profound clinical impact: the associated adverse subjective experience may have a negative influence on treatment compliance, and may confound the clinical assessment of the mental state because of symptomatic overlap between movement disorder and the psychotic illness for which the antipsychotic drugs are prescribed. Furthermore, anticholinergic drugs, prescribed to prevent or treat extrapyramidal side-effects, produce their own unwanted effects.

Tardive dyskinesia is the most common motor problem in patients receiving long-term antipsychotic treatment. Like the acute movement disorders, tardive dyskinesia has a clinical impact, with physical disability related directly to the specific movements, and a social handicap related to the nature of the movements. While abnormalities of movement similar to tardive dyskinesia were described in schizophrenia prior to the advent of antipsychotic drugs, their frequency is certainly increased by such treatment. Questions that remain pertinent are: first, whether a given patient developing dyskinetic movements while receiving antipsychotic medication would have developed such movements inevitably, as part of their schizophrenic illness; and second, whether such movements are the direct, iatrogenic effect of exposure to the drug therapy, or whether their emergence is, in fact, the manifestation of an interaction between an abnormally predisposed locomotor system, age-related cerebral changes, and an adverse environmental factor – the drug.

This chapter will address the acute and chronic motor disorders associated with antipsychotic drugs, their objective and subjective clinical features, implications for clinical practice, and theories regarding their pathophysiology.

Parkinsonism

Signs of parkinsonism may develop within days of starting antipsychotic medication. The reported prevalence of the disorder ranges widely, with figures around 40% being cited for parkinsonism severe enough to warrant treatment (Tonda and Guthrie 1994). The most obvious clinical features are muscle rigidity, tremor and bradykinesia. The muscle rigidity can be tested by passive movement of the limbs, when two types of stiffness can be detected. The first is 'lead pipe' rigidity, where the resistance is steady and even. The second is 'cogwheel' rigidity, where resistance is overcome in a ratchet-like fashion: the result of tremor being superimposed upon the stretch reflex. Other characteristic signs are impaired postural reflexes, seborrhoea of the face, excessive salivation and failure to habituate to the glabellar tap.

CONFOUNDING CLINICAL ASSESSMENT

The manifestations of the bradykinetic component of parkinsonism include diminished arm swing and narrow gait, a lack of facial expression, paucity of gesture, mask-like facies and slow monotonous speech (Rifkin *et al.*, 1975). These features overlap with the symptoms of retarded depression and negative symptoms of schizophrenia and can confound clinical assessment of the mental state (Lavin and Rifkin, 1992; Barnes and McPhillips, 1995). Particularly, the objective assessment of blunting of affect during an interview will be based on factors such as the patient's use of expressive gestures, modulation of the voice and facial mobility and expressiveness, all of which can be compromised by the presence of bradykinesia.

SUBJECTIVE BURDEN

There is an associated subjective burden with drug-induced parkinsonism. Bradykinesia is accompanied by decreased and slowed mental activity (Casey, 1995). Some patients complain of depressive feelings while others report apathy, listlessness and a sense of sedation; experiences that can be socially disabling (Lavin and Rifkin, 1992; De Leon and Simpson, 1992).

The influence of the experience of parkinsonism on compliance remains uncertain (Hummer and Fleischhacker, 1996). Equivocal findings in this area may partly reflect that measures of parkinsonism tend to reflect rigidity and tremor rather than the subjective, psychological effects, which may be more relevant to compliance.

PATHOPHYSIOLOGY

In common with the other movement disorders described in this chapter, neuroleptic-induced parkinsonism is at least partly attributable to a disorder of dopamine neurotransmission. It is therefore necessary to address some aspects of the functioning of the normal dopaminergic system.

There are four dopaminergic pathways in the brain (Table 10.1) of which the most relevant to the control of movement is the nigrostriatal pathway. The latter projects to the basal ganglia where it exerts a facilitatory tone. The basal ganglia are important for two reasons in this context: (i) they are directly involved in the control of movement, and (ii) they play a role in the modulation of frontal lobe function via their participation in parallel circuits (or 'loops') which project specifically to discrete regions of the thalamus and back to the frontal lobe (Table 10.2). These loops

Table 10.1. Dopamine pathways

DA pathway	Arises from:	Projects to:
Mesolimbic	Midbrain VTA	N. accumbens
Nigrostriatal	Substantia nigra	Basal ganglia
Mesocortical	Midbrain VTA	Limbic cortex
Tuberoinfundibular	Hypothalamus	Anterior pituitary

Abbreviations: DA = dopamine; VTA = ventral tegmental area; N. accumbens = nucleus accumbens.

Table 10.2. Basal ganglia-thalamocortical circuits

Circuit	Components	Cortical projection
Motor	SMA, PMC, SMC; PUT; GP/SNr; Thalamus	SMA
Occulomotor	FEF, DLPFC; PPC; CAUD; GP/SNr; Thalamus	FEF
Dorsolateral prefrontal	DLPFC, PPC, PMC; CAUD; GP/SNr; Thalamus	DLPFC
Lateral orbitofrontal	LOFC, STG, ITG, AC; CAUD; GP/SNr; Thalamus	LOFC
Anterior cingulate	AC, H, EC, STG, ITG; Vent S; GP/SNr; Thalamus	AC

A much simplified account of the five circuits described by Alexander *et al.* (1986). It should be noted that there is further subdivision into discrete projections within caudate, pallidum, substantia nigra, and thalamic nuclei (*see* reference).
Abbreviations: SMA = supplementary motor area; PMC = premotor cortex; SMC = sensorimotor cortex; PUT = putamen; GP/SNr = globus pallidum / substantia nigra; FEF = frontal eye fields; DLPFC = dorsolateral prefrontal cortex; PPC = posterior parietal cortex; CAUD = caudate nucleus; LOFC = lateral orbitofrontal cortex; STG & ITG = superior & inferior temporal gyrus respectively; AC = anterior cingulate; H = hippocampus; EC = entorrhinal cortex; Vent S = ventral striatum.

are 'funnelled' through the basal ganglia (Alexander *et al.*, 1986) and are described as neuroanatomically discrete and separate circuits, although some connection between them may be postulated. Thus, disordered functioning of this region, whether 'organic' or pharmacological in aetiology, may not only affect the execution of movement directly but may also exert indirect effects upon other brain regions, and their instantiated cognitive functions.

The role of the basal ganglia in motor control has been reviewed by Brooks (1995). Studies of non-human primates and of normal humans using functional neuroimaging suggest that the basal ganglia play a role in movement preparation and execution. The lentiform nuclei are activated equally by imagined or executed movement, varying rates and forces of movement, and by both self-selected and stereotypic movement sequences. Similarly, they are equally active during old and newly learned motor routines. Thus, Brooks (1995) concludes that their role lies in facilitating movements which have already been selected by 'higher' cortical centres, specifically the supplementary motor area (SMA) and dorsolateral prefrontal cortex (DLPFC). Neurons in the SMA fire on average around 270 ms before striatal cells when self-initiated actions are performed, and the time for neuronal impulses to travel around the 'motor' basal ganglia loop has been estimated to be of the order of 35 ms. Information could be transported between the SMA and striatum many times before the onset of a movement (Romo and Schultz, 1992), and thus the basal ganglia may optimize the motor programme 'in some fashion before it is transmitted to the motor cortex and the spinal cord' for execution (Brooks, 1995).

The anatomy of the local circuits found within the basal ganglia themselves is complex. The output from putamen or caudate to globus pallidus interna (GPi; Table 10.2) comprises both a direct and an indirect pathway, the latter via the globus pallidus externa and subthalamic nucleus. The net effect of a loss of nigrostriatal dopamine is excessive inhibitory output (via GPi) of the ventral thalamus, with subsequent excessive inhibition of SMA and DLPFC (*see* Table 10.2). The observable results are the rigidity and bradykinesia seen in the parkinsonian patient. Lesioning GPi or the subthalamic nucleus has predictable consequences upon movement output, that is, disinhibition. PET activation studies in Parkinson's disease have demonstrated hypo-activation of SMA, DLPFC, and anterior cingulate cortex, with preservation of primary motor, and lateral premotor cortical activity (Brooks, 1995). Jenkins and colleagues (1992) have demonstrated recovery of SMA activity when patients with Parkinson's disease are 'switched on' using the dopaminergic agent apomorphine. Thus, it can be seen that loss of dopaminergic function in the basal ganglia may lead to potentially reversible hypo-activation of distant cortical regions receiving thalamic 'loop' projections (Table 10.2).

The parkinsonian features seen with antipsychotic drugs are thought to be due to antagonism of postsynaptic dopamine (D2) receptors in the basal ganglia, causing a functional block to dopamine released by the nigrostriatal system (Marsden and Jenner, 1980). This contention is supported by the predictive relationship existing between the effects of antipsychotics on the dopaminergic systems of rodents and their clinical effects in psychotic human patients. The potential of individual neuroleptics to produce extrapyramidal side-effects in the latter correlates with their propensity for inducing 'depolarization block' (inactivation) of dopamine neuron firing in the *nigrostriatal* system of the former (Grace *et al.*, 1997). However, their therapeutic effect upon psychotic symptoms correlates with their ability to induce such depolarization block in the rodent *mesolimbic* system (Table 10.1). Therefore the therapeutic and acute extrapyramidal effects of antipsychotic drugs are, potentially, neurobiologically distinct. This offers the possibility of developing limbic-selective drugs that are effective antipsychotics with a low risk of inducing acute motor disturbance.

In this regard, it is of interest that clozapine, which has a low liability for acute extrapyramidal side-effects, preferentially blocks the mesolimbic dopamine system, but has a minimal effect, in terms of depolarization block, in the nigrostriatal system (Grace *et al.*, 1997). The nature of this difference at a pharmacological level may relate to relative affinities for D2 and D4 dopamine receptors. For example, new drugs such as clozapine and seroquel have low affinities for D2 but higher affinities for D4 receptors, relative to conventional antipsychotics. Whereas the D2 subtype is expressed in subcortical regions (the dopamine neurons of the substantia nigra and ventral tegmental area, the enkephalin neurons of the neostriatum and nucleus accumbens, and the neurotensin neurons of the latter), the D4 sub-type is expressed in frontal cortex (and the granule and pyramidal cells of the hippocampus, and the granule cells of the cerebellum) (Sokoloff and Schwartz, 1996). The possible limitations of animal studies, with respect to human extrapyramidal side-effects, have been reviewed elsewhere by Waddington (1992).

The role of anticholinergics in the treatment of parkinsonism may be understood in terms of the normal balance which pertains between dopaminergic and cholinergic systems at the level of the basal ganglia. Nigrostriatal dopamine neurons exert a (postsynaptic) inhibition of cholinergic neurons in this region. Blockade (or loss) of dopaminergic receptors, for example by antipsychotic drugs, leads to a functional excess of cholinergic activity, associated with parkinsonism. Such an excess is most marked when the antipsychotic involved does not possess inherent anticholinergic activity, but this may be compensated by the use of antimuscarinic agents (Stahl, 1996).

Although the account given above has focused upon the role of dopaminergic blockade in neuroleptic-induced parkinsonism, full consideration of the evidence must leave open the possible participation of other neurotransmitter systems. Although dopaminergic receptor blockade occurs within hours of such treatment being initiated, parkinsonism may not occur for days or weeks. Also, patients may develop tolerance to such side-effects over time. Hence, adaptation may be occurring both initially and over time within other neurotransmitter systems.

TREATMENT

Anticholinergic agents

The mainstay of treatment for antipsychotic-induced parkinsonism is the antimuscarinic agent, e.g. procyclidine or orphenadrine. The condition tends to improve spontaneously, so that after three months or so, anticholinergics may be successfully discontinued in a proportion of patients. The need for continued administration of anticholinergic treatment should be regularly tested by withdrawal, and monitoring of any emergent parkinsonism.

There is a continuing controversy regarding the routine use of anticholinergic drugs prophylactically for extrapyramidal side-effects (Barnes and McPhillips, 1996). The arguments mounted in favour include a potential positive influence on compliance related to a reduced incidence and severity of extrapyramidal side-effects, and the avoidance of any difficulties of clinical assessment related to the need to distinguish clinically between the psychological components of these side-effects and symptoms of the psychiatric illness being treated. Those arguing against such a strategy point out that many patients administered antipsychotic medication, particularly in modest dosage, will not develop extrapyramidal side-effects. Thus, the routine use of anticholinergic agents results in a proportion of patients receiving these drugs unnecessarily. Furthermore, these agents are associated with a host of unwanted effects, including dry mouth, constipation, tachycardia, urinary hesitancy or retention, and blurred vision with paralysis of accommodation and pupillary dilatation. The emerging consensus seems to be against prophylactic use, except for the prevention of acute dystonia in those at risk (Barnes, 1990a; Lavin and Rifkin, 1992). A statement by the WHO (1990) on this issue did not recommend prophylaxis, and concluded that these agents should only be prescribed when parkinsonism develops, although the clinician might first wish to try other treatment strategies, such as reducing the dosage of the antipsychotic drug or switching to one with a lower liability for extrapyramidal side-effects.

New (atypical) antipsychotic drugs

The double-blind, six-week study of Kane *et al.* (1988), which established clozapine as a superior antipsychotic for severely ill patients with neuroleptic-unresponsive schizophrenia, also indicated that the drug had a low liability for extrapyramidal side-effects. Parkinsonism ratings were significantly lower in the clozapine-treated patients compared with the other treatment group, receiving a combination of chlorpromazine and benztropine. The lower incidence of parkinsonian features such as bradykinesia and tremor with clozapine, compared with conventional antipsychotic treatment, has been confirmed in the longer term (Gerlach and Peacock, 1995; Kurz *et al.*, 1995).

Analysis of the double-blind, randomized, controlled trials of risperidone suggests that, within the optimum daily dose range of 4 to 8 mg, risperidone is associated with fewer extrapyramidal problems than conventional antipsychotics, and significantly less use of concomitant antiparkinsonian medication (Song, 1997). However, the data from these clinical studies suggest that the propensity of risperidone to cause extrapyramidal side-effects is dose-dependent; at higher doses the advantage appears to be lost (Chouinard *et al.*, 1993; Marder and Meibach, 1994).

A key study examining the efficacy and safety of sertindole in schizophrenia compared three doses of the drug (12, 20 and 24 mg/day) with three doses of haloperidol (4, 8 and 16 mg/day) and placebo (Daniel *et al.*, 1996; Tamminga *et al.*, 1997). All doses of sertindole produced improvement in parkinsonism ratings, while all doses of haloperidol produced a worsening. Parkinsonism ratings in the three sertindole-treated groups were significantly lower than for all the haloperidol-treated groups, and not significantly different from placebo. Similar findings have been reported for olanzapine. Beasley *et al.* (1996) compared three dosage ranges of olanzapine (5 ± 2.5 mg/day; 10 ± 2.5 mg/day; or 15 ± 2.5 mg/day) with a single haloperidol dose range (15 ± 2.5 mg/day) and placebo. Parkinsonism ratings improved in the placebo group and all three olanzapine dosage groups, but worsened significantly in the patients receiving haloperidol. This was despite the use of significantly more antiparkinsonian medication in the haloperidol group compared with all the other treatment groups.

Clinical studies with amisulpride suggest that while it causes extrapyramidal side-effects on a dose-related basis, the relative liability for such problems within the recommended dose range is lower than with conventional antipsychotics (Coukell *et al.*, 1996; Freeman, 1997). The incidence of parkinsonism with low dosage, 300 mg/day or less, would seem to be similar to that seen with placebo (Boyer *et al.*, 1995; Loo *et al.*, 1997). A lower risk of parkinsonism has also been demonstrated for quetiapine (Small *et al.*, 1997; Arvanitis *et al.*, 1997; Peuskens and Link, 1997).

Dystonia

ACUTE DYSTONIA

Acute dystonia presents as sustained muscle contraction causing contorting, twisting, repetitive movements or abnormal postures. The reactions usually occur dramatically, often within 24 to 48 hours of starting antipsychotic treatment, or following abrupt increase in dosage. Less commonly, they are seen as withdrawal phenomena, sometimes occurring 24 hours or more after antipsychotic drug withdrawal. The muscles of the head and neck are most commonly affected, with sustained contraction of the masticatory muscles (trismus), forceful, sustained eye closure (blepharospasm), facial grimacing, oculogyric spasm (characterized by a brief, fixed stare, followed by upward and lateral rotation of the eyes so that only the sclera are visible), dysarthria and dysphagia (due to glossopharyngeal contractions) and torticollis. The extremities may be involved with dystonic limb and trunk movements and bizarre postures and gait (Rupniak *et al.*, 1986; Burke, 1992). Less obvious forms of dystonia, such as tightness of the neck and shoulder muscles or mild lingual or laryngeal dystonia causing difficulties in speaking or chewing, may go unnoticed.

Acute dystonia has been considered as a relatively rare problem, with a reported incidence of around 2–5% in patients receiving antipsychotic drugs (Ayd, 1961; Rupniak *et al.*, 1986). However, the reported frequency seems to have increased recently, with Addonzio and Alexopoulos (1988) finding the much higher overall figure of 25%. Children and young adults are the most vulnerable to develop acute dystonia, with the highest prevalence being found in young men (Swett, 1975).

TARDIVE DYSTONIA

While acute dystonia has long been recognized as a distinct side-effect, the occurrence of persistent dystonia in association with long-term neuroleptic treatment has only been widely acknowledged for a decade or so. Diagnosis is based on the following criteria: the presence of chronic dystonia; exposure to antipsychotic drugs prior to the onset; exclusion of other known causes of dystonia; and a negative family history for dystonia (Burke *et al.*, 1982). The reported prevalence is around 1.5 to 4% (Drug and Therapeutics Bulletin, 1988; Raja, 1995). The condition is apparently identical to idiopathic torsion dystonia or secondary dystonia associated with conditions such as Huntington's disease, Wilson's disease, Meige's syndrome and Hallevorden–Spatz disease associated with abnormal iron deposition in the basal ganglia (Marsden and Quinn, 1990; Burke, 1992). The condition also needs to be distinguished from tardive dyskinesia, with which it may co-exist (Barnes, 1990b; Wojcik *et al.*, 1991). Patients with tardive dyskinesia will commonly have dystonic movements as part of the clinical picture.

There are no established risk factors for the development of tardive dystonia, although the majority of cases are under 50 years of age and most are male (Wojcik *et al.*, 1991). Even the appearance of acute dystonia does not appear to predict the later development of the disorder (Drugs and Therapeutics Bulletin, 1988). Clinically, the features are not clearly distinguishable from acute dystonia except by their duration. As with acute dystonia, the muscles of the face and neck are characteristically involved, with blepharospasm, torticollis, retrocollis and oculogyric spasm being common presentations. The trunk and limbs are less commonly involved (Kang *et al.*, 1986),

SUBJECTIVE BURDEN/ADVERSE CLINICAL CONSEQUENCES

The muscle spasms of acute dystonia may last from a few seconds to several hours. They are often painful and distressing, being a source of concern for both patients and carers. However, serious adverse clinical consequences would seem to be rare. Dislocation of the jaw has occurred on occasion, and other reports suggest that laryngeal dystonia can lead to respiratory distress and asphyxia, while acute dystonia of respiratory muscles can cause life-threatening dyspnoea (Flaherty and Lahmeyer, 1978; Modestin *et al.*, 1981; Brown and Kocsis, 1984).

Tardive dystonia rarely remits, and can be a substantial handicap. Persistent dystonia of the trunk and limbs can cause severe physical and social disability, with problems such as neck hyperextension, arching of the back, excessive lordosis and axial dystonia (Burke, 1992) Constant blepharospasm can produce functional blindness. Laryngospasm and spasmodic dysphonia are rare presentations of tardive dystonia, and can interfere with speech, reducing it to a hoarse whisper or guttural inflections (Davis *et al.*, 1988).

CONFOUNDING OF CLINICAL ASSESSMENT

Dystonic reactions have been misdiagnosed as dissociative phenomena, malingering, seizures, tetany or posturing associated with psychosis (Klein *et al.*, 1980). They may even be misinterpreted on occasion as an attempt by the patient to persuade the doctor to prescribe anticholinergic agents.

PATHOPHYSIOLOGY

Marsden and Jenner (1980) proposed that drug-induced dystonia was due to a compensatory increase in dopamine synthesis and presynaptic release, provoked by the acute administration of antipsychotic drugs, in addition to an acute hypersensitivity of (upregulated) postsynaptic dopamine receptors. Decreases in the concentration of antipsychotic drug present in the synapse, following a single dose or between doses, might lead to the supersensitive receptor being exposed to increased dopamine. According to this theory, dystonic reactions are a consequence of the enhanced dopamine response.

Such an explanation would account for these events arising transiently, early on in treatment, and as withdrawal phenomena later on. Thus, they may be conceptualized as hyper-dopaminergic phenomena as opposed to the hypo-dopaminergic state of parkinsonism. However, such an account is incongruent with the clinically efficacious treatment of dystonic reactions using anticholinergic agents. The use of the latter suggests that a disturbance of dopaminergic–cholinergic balance might be the relevant mechanism, and is supported by reports of successful treatment using apomorphine and methylphenidate (Fann, 1966; Gessa *et al.*, 1972).

The neurobiology of neuroleptic-induced dystonia awaits explication, but some clues to its functional anatomy may be gained by considering the idiopathic dystonias. Indeed, the latter may be especially relevant in view of the propensity (recognized before the introduction of neuroleptics) of schizophrenic patients to develop movement disorders. The majority of idiopathic dystonias are now considered to be dominantly inherited, with 40% penetrance and variable clinical manifestations (Brooks, 1995). When patients exhibiting such phenomena are studied using functional imaging, characteristic abnormalities of cortical activation are seen. Specifically, these are hyper-activation of the SMA and DLPFC areas (Playford *et al.*, 1992; Ceballos-Baumann *et al.*, 1995; *see* Brooks, 1995, for review). On this basis, the profiles of patients with dystonia appear to be the opposite of parkinsonian patients, who exhibit hypo-activation of these same cortical regions.

The cause of such hyper-activation in higher motor planning areas is likely to be an excessive thalamic input (Table 10.2). This in turn may be due to a striatal dysfunction. Dystonic movements may be induced in primates by the injection of muscimol, a GABA agonist, into the globus pallidus, disrupting inhibitory input into the ventral thalamus. Also, intra-operative recordings taken from dystonic patients have shown abnormal overactivity of posterior thalamus (Brooks, 1995). Hence, thalamic hyper-activation may in turn lead to hyper-activation of cortical projection areas.

Whether such findings are of relevance to schizophrenic patients experiencing dystonic symptoms on medication awaits further study. Clearly there is still an unresolved issue as to the effectiveness of anticholinergics in treating both parkinsonism and dystonia secondary to neuroleptic exposure.

TREATMENT

Anticholinergic agents are an effective treatment for acute dystonic reactions, and may be given intramuscularly or intravenously for rapid relief. Further, a preventive value for these agents has been demonstrated (Winslow *et al.*, 1986). Some clinicians routinely use anticholinergics prophylactically, while others would limit such use to the patients they judge to be at greater risk of developing dystonia. The condition is more likely in younger patients, those administered high initial doses of antipsychotic medication, and those with a history of acute dystonia with previous antipsychotic treatment (Rupniak *et al.*, 1986). As the majority of acute dystonic reactions occur in the first few days of antipsychotic treatment, the period of prophylactic therapy is short and the dose of anticholinergic medication can start to be reduced after a week.

There are no consistently effective treatments for tardive dystonia, and the first consideration should be whether to reduce or withdraw the offending antipsychotic medication. Even after discontinuation, the condition may persist for years without remission (Wojcik *et al.*, 1991; Burke, 1992). Specific treatments that have been tried include the dopamine depleters, tetrabenazine and reserpine, and anticholinergic drugs, although the response to the latter may be only partial, and is generally less impressive than that seen with acute dystonia. Switching from a conventional antipsychotic to clozapine has been reported to produce dramatic improvement in tardive dystonia in several case reports (Factor and Friedman, 1997), and controlled trials are warranted. If the condition fails to respond to such treatment, local botulinum toxin injections may provide symptomatic relief, where the affected muscle groups can be targeted (Jankovic and Schwartz, 1990; Anderson *et al.*, 1992).

Akathisia

ACUTE AKATHISIA

Acute akathisia is a dose-related syndrome of motor restlessness with a reported incidence of 20–30% (Braude *et al.*, 1983; Gibb and Lees, 1986). The condition differs from the other acute extrapyramidal side-effects in that, first, the observed movements are not dyskinetic in nature but more akin to normal, restless movement. Second, it may be conceived of as essentially an abnormal subjective state, as the signs of motor restlessness are not invariably present, particularly in milder cases. At a certain threshold of intensity, the subjective feelings of restlessness drive a patient to agitated, restless movement in an attempt to gain subjective relief.

Clinical diagnosis is based on the patient's report of a subjective sense of inner restlessness, mental unease, irritability or dysphoria (Braude *et al.*, 1983; Marder *et al.*, 1991). This experience, which can be intense, is associated with feeling unable to keep still or an irresistible urge to move, particularly when they are required to stand, sit or lie still. Also relevant are characteristic patterns of restless movement, such as rocking from foot to foot and walking on the spot when standing, and shuffling or tramping of feet and swinging one leg on the other when sitting (Braude *et al.*, 1983; Barnes and Braude, 1985). Rocking of the trunk and fidgety movements of the upper limbs may be seen, although they are less typical (Walters *et al.*, 1989). In severe cases, patients are unable to stand without walking or pacing. Characteristic accelerometric readings of relatively low frequency have also been reported in patients with akathisia (Braude *et al.*, 1984; Rapoport *et al.*, 1994).

CHRONIC AKATHISIA

The term chronic akathisia is applied if restlessness has persisted for more than six months after the last increment in antipsychotic medication (Barnes and Braude, 1985). Prevalence figures of around a third have been reported for samples of schizophrenic outpatients receiving maintenance neuroleptic treatment (Barnes and Braude, 1985; Gibb and Lees, 1986; Kahn *et al.*, 1992). In an epidemiological sample of schizophrenic patients in Scotland the prevalence was 18% (McCreadie *et al.*, 1992). The condition may develop after a relatively short exposure to antipsychotic medication (Stein and Pohlman, 1987; Burke *et al.*, 1989).

In some cases, akathisia may appear when maintenance antipsychotic drug treatment is withdrawn or the dose reduced (Fahn, 1983; Braude and Barnes, 1983). This has been termed tardive or withdrawal akathisia on the basis that it shares the pharmacological characteristics of tardive dyskinesia, that is, it seems to be exacerbated or provoked by antipsychotic drug reduction or withdrawal and improved at least temporarily when medication is restarted or the dose increased.

Some patients may exhibit the repetitive, complex movements characteristic of acute akathisia but deny any subjective symptoms. This condition has been called pseudoakathisia, and has a reported prevalence of 5-18% (McCreadie *et al.*, 1992, Halstead *et al.*, 1994). It is more likely to be seen in older patients, and in those with negative schizophrenic symptoms, and commonly co-exists with orofacial dyskinesia (Barnes and Braude 1985; Brown and White, 1991). It has been suggested that pseudoakathisia represents an end-stage, where the subjective sense of restlessness has faded. Another possibility is that patients with akathisia learn to avoid the dysphoric experience by adopting a regime of repetitive movement. Another view is that it is a variant of tardive dyskinesia (Munetz, 1986). However, according to this notion, non-dyskinetic limb movements are being included within the tardive dyskinesia syndrome which traditionally comprises dyskinetic, choreiform movements.

RISK FACTORS

Risk factors for akathisia include no previous exposure to antipsychotic drugs, and a rapid increase in drug dose (Braude *et al.*, 1983; Sachdev, 1995). Curiously, intravenous administration of haloperidol to healthy volunteers, which would seem to combine these risk factors, seems to be free of the adverse subjective effects typical of akathisia (Williams *et al.*, 1997).

SUBJECTIVE BURDEN

The subjective experience of akathisia can be intense and distressing. Halstead *et al.* (1994) found that the characteristic feelings of inner restlessness were associated with symptoms of anxiety and dysphoria (tension, panic, irritability and impatience). This discomfort may become intolerable, and may contribute to aggressive behaviour or impulsive suicidal or homicidal behaviour although this remains a controversial area (Van Putten and Marder, 1987; Ayd, 1988; Sachdev, 1995). It has been suggested that akathisia may be responsible for aggravating the psychosis being treated (Van Putten *et al.*, 1987, Duncan *et al.*, 1989) and that patients developing akathisia show a poorer response to antipsychotic medication (Levinson *et al.*, 1990). Such findings may be partly explained by the symptoms of akathisia, particularly the dysphoria, contributing to the ratings of residual psychopathology used to measure treatment outcome (Newcomer *et al.*, 1994).

CLINICAL IMPLICATIONS

Effect on compliance with medication

Subjective dysphoria has been implicated as a cause of poor compliance with acute antipsychotic treatment (Van Putten and Marder, 1987). However, while the condition has been linked with inpatient non-compliance, the relationship has not been convincing in outpatient studies (Weiden *et al.*, 1991; Buchanan, 1992).

Risk factor for tardive dyskinesia

Crane (1972) was the first to suggest that tardive dyskinesia was more likely to develop in patients who had exhibited acute extrapyramidal side-effects, akathisia or parkinsonism, than in those who had not. There is now evidence from prospective studies of tardive dyskinesia to support this view (Umbricht and Kane, 1996a).

PATHOPHYSIOLOGY

As with parkinsonism and dystonia, the pathophysiological theory for akathisia put forward by Marsden and Jenner in 1980 remains credible. They proposed that the underlying mechanism was dopamine receptor blockade in the mesocortical dopamine system (Table 10.1). Animal experiments suggest that the prefrontal systems may regulate subcortical dopamine activity, exerting an inhibitory effect on spontaneous locomotor behaviour (Iversen, 1971; Tassin *et al.*, 1978). Lesions of the prefrontal cortex can lead to increased activity in the subcortical dopamine systems, with an associated increase in locomotor activity (Pycock *et al.*, 1980). Lesions in the ventral tegmental area (VTA) in rats reduce frontal cortex dopamine concentrations, and significantly increase locomotion (Tassin *et al.*, 1978). Marsden and Jenner (1980) suggested that the equivalent result in humans, following mesocortical dopamine receptor blockade by antipsychotic drugs, is the psychological and motor syndrome of akathisia.

The evidence for the above theory has been reviewed critically by Sachdev (1995). He points out that it derives from studies of the relevant dopamine projections in rodents, which are different in some critical respects from those in primates. There is also a problem with regard to the modelling of the subjective distress component of akathisia in animals. Further, other measures tend to suggest that these animals are hypo-aroused despite being hyper-active, which would appear to be in conflict with the human experience of akathisia.

There is a great deal of clinical evidence linking akathisia with so-called high-potency antipsychotic drugs and their use in high doses. PET studies of normal controls and schizophrenic patients given antipsychotics suggest a link between the extent of dopamine receptor occupancy in the striatum and the development of extrapyramidal side-effects, including akathisia (Farde, 1992; Farde *et al.*, 1992). Akathisia was found to correlate with the time course of occupancy of D2 striatal receptors by neuroleptics, although similar results were also obtained with a highly selective D1 antagonist. One interpretation of these data is that blockade of either D1 or D2 receptors may be necessary for akathisia to occur. D1 receptors are expressed in both the neostriatum and nucleus accumbens, on Substance P and neurotensin neurons (Sokoloff and Schwartz, 1996).

The role of dopaminergic systems in akathisia seems clear, although not restricted to a particular dopamine receptor or pathway. Many drugs may produce akathisia and most that do so, such as selective serotonin reuptake inhibitor (SSRI) antidepressants and calcium channel blockers, exert some influence over dopaminergic function. Hence, antidepressants which enhance serotonergic function affect dopaminergic systems, possibly because serotonin inhibits dopamine in the VTA (Lipinski *et al.*, 1988). Calcium channel antagonists may also cause akathisia and affect dopaminergic function: in some cases by competing for D2 receptor occupancy, and in others by inhibiting dopamine release (*see* Sachdev, 1995).

The response of akathisia to beta-adrenergic receptor blockers such as propranolol has led to explanatory notions involving noradrenergic pathways. De Keyser *et al.* (1987) suggested that akathisia may be an expression of an over-active beta-adrenergic state, possibly generated by the blockade of presynaptic dopamine terminals on noradrenergic pathways by antipsychotic drugs. Other investigators have hypothesized that an imbalance between central dopaminergic and noradrenergic systems may be involved (Yassa *et al.*, 1988). Lipinski *et al.* (1988) postulated that beta-blockers alleviate akathisia by antagonizing the inhibitory effect of noradrenergic input to the VTA, the origin of the mesocortical dopamine system (Table 10.1). The result of such an action would be enhanced dopamine release, the opposite effect to antidepressant drugs which potentiate serotonin, such as SSRIs, as noted above.

Akathisia associated with SSRI antidepressants (Sandyk, 1984; Zubenko *et al.*, 1987; Lipinski *et al.*, 1989) could be explained by enhanced 5HT-mediated inhibition of dopamine neurons in the VTA, leading to decreased dopamine activity, and hence the secondary effects upon cortical and locomotor function noted above. The serotonergic contribution to akathisia may specifically involve the 5HT2 receptor. Evidence for this view is the finding that antidepressants which elevate serotonin but also specifically block 5HT2 (the serotonin-2 antagonist/ re-uptake inhibitors; SARIs) lack the activating side-effects of the SSRIs (Stahl, 1996). Further, akathisia may be treated effectively with the selective 5HT2 antagonist ritanserin (Miller *et al.*, 1990, 1992), and newer antipsychotics, with relatively potent 5HT2 receptor antagonism, such as risperidone, olanzapine and sertindole, have less liability to produce akathisia. The role of the VTA in akathisia is further supported by the finding that ritanserin enhances the firing rate of dopaminergic neurons in the VTA but not the substantia nigra (Baldwin *et al.*, 1991).

TREATMENT

Antipsychotic drug strategies

Neuroleptic-induced akathisia is likely to improve if the antipsychotic medication is reduced or stopped. This may not be a realistic clinical option for many acute psychiatric patients. It may be worthwhile switching to one of the newer antipsychotics which have a lower liability for akathisia. Low rates of akathisia around 6–7% have been found with clozapine treatment (Chengappa *et al.*, 1994; Kurz *et al.*, 1995). Where prevalence figures comparable to those of conventional antipsychotics have been reported in clinical studies, they have been attributed to carry-over effects from previous medication (Umbricht and Kane, 1996b). Clinical studies of risperidone (Moller, 1996), sertindole (Daniel *et al.*, 1996; Tamminga *et al.*, 1997), olanzapine (Beasley *et al.*, 1996) and quetiapine (Small *et al.*, 1997) all suggest that within their optimum dose ranges, these drugs produce a significantly lower incidence of akathisia compared to a conventional antipsychotic, usually haloperidol. Akathisia would also appear to be a relatively infrequent problem with amisulpride (Loo *et al.*, 1997).

Anticholinergic agents

Anticholinergic drugs have an uncertain reputation for the treatment of acute akathisia, being only partially effective, or only effective in a proportion of patients

(Barnes, 1992). However, there is some logic to prescribing an anticholinergic drug in cases where akathisia and parkinsonism are both present, as both may respond. Indeed, there is some evidence that akathisia accompanied by parkinsonism may be more likely to respond to an anticholinergic agent than akathisia alone (Braude *et al.*, 1983; Friis *et al.*, 1983; Adler *et al.*, 1987).

Beta-adrenergic blockers

Catecholamine agonists such as methylphenidate and amantadine, the alpha2-agonist clonidine, and benzodiazepines such as diazepam and lorazepam, have all been shown to produce some benefit in akathisia. However, beta-adrenergic blocking agents seem to offer the most consistently effective treatment (Fleischhacker *et al.*, 1990). The majority of clinical studies have used propranolol at doses of 20–80 mg/day. Benefit can be seen within hours of the first dose, with the maximum clinical response occurring within 24 to 48 hours. With regard to the mechanism of action of beta-blockers in akathisia, the evidence suggests that this is via a central rather than peripheral action, but there are claims for efficacy with both selective beta1 and beta2 adrenoceptor blockers (Zubenko *et al.*, 1984b; Adler *et al.*, 1989). Tolerance to the therapeutic effect does not seem to develop, but symptoms may reappear within a few days when the beta-blocker is withdrawn (Zubenko *et al.*, 1984a).

Treatment of chronic akathisia

The treatment of chronic akathisia has not been subjected to systematic study. On the basis of their clinical experience with chronic akathisia, Burke *et al.* (1989) found the best response with reserpine and tetrabenazine, while anticholinergics were generally ineffective and levodopa aggravated the condition. They found little benefit with beta blockers, in contrast to other case reports (Stein and Pohlman, 1987; Yassa *et al.*, 1988). Anticholinergic drugs have been used in different studies with contradictory results, that is, efficacy in some studies but not others.

Tardive dyskinesia

CLINICAL FEATURES

Tardive dyskinesia is a syndrome of abnormal, involuntary, repetitive movements, principally of a choreiform nature. Most descriptions have emphasized orofacial movements, including protrusion or twisting of the tongue, smacking, pursing and sucking movements of the lips, puffing of the cheeks and chewing and lateral motion of the jaw. Although orofacial dyskinesia is the most prevalent and characteristic component, the trunk and limbs are frequently involved. The involuntary limb movements seen are purposeless, jerky and often rather stereotypic in nature, and usually described as choreiform or choreoathetoid. Athetoid and dystonic movements are also included sometimes as part of the syndrome, as are grunting and respiratory arrhythmias and abnormalities of gait and trunk posture.

Early evidence that orofacial and trunk and limb dyskinesia should be considered as distinct sub-syndromes of tardive dyskinesia (Barnes and Kidger, 1979; Kidger *et al.*, 1980) has been supported by subsequent studies examining the clinical correlates, risk factors and drug responses of the two sub-syndromes (Barnes, 1990b; Paulsen *et al.*, 1996). Therefore, it may be appropriate to analyse ratings from the two regions separately, on the basis that they may be pathophysiologically distinct. However, a more prosaic explanation for some of these findings may be that orofacial dyskinesia is a more discrete, rateable entity than trunk and limb dyskinesia. Ratings for the latter may be more likely to be contaminated by other phenomena such as stereotypies and mannerisms, fidgety, agitated movements and the restless movements of akathisia (Barnes, 1990b).

The mean reported prevalence seems to be around 15–20% world-wide (Kane *et al.*, 1992; Koshino *et al.*, 1992; Pandurangi and Aderibigbe, 1995). A major prospective study found a 3–4% incidence each year in the first eight years or so of drug treatment (Kane and Lieberman, 1992). Tardive dyskinesia is not usually progressive, but rather follows a fluctuating course with spontaneous remissions being relatively common, particularly in younger patients. The results from two 10-year follow-up studies (Yagi and Itoh, 1987; Casey and Gardos 1990) provide further support for this view, although there are occasional reports of tardive dyskinesia worsening during continued drug therapy. If antipsychotic drug treatment is stopped, tardive dyskinesia may have a more favourable outcome than is often assumed (Casey, 1985; Casey and Gerlach, 1986). The condition may rapidly improve, or follow a course of gradual improvement or stabilization over many years. In those patients whose abnormal involuntary movements appear irreversible, in that they persist for years despite the discontinuation of antipsychotic drugs, the movements may represent manifestations of the psychotic illness or spontaneous dyskinesia of the elderly (Marsden, 1985).

SUBJECTIVE BURDEN AND PHYSICAL DISABILITY

While patients usually seem to be unaware of the condition (Macpherson and Collis, 1992), it can still stigmatize patients in the community. Orofacial dyskinesia can look odd, and even grotesque in severe cases, and can have an adverse influence on a patient's social acceptability (Boumans *et al.*, 1994).

In the more severe cases, tardive dyskinesia can also constitute a physical handicap. Disability may be directly related to abnormal pharyngeal and laryngeal movements which can interfere with eating and swallowing, and cause speech disorders and breathing difficulties, sometimes leading to dysphagia or choking (Yassa and Lal, 1986; Gregory *et al.*, 1992, Khan *et al.*, 1994; Feve *et al.*, 1995). Respiratory dyskinesia in patients with tardive dyskinesia is said to be characterized by irregularity in rate, rhythm and depth of breathing, and is likely to be overlooked by clinicians (Chiu *et al.*, 1993). Wilcox *et al.* (1994) found that patients with tardive dyskinesia had irregular shallow breathing but this did not appear to limit their exercise performance. However, more dramatically, Kruk *et al.* (1995) described five cases of a respiratory dyskinesia variant, manifesting as irregular respiration, dyspnoea, with gasping or grunting noises and abnormal chest movements. Patients with tardive dyskinesia may carry an excess burden of mortality and morbidity related to respiratory tract infections and cardiovascular disorders (Youssef and Waddington, 1987).

RISK FACTORS

Age

Advancing age is a major predisposing factor for tardive dyskinesia, being associated with not only an increased occurrence of tardive dyskinesia but also greater severity and a reduced likelihood of spontaneous remission (Kane *et al.*, 1992; Jeste *et al.*, 1995). Although age and duration of drug exposure to antipsychotic drugs are likely to be linked, studies using regression methodologies have found age to be the only consistent predictor of tardive dyskinesia when other cumulative variables, such as duration of antipsychotic exposure, lifetime hospital admission and ECT have been accounted for (Brown *et al.*, 1992; Waddington *et al.*, 1993).

Antipsychotic drug treatment variables

The majority of clinical studies examining the relationship between tardive dyskinesia and antipsychotic drug dosage or duration of treatment have not found any significant association between the development of tardive dyskinesia and variables such as the length of time on medication, the total amount administered, the type or class of drug, current dosage, or plasma drug concentrations (Kane and Smith, 1982; Gardos *et al.*, 1988). The general failure to find such an association may partly reflect the retrospective nature of most studies. However, there are other plausible reasons. First, a dose–response relationship would only be apparent in the minority of patients who are vulnerable to the disorder and this subgroup is difficult to identify and study separately (Kane and Lieberman, 1992). Second, Baldessarini *et al.* (1988) argued that the high doses of antipsychotic medication prescribed to most patients would tend to obscure any relationship that might exist between the risk of tardive dyskinesia and dosage within a more modest range. Third, older patients are not only at greater risk of developing tardive dyskinesia but invariably they are prescribed lower doses of antipsychotic medication.

Where a relationship between drug dose and tardive dyskinesia has been reported, it has generally been over the first few years of treatment (Morgenstern and Glazer, 1993; Kane *et al.*, 1994). For example, Chakos *et al.* (1996) studied a sample of patients with first-episode schizophrenia prospectively for a period of up to eight and a half years. They found that both antipsychotic drug dose and poor response to treatment of the first psychotic episode were significant predictors of time to the development of tardive dyskinesia.

All the conventional antipsychotic drugs would seem to have the capacity to induce tardive dyskinesia, but the large, prospective cohort studies necessary to establish their relative liability for the condition have not been carried out. There is now the prospect that the newer antipsychotic drugs, which have a lower liability for acute extrapyramidal side-effects, may be associated with a lower incidence of tardive dyskinesia in the long term (Umbricht and Kane, 1996a). The clinical trials conducted so far have not lasted long enough to allow for any predictions regarding the relative risk of tardive dyskinesia with chronic treatment with new and conventional drugs. Nevertheless, published reports of tardive dyskinesia developing in association with clozapine are scarce, suggesting that if the condition occurs, the incidence is significantly lower than is seen with conventional antipsychotics (Umbricht and Kane, 1996b). There is also emerging evidence for a lower risk of tardive dyskinesia with risperidone (Gutierrez-Esteinou and Grebb, 1997) and olanzapine (Beasley *et al.*, 1999).

Patients whose drug treatment has been regularly interrupted may be at greater risk of developing persistent tardive dyskinesia than those who have received continuous treatment (Jeste *et al.*, 1979; Yassa *et al.*, 1985, 1990). However, controlled studies of intermittent, targeted antipsychotic treatment versus continuous treatment have not found any significant differences in tardive dyskinesia between the groups (Jolley *et al.*, 1990; Herz *et al.*, 1991). A prospective follow-up study of patients who had developed tardive dyskinesia found that the modal dose of antipsychotic, and the proportion of time on medication after the condition had been diagnosed appeared to be associated with outcome (Kane *et al.*, 1994). One interpretation of the data is that intermittent treatment is a risk factor for the persistence of tardive dyskinesia.

Anticholinergic agents

It is well known that anticholinergic drugs worsen tardive dyskinesia, and that stopping such medication usually improves the condition. Studies have generally found a positive relationship between the administration of these drugs and the severity of tardive dyskinesia, although not invariably (Kane and Smith, 1982; Silver *et al.*, 1995). However, it has not been established that patients receiving antiparkinsonian medication in addition to antipsychotic medication have an increased risk of developing the condition (Klawans *et al.*, 1980; Gardos and Cole, 1983).

Gender

There is some evidence that women have a greater prevalence of severe dyskinesia, although this may only be true in those patients over 70 years of age (Kane and Smith, 1982). Yassa and Jeste (1992) reviewed 76 selected studies, and concluded that, overall, the prevalence in women (27%) was significantly higher than that in men (22%). In men, prevalence seems to peak between 50 and 70 years of age, while for women the prevalence continues to rise after the age of 70 years. However, a prospective study of tardive dyskinesia in the elderly (Saltz *et al.*, 1991) not only failed to find a significant relationship between sex and incidence but actually reported a slightly higher incidence for the males in the sample, who were significantly younger than the females.

No clear explanation has emerged for this gender effect, although neuroendocrine factors have been postulated (Hruska and Silbergeld, 1980; Davila *et al.*, 1991, Yassa and Jeste, 1992).

Alcohol abuse

Alcohol abuse may be a risk factor for orofacial dyskinesia. For example, Paulsen *et al.* (1996) found this to be the case in a prospective study of 266 middle-aged and elderly outpatients receiving antipsychotic medication for two years. In an epidemiologically-based prevalence study of schizophrenia, Duke *et al.* (1994) found no difference between patients with or without a history of problem drinking in their ratings for tardive dyskinesia, although the former group had a significantly shorter duration of illness. However, peak alcohol consumption showed a significant, positive correlation with orofacial dyskinesia. Dixon *et al.* (1992) studied 75 consecutive admissions with schizophrenia, assessing tardive dyskinesia and lifetime diagnosis of alcohol and drug use. Patients with a lifetime diagnosis of drug or alcohol abuse had significantly higher scores for tardive dyskinesia compared with non-abusers, and this association seemed to be independent of other known risk factors for tardive dyskinesia.

Schizophrenia

In patients with schizophrenia treated with antipsychotic medication, the designation of abnormal involuntary movements as signs of tardive dyskinesia should take into account the possible presence of spontaneous dyskinesia related to both age and the schizophrenic illness. Spontaneous or idiopathic orofacial dyskinesia, apparently indistinguishable from tardive dyskinesia, has been observed in between 1% and 15% of elderly individuals who have never received antipsychotic drugs (Blowers *et al.*, 1981; Kane *et al.*, 1982).

In respect of illness-related motor disturbance, descriptions of people with schizophrenia before the advent of antipsychotic drugs refer to motor phenomena such as stereotypies and mannerisms, perseverative movements, tics, grimaces and lack of co-ordination (Kraepelin, 1919; Farran-Ridge, 1926). These movements were generally conceptualized as secondary to the disturbance of will, thought and emotion that occurs in psychotic illness (Kraepelin, 1919; Bleuler, 1950). More recently, abnormal, involuntary movements have been identified in chronic schizophrenic patients never treated with antipsychotic drugs (Owens *et al.*, 1982). Studies examining relatively small samples of drug-naïve patients at the time of their first-episode of psychosis have yielded inconsistent findings in terms of the presence and severity of orofacial and trunk and limb dyskinesia. Some have found no evidence of abnormal movements (Chorfi and Moussaoui, 1985; Hernan-Silva *et al.*, 1994) or only a very low prevalence (Chatterjee *et al.*, 1995). Nevertheless, the higher prevalence figures of up to 26% reported in several studies (Fenn *et al.*, 1996; Hoffman *et al.*, 1996; Fenton *et al.*, 1997; Puri *et al.*, 1999) support the notion that movement disorder, particularly orofacial dyskinesia, appears to be part of the clinical presentation of schizophrenia.

Current hypotheses regarding the underlying mechanisms of tardive dyskinesia suggest that the schizophrenic illness itself confers a vulnerability to develop the condition (Barnes and Liddle, 1985; Waddington, 1989). There would seem to be a complex interaction between the ageing process, exposure to antipsychotic drug treatment and the pathological changes underlying the schizophrenic illness, particularly those implicated in negative symptoms, which serves to hasten or provoke the appearance of the abnormal movements (Liddle *et al.*, 1993). Collinson *et al.* (1996) suggest that dyskinesia may occur because of failure to inhibit an inherent motor pattern, akin to a primitive reflex. Loss of control of such reflexes occurs with ageing, but the relevant inhibitory systems may also be compromised by the schizophrenic state, and antipsychotic drugs may further accelerate this process, bringing forward in time the emergence of tardive dyskinesia.

COGNITIVE IMPAIRMENT

Cognitive impairment, as measured on short form measures of global cognition, appears to be more common in schizophrenic patients who develop tardive dyskinesia than their non-dyskinetic fellows (Waddington, 1989; Collinson *et al.*, 1996). This association has generally been more robust in relation to orofacial dyskinesia rather than trunk and limb dyskinesia (Waddington *et al.*, 1990) and in relation to persistent rather than transient dyskinesia (Struve and Wilner, 1983).

This relationship between dyskinesia and cognitive impairment could be explained on the basis that pre-existing dementia or brain dysfunction renders patients vulnerable to develop tardive dyskinesia or by both conditions being manifestations of neuroleptic toxicity. However, the association between tardive dyskinesia, cognitive impairment and negative symptoms of schizophrenia, particularly blunted affect and poverty of speech, led to notions of a shared pathophysiological basis, referring specifically to frontal-subcortical systems (Brown and White, 1992; Pantelis *et al.*, 1992; Collinson *et al.*, 1996). Subsequent studies of patients with tardive dyskinesia have revealed more specific cognitive deficits on tasks of executive functioning, learning and memory. This pattern of neuropsychological impairment can be likened to that seen in patients with basal ganglia pathology, such as Parkinson's disease and Huntington's disease, and is consistent with theories implicating disturbances of basal ganglia thalamo-cortical circuits (Collinson *et al.*, 1996).

PATHOPHYSIOLOGY

The dopamine supersensitivity theory

Pathophysiological theories for tardive dyskinesia were derived by analogy with the spontaneous movement disorders such as Huntington's disease and levodopa-induced dyskinesia. An underlying mechanism in these conditions is thought to be hyperactivity within central dopaminergic systems. For tardive dyskinesia, the hypothesis generated was that the condition was related to striatal dopaminergic hyperfunction, consequent upon an increase in number (supersensitivity) of post-synaptic D2 receptors (Klawans, 1973). The explanation was that this supersensitivity represented a response to chronic blockade of these receptors by neuroleptics, so-called 'denervation' supersensitivity.

The validity of this hypothesis has been challenged by the findings of post-mortem investigations, work in clinical pharmacology, and latterly, in-vivo neuroimaging (Jeste and Wyatt, 1981; Blin *et al.*, 1989; Andersson *et al.*, 1990). An obvious inconsistency is that the majority of patients receiving long-term antipsychotic medication will not manifest dyskinesia, even though the development of dopamine receptor supersensitivity appears to be an inevitable consequence of such treatment (Reynolds and Cutts, 1992).

D1 receptor agonists have been shown to cause tongue protrusion and chewing movements in animals. This prompted Gerlach (1991) to propose a modification of the supersensitivity theory. Neuroleptics block postsynaptic D2 receptors, inducing parkinsonism. The simultaneous blockade of presynaptic D2 autoreceptors leads to increased synthesis and release of dopamine which, in turn, stimulates the unblocked postsynaptic D1 receptor, causing dyskinesia in predisposed individuals. However, as has been previously demonstrated, animal models may be of limited application to human movement disorders. For example, while the oral dyskinesias induced in primates remit upon withdrawal of antipsychotic drugs, this is frequently not the case in humans. The persistence of tardive dyskinesia in schizophrenic patients may imply structural, as well as pharmacological, change in some patients. Indeed, the latter may explain the apparent association between tardive dyskinesia and cognitive impairment.

One prediction from the supersensitivity theory would be an association between the presence and severity of dyskinesia and the number of postsynaptic receptors found in critical brain areas. However, post-mortem studies in schizophrenia, using radiolabelled, ligand-binding techniques have failed to reveal any clear relationship between the presence of dyskinesia in life and dopamine D1 or D2 receptor numbers in the basal ganglia (Cross *et al.*, 1985; Seeman, 1985). Furthermore, Kornhuber *et al.* (1989) found no differences in D2 receptor binding in the putamen between patients with or without tardive dyskinesia in life. In-vivo studies of tardive dyskinesia patients have demonstrated unchanged D2 receptor densities in striatum (Blin *et al.*, 1989; Andersson *et al.*, 1990). Reynolds *et al.* (1989) reported a decrease in caudate D2 receptors in the brains of some patients with tardive dyskinesia compared with controls, although further studies from these investigators have suggested that D2 receptor changes in pallidum, rather than striatum as a whole, may be more relevant to the production of dyskinesias (Reynolds and Cutts, 1992; Reynolds *et al.*, 1992).

Despite the evidence against the supersensitivity theory, it remains a plausible explanation for a number of clinical observations. First, dyskinesia may worsen or appear for the first time following neuroleptic dose reduction or withdrawal. This would be explained by exposure of supersensitive receptors to dopamine. Second, reinstitution of neuroleptic, or an increase in dose, will temporarily relieve the symptoms. The eventual re-emergence of dyskinesia may be seen as a consequence of further supersensitivity (Kazamatsuri *et al.*, 1972). Third, the administration of anticholinergic agents may uncover or aggravate the condition, a result of tipping the postulated balance between cholinergic and dopaminergic activity in the striatum further towards relative dopamine dominance.

The GABAergic theory

Refinements to the dopamine supersensitivity theory have addressed the changes occurring in the basal ganglia secondary to neuroleptic treatment, starting with dopamine blockade and extending to secondary biochemical and functional changes in the striatal projection areas. One theory has been that while changes in dopamine receptors may not differentiate between affected and non-affected patients, perhaps changes in GABA content or metabolism might (Thaker *et al.*, 1987). As alluded to above, GABA plays an inhibitory role in the modulation of striatal output (via the substantia nigra) to the thalamus (*see* Table 10.2). Thus, depletion of GABA might, simplistically, be expected to result in hyperkinetic disorders. Neurochemical studies on a primate tardive dyskinesia model have reported severe depletion of subthalamic and pallidal levels of GABA (Gunne *et al.*, 1984). Congruent with these findings are reports that clonazepam, either alone or in combination with clozapine, may abolish tardive dyskinesia in some patients (Thaker *et al.*, 1990; Shapleske *et al.*, 1996), a response which is reversed by swapping to placebo, diminished by drug tolerance, and re-established upon reintroduction of clonazepam after a cessation of treatment (Thaker *et al.*, 1990).

A present formulation of a combined 'dopamine-GABA' hypothesis of tardive dyskinesia might be the following (Tamminga and Thaker, 1989): that the pathophysiology of tardive dyskinesia stems from chronic blockade of dopamine receptors in the striatum, with subsequent mediation via the striatonigral–GABAergic pathway, finally manifesting itself as a disturbance of GABA transmission in the substantia nigra.

As in the other movement disorders (considered above) it is clear that dopaminergic function is involved in the pathophysiology of tardive dyskinesia, but it does not provide an exhaustive account of this disorder. Investigation of other neurotransmitter systems is necessary, as is the study of remote effects (outside the basal ganglia). Recent reports have emphasized the cognitive impairment that may accompany the onset of tardive dyskinesia in schizophrenic patients together with the stigmata of craniofacial dysmorphogenesis which may distinguish those patients predisposed to the disorder (Waddington *et al.*, 1995, Waddington and Youssef, 1996). Hence, tardive dyskinesia must be considered in the context of a dysfunctional, predisposed, locomotor system which (perhaps through striatal 'loop' projections) exerts an abnormal modulatory tone upon distant, cortical, projection sites. In this regard, abnormal performance on the Wisconsin Card Sort Test may implicate DLPFC dysfunction as a result of disturbed thalamic tone.

TREATMENT

Specific antidyskinetic drugs with some claims for efficacy in tardive dyskinesia include dopamine depleters (such as tetrabenazine, reserpine, oxypertine), cholinomimetic agents (choline, lecithin, deanol), GABA agonists (sodium valproate, gamma-vinyl GABA), calcium channel blockers (diltiazem, verapamil) and vitamin E (alpha-tocopherol) (Jeste *et al.*, 1988; Shriqui and Annable, 1995). Most treatment studies have been of relatively short duration, with no demonstration of long-term efficacy. A survey of these putative treatments in the American Psychiatric Association Task Force report on tardive dyskinesia (Kane *et al.*, 1992) concluded that despite the numerous clinical trials, no consistently effective treatment had been identified. Detailed review of the various pharmacological treatments is beyond the scope of this review.

Antipsychotic drug strategies

Shriqui and Annable (1995) suggest that the best management strategy is gradual reduction in antipsychotic dosage whenever possible, but such a strategy poses problems clinically because of the increased risk of worsening or relapse of the psychotic illness. Withdrawal of any concomitant anticholinergic medication is also recommended, and usually improves the tardive dyskinesia.

For some of the newer antipsychotics, preliminary data point to a relatively low liability for tardive dyskinesia (see above) and there is also evidence that clozapine can have an ameliorating effect on tardive dyskinesia which has developed during previous treatment with conventional antipsychotics (Lamberti and Bellnier, 1993). Reviewing eight published studies of clozapine's effect on tardive dyskinesia, Lieberman *et al.* (1991) concluded that approximately 43% of patients with pre-existing tardive dyskinesia show a reduction in symptoms of least 50% when switched to clozapine. Factor and Friedman (1997) critically reviewed 13 studies, varying from single-case reports to larger controlled studies, addressing the therapeutic value of clozapine in tardive dyskinesia. Their opinion was that most of the studies had methodological limitations and that controlled, double-blind studies were necessary before a definitive conclusion could be reached. Nevertheless, the available evidence indicated that in some patients the condition improves with clozapine, although the mechanism of such an effect was uncertain. Further, the variability of response might possibly relate to the heterogeneity of tardive dyskinesia. Specifically, the response may be greater when dystonic phenomena are present (Lieberman *et al.*, 1991), although there are conflicting case reports (Factor and Friedman, 1997).

Conclusion

Although conventional antipsychotic drugs have been the mainstay of treatment for acute and chronic psychotic illness, a major limitation has been the production of movement disorders. This chapter has reviewed their clinical manifestations, clinical implications, pathophysiology, risk factors and treatment. A major advantage of the new, so-called atypical antipsychotic drugs is their lower liability for acute extrapyramidal side-effects and in some cases, indications of a reduced risk of developing tardive dyskinesia. Patients should find these new drugs more tolerable and acceptable, although whether or not this will translate into better compliance in the longer term has yet to be established.

Dopaminergic systems seem important to all the movement disorders described with antipsychotic drug treatment. But in each case different receptors, pathways, and imbalances of (hypo- or hyper-) function seem relevant. Increasingly, other neurotransmitter systems are being invoked (and modulated pharmacologically) in attempts to understand, treat, and hopefully prevent these drug effects. It seems likely that a clear explanation of the pathophysiology of any of these disorders will involve consideration of brain regions outside the striatum, and a knowledge of basal ganglia-thalamocortical circuitry seems essential. We are still only beginning to understand why certain patients might be predisposed to some of these disorders and a full account of these factors might inform not just our understanding of psychopharmacology, but also our understanding of schizophrenia itself.

References

Adler, L., Angrist, B., Reiter, S. *et al.* (1989) Neuroleptic-induced akathisia: a review. *Psychopharmacology,* **97**, 1–11.

Adler, L., Reiter, S., Corwin, J. *et al.* (1987). Differential effects of benztropine and propranolol in akathisia. *Psychopharmacol Bull,* **23**, 519–21.

Addonzio, G. and Alexopoulos, G.S. (1988) Drug-induced dystonia in young and elderly patients. *Am J Psychiatry,* **145**, 869–71.

Alexander, G.E., DeLong, M.R. and Strick, P.L. (1986) Parallel organization of functionally segregated circuits linking basal ganglia and cortex. *Ann Rev Neurosci,* **9**, 357–81.

Anderson T.J., Rivest, J., Stell, R. *et al.* (1992) Botulinum toxin treatment of spasmodic torticollis. *J Roy Soc Med,* **85**, 525–9.

Andersson, U., Eckernas, S.A., Hartvig, P. *et al.* (1990) Striatal binding of ^{11}C-NMSP studied with positron emission tomography in patients with persistent tardive dyskinesia: no evidence for altered dopamine receptor binding. *J Neural Transm,* **79**, 215–26.

Arvanitis, L.A., Miller, B.G., and the Seroquel Trial 13 Study Group.(1997) Multiple fixed doses of 'Seroquel' (quetiapine) in patients with acute exacerbation of schizophrenia: a comparison with haloperidol and placebo. *Biol Psychiatry,* **42**, 233–46.

Awad, A.G., Hogan, T.P., Vorungati, L.N.P. *et al.* (1995) Patients' subjective experiences on antipsychotic medications: implications for outcome and quality of life. *Int Clin Psychopharmacol,* **10** (Suppl. 3), 123–32.

Ayd, F.J. (1961) A survey of drug-induced extrapyramidal reactions. *J Am Med Assoc,* **175**, 1054–60.

Ayd, F.J. Jr. (1988) Akathisia and suicide: fact or myth?. *Int Drug Therapy Newslett,* **23**, 37–8.

Baldessarini, R.J., Cohen, B.M. and Teicher, M.H. (1988) Significance of neuroleptic dose and plasma level in the pharmacological treatment of psychosis. *Arch Gen Psychiatry,* **45**, 79–91.

Baldwin, D., Fineberg, N. and Montgomery, S. (1991) Fluoxetine, fluvoxamine and extrapyramidal tract disorders. *Int Clin Psychopharmacol,* **6**, 51–8.

Barnes, T.R.E. (1990a) Comment on the WHO Consensus Statement. *Br J Psychiatry,* **156**, 413–14.

Barnes, T.R.E. (1990b) Movement disorder associated with antipsychotic drugs: the tardive syndromes. *Int Rev Psychiatry,* **2**, 355–66.

Barnes, T.R.E. (1992) Neuromuscular effects of neuroleptics: Akathisia. In J.M. Kane, J.A. Lieberman (eds), *Adverse effects of psychotropic drugs.* New York: Guilford Press, 201–17.

Barnes, T.R.E. and Braude, W.M. (1984). Persistent akathisia associated with early tardive dyskinesia. *Postgrad Med J,* **60**, 51–3.

Barnes, T.R.E. and Braude, W.M. (1985) Akathisia variants and tardive dyskinesia. *Arch Gen Psychiatry,* **42**, 874–8.

Barnes, T.R.E. and Edwards, J.G. (1993) The side-effects of antipsychotic drugs. I. Neuropsychiatric effects. In T.R.E. Barnes (ed.), *Antipsychotic drugs and their side-effects.* London: Academic Press, 213–47.

Barnes, T.R.E. and Kidger, T. (1979) The concept of tardive dyskinesia. *Trends Neurosci,* **2**, 135–6.

Barnes, T.R.E. and Liddle, P.F. (1985) Tardive dyskinesia: implications for schizophrenia? In A.A. Schiff, M. Roth and H.L. Freeman (eds), *Schizophrenia: new pharmacological and clinical developments.* London: Royal Society of Medicine Services (International Congress and Symposium Series, No. 94), 81.

Barnes, T.R.E. and McPhillips, M.A. (1995) How to distinguish between the neuroleptic-induced deficit syndrome, depression and disease-related negative symptoms in schizophrenia. *Int Clin Psychopharmacol*, **10**, 115–21.

Barnes, T.R.E. and McPhillips, M.A. (1996) Antipsychotic-induced extrapyramidal symptoms: Role of anticholinergic drugs in treatment. *CNS Drugs*, **6**, 315–30.

Barnes, T.R.E., McPhillips, M.A., Hillier, R. *et al.* (1997) Compliance with maintenance medication in first-episode schizophrenia. *Schizophr Res*, **24**, 205.

Beasley, C.M., Tollefson, G., Tran, P. *et al.* (1996) Olanzapine versus placebo and haloperidol: acute phase results of the North American double-blind olanzapine trial. *Neuropsychopharmacology*, **14**, 111–23.

Beasley, C.M., Dellva, M.A., Tamura, R.N. *et al.* (1999) Randomized double-blind comparison of the incidence of tardive dyskinesia in patients with schizophrenia during long-term treatment with olanzapine or haloperidol. *Br J Psychiatry*, **174**, 23–30.

Bleuler, E. (1950) *Dementia Praecox or the Group of Schizophrenias*. 1911 Edition, translated by J. Zinkin. New York: International Universities Press.

Blin J., Baron J.C., Cambon H. *et al.* (1989) Striatal dopamine D2 receptors in tardive dyskinesia: PET study. *J Neurol Neurosurg Psychiatry*, **52**, 1248–52.

Blowers, A.J., Borison, R.L., Blowers, C.M. *et al.* (1981) Abnormal involuntary movements in the elderly. *Br J Psychiatry*, **139**, 363–4.

Boyer, P., Lecrubier, Y., Puech, A.J. *et al.* (1995) Treatment of negative symptoms in schizophrenia with amisulpride. *Br J Psychiatry*, **166**, 68–72.

Boumans, C.E., de Mooij, K.J., Koch, P.A.M. *et al.* (1994) Is the social acceptability of psychiatric patients decreased by orofacial dyskinesia? *Schizophr Bull*, **20**, 339–44.

Braude, W. M., Barnes, T.R.E. and Gore, S.M. (1983). Clinical characteristics of akathisia. A systematic investigation of acute psychiatric inpatient admissions. *Br J Psychiatry*, **143**, 139–50.

Braude, W.M., Charles, I.P. and Barnes, T.R.E. (1984) Course, jerky, foot tremor: tremographic investigation of an objective sign of acute akathisia. *Psychopharmacology*, **82**, 95–101.

Brooks, D.J. (1995) The role of basal ganglia in motor control: contributions from PET. *J. Neurol. Sci.*, **128**, 1–13.

Brown, K.W. and White, T. (1991) Pseudoakathisia and negative symptoms in schizophrenic subjects. *Acta Psychiat Scand*, **84**, 107–9.

Brown, K.W. and White, T. (1992) Sub-syndromes of tardive dyskinesia and some clinical correlates. *Psychol Med*, **22**, 923–7.

Brown, K.W., White, T. and Palmer, D. (1992) Movement disorders and psychological tests of frontal lobe function in schizophrenic patients. *Psychol Med*, **22**, 69–77.

Brown, R.P. and Kocsis, J.H. (1984) Sudden death and antipsychotic drugs. *Hosp Comm Psychiatry*, **35**, 486–91.

Buchanan, A. (1992) A two-year prospective study of treatment compliance in patients with schizophrenia. *Psychol Med*, **22**, 787–97.

Burke, R.E., Fahn, S., Jankovic, J. *et al.* (1982) Tardive dystonia: late-onset and persistent dystonia caused by antipsychotic drugs. *Neurology*, **32**, 1335–46.

Burke, R.E., Kang, U.J., Jankovic, J. *et al.* (1989) Tardive akathisia: an analysis of clinical features and response to open therapeutic trials. *Movement Disorders*, **4**, 157–75.

Burke, R.E. (1992) Neuromuscular effects of neuroleptics: dystonia. In J.M. Kane and J.A. Lieberman. *Adverse effects of psychotropic drugs*. New York: Guilford Press, 189–200.

Casey, D.E. (1985) Tardive dyskinesia: reversible and irreversible. In D.E. Casey, T.N. Chase, A.V. Christensen and J. Gerlach (eds), *Dyskinesia – research and treatment*. Berlin: Springer-Verlag, 88–97.

Casey, D.E. (1995) Motor and mental aspects of extrapyramidal syndromes. *Int Clin Psychopharmacol*, **10** (Suppl 3), 105–14.

Casey, D.E. and Gerlach, J. (1986) Tardive dyskinesia: what is the long-term outcome? In D.E. Casey and G. Gardos (eds), *Tardive dyskinesia and neuroleptics: from dogma to reason*. Washington, DC: American Psychiatric Press, 75–97.

Casey, D.E. and Gardos, G. (1990) Tardive dyskinesia: outcome at 10 years. *Schizophr Res*, **3**, 11.

Ceballos-Baumann, A.O., Passingham, R.E., Warner, T. *et al.* (1995) Overactive prefrontal and underactive motor cortical areas in idiopathic dystonia. *Ann Neurol*, **37**, 363–72.

Chakos, M.H., Alvir, J.M.J., Woerner, M.G. *et al.* (1996) Incidence and correlates of tardive dyskinesia in first episode of schizophrenia. *Arch Gen Psychiatry*, **53**, 313–19.

Chatterjee, A., Chakos, M., Koreen, A. *et al.* (1995) Prevalence and clinical correlates of extrapyramidal signs and spontaneous dyskinesia in never-medicated schizophrenic patients. *Am J Psychiatry*, **152**, 1724–9.

Chengappa, K.N., Shelton, M.D., Baker, R.W. *et al.* (1994) The prevalence of akathisia in patients receiving stable doses of clozapine. *J Clin Psychiatry*, **55**, 142–5.

Chiu, H.F., Lam, L.C., Chan, C.H. *et al.* (1993) Clinical and polygraphic characteristics of patients with respiratory dyskinesia. *Br J Psychiatry*, **162**, 828–30.

Chorfi, M. and Moussaoui, D. (1985) Never treated schizophrenic patients have no abnormal movements such as tardive dyskinesia. *Encephale*, **11**, 263–5.

Chouinard, G., Jones, B., Remington, G. *et al.* (1993) A Canadian multi-center placebo-controlled study of fixed doses of risperidone and haloperidol in the treatment of chronic schizophrenic patients. *J Clin Psychopharmacol*, **130**, 25–40.

Collinson, S.L., Pantelis, C. and Barnes, T.R.E. (1996) Abnormal involuntary movements in schizophrenia and their association with cognitive impairment. In C. Pantelis, H.E. Nelson, T.R.E. Barnes (eds), *Schizophrenia: a neuropsychological perspective*. Chichester: John Wiley, 237–58.

Coukell, A.J., Spencer, C.M. and Benfield, P. (1996) Amisulpride: a review of its pharmacodynamic and pharmacokinetic properties and therapeutic efficacy in the management of schizophrenia. *CNS Drugs*, **6**, 237–56.

Crane, G.E. (1972) Pseudoparkinsonism and tardive dyskinesia. *Arch Neurol*, **27**, 426–30.

Cross, A.J., Crow, T.J., Ferrier, I.N. *et al.* (1985) Chemical and structural changes in the brain in patients with movement disorder. In D.E. Casey, T.N. Chase and A.V. Christenson (eds), *Dyskinesia: research and treatment*. Berlin: Springer-Verlag, 104–10.

Daniel, D., Targum, S., Zimbroff, S. *et al.* (1996) Efficacy, safety and dose response of three doses of sertindole and three doses of haldol in schizophrenic patients. Poster presented at 149th American Psychiatric Association meeting.

Davila, R., Andia, I., Miller, J.C. *et al.* (1991) Evidence of low dopaminergic activity in elderly women with spontaneous orofacial dyskinesia. *Acta Psychiat Scand*, **83**, 1–3.

Davis, R.J., Cummings, J.L. and Hierholzer, R.W. (1988) Tardive dystonia: clinical spectrum and novel manifestations. *Behav Neurol*, **1**, 41–7

De Keyser, J., Ebinger, G. and Herregodts, P. (1987) Pathophysiology of akathisia. *Lancet*, **ii**, 336.

De Leon, J. and Simpson, G.M. (1992) Assessment of neuroleptic-induced extrapyramidal symptoms. In J.M. Kane and J.A. Lieberman (eds), *Adverse effects of psychotropic drugs*. New York: Guilford Press, 218–34.

Dixon, L., Weiden, P.J., Haas, G. *et al.* (1992). Increased tardive dyskinesia in alcohol-abusing schizophrenic patients. *Comp Psychiatry*, **33**, 121–2.

Drug and Therapeutics Bulletin. (1988) Dystonia: underdiagnosed and undertreated? Vol. 26, 33–6.

Duke, P.J., Pantelis, C. and Barnes, T.R.E. (1994) South Westminster Schizophrenia Survey: alcohol use and its relationship to symptoms, tardive dyskinesia and illness onset. *Br J Psychiatry*, **164**, 630–6.

Duncan, E., Angrist, B., Adler, L. *et al.* (1989). Pharmacologic challenge in akathisia variants (abstract). *Schizophr Res*, **2**, 242.

Edwards, J.G. and Barnes, T.R.E. (1993) The side-effects of antipsychotic drugs. II. Effects on other physiological systems. In T.R.E. Barnes (ed.), *Antipsychotic drugs and their side-effects*. London: Academic Press, 249–75.

Factor, S.A. and Friedman, J.H. (1997) The emerging role of clozapine in the treatment of movement disorders. *Movement Disorders, 12*, 483–96.

Fahn, S. (1983). Long-term treatment of tardive dyskinesia with presynaptically acting dopamine-depleting agents. In S. Fahn, D.B. Calne. and I. Shoulson (eds), *Advances in Neurology, Vol. 37: Experimental Therapeutics of Movement Disorders*. (eds) New York: Raven Press.

Fann, W.E. (1966) Use of methylphenidate to counteract acute dystonic effects of phenothiazines. *American Journal of Psychiatry, 122*, 1293.

Farde, L. (1992) Selective D_1– and D_2–dopamine receptor blockade both induces akathisia in humans – A PET study with [^{11}C]-SCH 23390 and [^{11}C]raclopride. *Psychopharmacology, 107*, 23–9.

Farde, L., Norstrom, A-L., Wiesel, F-A. *et al.* (1992) Positron emission tomographic analysis of central D_1 and D_2 dopamine receptor occupancy in patients treated with classical neuroleptics and clozapine: relation to extrapyramidal side effects. *Arch Gen Psychiatry, 49*, 538–44.

Farran-Ridge, C. (1926) Some symptoms referable to the basal ganglia occurring in dementia praecox and epidemic encephalitis. *J Mental Sci, 72*, 513–23.

Fenn, D.S., Moussaoui, D., Hoffman, W.F. *et al.* (1996) Movements in never-medicated schizophrenics: a preliminary study. *Psychopharmacology, 123*, 206–10.

Fenton, W.S., Blyler, C.R., Wyatt, R.J. *et al.* (1997) Comparison of the prevalence of spontaneous dyskinesia in schizophrenic and nonschizophrenic psychiatric patients. *Br J Psychiatry, 171*, 265–8.

Feve, A., Angelard, B. and Lacau-St-Guily, J. (1995) Laryngeal tardive dyskinesia. *J Neurol, 242*, 455–9.

Flaherty, J.A. and Lahmeyer, H.W. (1978) Laryngeal–pharyngeal dystonia as a possible cause of asphyxia with haloperidol treatment. *Am J Psychiatry, 135*, 1414–15.

Fleischhacker, W.W., Roth, S.D. and Kane, J.M. (1990) The pharmacologic treatment of neuroleptic-induced akathisia. *J Clin Psychopharmacol, 10*, 12–21.

Freeman, H.L. (1997) Amisulpride compared with standard neuroleptics in acute exacerbations of schizophrenia. *Int Clin Psychopharmacol, 12* (Suppl 2), 11–17.

Friis, T., Rosted Christensen, T. and Gerlach, J. (1983). Sodium valproate and biperiden in neuroleptic-induced akathisia, parkinsonism and hyperkinesia. *Acta Psychiat Scand, 67*, 178–87.

Gardos, G. and Cole, J.O. (1983) Tardive dyskinesia and anticholinergic drugs. *Am J Psychiatry, 140*, 200–2.

Gardos, G., Cole, J.O., Haskell, D. *et al.* (1988) The natural history of tardive dyskinesia. *J Clin Psychopharmacol, 8* (Suppl), 31–7.

Gerlach, J. (1991) Current views on tardive dyskinesia. *Pharmacopsychiatry, 24*, 47–8.

Gerlach, J. and Peacock, L. (1995) Intolerance to neuroleptic drugs: the art of avoiding extrapyramidal syndromes. *Eur Psychiatry, 10* (Suppl 1), 27–3.

Gessa, R., Tagliamonte, A. and Gessa, G.L. (1972) Blockade by apomorphine of haloperidol-induced dyskinesia in schizophrenic patients. *Lancet, ii*, 981.

Gibb, W.R.G. and Lees, A.J. (1986). The clinical phenomenon of akathisia. *J Neurol, Neurosurg Psychiatry, 49*, 861–6.

Grace, A.A., Bunney, B.S., Moore, H. *et al.* (1997) Dopamine-cell depolarization block as a model for the therapeutic actions of antipsychotic drugs. *Trends Neurosci, 20*, 31–7.

Gregory, R.P., Smith, P.T. and Rudge, P. (1992) Tardive dyskinesia presenting as severe dysphagia. *J Neurol Neurosurg Psychiatry, 55*, 1203–4.

Gunne, L.M., Haggstrom, J-E. and Sjoquist, B. (1984) Association with persistent neuroleptic-induced dyskinesia of regional changes in brain GABA synthesis. *Nature*, **309**, 347–9.

Gutterrez-Esteinou, R. and Grebb, J.A. (1997) Risperidone: an analysis of the first three years in general use. *Int. Clin Psychopharmacol*, **12** (Suppl 4), 3–10.

Halstead, S.M., Barnes, T.R.E. and Speller, J.C. (1994) Akathisia: prevalence and associated dysphoria in an inpatient population with chronic schizophrenia. *Br J Psychiatry*, **164**, 177–83.

Hernan-Silva, I., Jerez, C.S., Ruiz, T.A. *et al*. (1994) Lack of involuntary abnormal movements in untreated schizophrenic patients. *Actas Luso Esp Neurol Psiquiatr Cienc Afines*, **22**, 200–2.

Herz, M.I., Glazer, W.M., Mostert, M.A. *et al*. (1991) Intermittent versus maintenance medication in schizophrenia. Two year results. *Arch Gen Psychiatry*, **48**, 333–9.

Hoffman, W., Kadri, N., Fenn, D. *et al*. (1996) Choreo-athetoid movements occur spontaneously in never-medicated patients with schizophrenia. *European Neuropsychopharmacol*, **6** (Suppl. 3), 223.

Hruska, R.E. and Silbergeld, E.K. (1980) Estrogen treatment enhances dopamine receptor sensitivity in the rat striatum. *Eur J Pharmacol*, **61**, 397–400.

Hummer, M. and Fleischhacker, W.W. (1996) Compliance and outcome in patients treated with antipsychotics. *CNS Drugs*, **5** (Suppl. 1), 13–20.

Iversen, S.D. (1971) The effect of surgical lesions to frontal cortex and substantia nigra on amphetamine responses in rats. *Brain Res*, **31**, 295–311.

Jankovic, J. and Schwartz, K. (1990) Botulinum toxin injection for cervical dystonia. *Neurology*, **40**, 277–80.

Jenkins, I.H., Fernandez, W., Playford, E.D. *et al*. (1992) Impaired activation of the supplementary motor area in Parkinson's disease is reversed when akinesia is treated with apomorphine. *Ann Neurol*, **32**, 749–57.

Jeste, D.V., Caligiuri, M.P., Paulsen, J.S. *et al*. (1995) Risk of tardive dyskinesia in older patients. A prospective longitudinal study of 266 outpatients. *Arch Gen Psychiatry*, **52**, 756–65.

Jeste, D.V., Lohr, J.B., Clark, K. *et al*. (1988) Pharmacological treatments of tardive dyskinesia in the 1980s. *J Clin Psychopharmacol*, **8** (Suppl), 38–48.

Jeste, D.V., Potkin, S.G., Sinha, S. *et al*. (1979) Tardive dyskinesia – reversible and persistent. *Arch Gen Psychiatry*, **36**, 585–90.

Jeste, D.V. and Wyatt, R.J. (1981) Changing epidemiology of tardive dyskinesia: an overview. *Am J Psychiatry*, **138**, 297–309.

Jolley, A.G., Hirsch, S.R., Morrison, E. *et al*. (1990) Trial of brief intermittent neuroleptic prophylaxis for selected schizophrenic outpatients: clinical and social outcome at two years. *Br Med J*, **301**, 837–42.

Kahn, E.M., Munetz, M.R., Davies, M.A. *et al*. (1992) Akathisia: clinical phenomenology and relationship to tardive dyskinesia. *Comp Psychiatry*, **33**, 233–6.

Kane, J.M. and Lieberman, J. (1992) Tardive dyskinesia. In J.M. Kane and J.A. Lieberman (eds), *Adverse effects of psychotropic drugs*. New York: Guilford Press, 235–45.

Kane, J.M. and Smith, J.M. (1982) Tardive dyskinesia: prevalence and risk factors 1959–1979. *Arch Gen Psychiatry*, **39**, 473–81.

Kane, J., Honigfeld, G., Singer, J. *et al*. (1988) Clozapine for the treatment-resistant schizophrenic. *Arch Gen Psychiatry*, **45**, 789–96.

Kane, J.M., Jeste, D.V., Barnes, T.R.E. *et al*. (1992) Tardive dyskinesia: a task force report of the American Psychiatric Association. Washington: APA.

Kane, J.M., Weinhold, P., Kinon, B. *et al*. (1982) Prevalence of abnormal involuntary movements ("spontaneous dyskinesias") in the normal elderly. *Psychopharmacology*, **77**, 105–8.

Kane, J.M., Woerner, M. and Borenstein, M. (1994) Tardive dyskinesia incidence and outcome (Abstract). *Schizophr Res*, **11**, 193.

Kang, U.J., Burke, R.E. and Fahn, S. (1986) Natural history and treatment of tardive dystonia. *Movement Disorders*, **1**, 193–208.

Kazamatsuri, H., Chien, C.P. and Cole, J.O. (1972) Treatment of tardive dyskinesia. 1. Clinical efficacy of a dopamine-depleting agent, tetrabenazine. *Arch Gen Psychiatry*, **27**, 95–9.

Khan, R., Jampala, V.C., Dong, K. *et al.* (1994) Speech abnormalities in tardive dyskinesia. *Am J Psychiatry, 151*, 760–2.

Kidger, T., Barnes, T.R.E., Trauer,T. *et al.* (1980) Subsyndromes of tardive dyskinesia. *Psychol Med*, **10**, 513–20.

Klawans, H.L. (1973) The pharmacology of tardive dyskinesia. *Am J Psychiatry*, **130**, 82–6.

Klawans, H.L., Goetz, C.G. and Perlik, S. (1980) Tardive dyskinesia: review and update. *Am J Psychiatry, 137*, 900–8.

Klein, D.F., Gittelman, R., Quitkin, F. *et al.* (1980) *Diagnosis and treatment of psychiatric disorders: adults and children*, 2nd edition. Baltimore: Williams and Wilkins, 174–81.

Koshino,Y., Madokoro, S., Ito, T. *et al.* (1992) A survey of tardive dyskinesia in psychiatric inpatients in Japan. *Clin Neuropsychopharmacol, 15*, 34–43.

Kornhuber, J., Riederer, P., Reynolds, G.P. *et al.* (1989) ^{3}H-spiperone binding sites in post-mortem brains from schizophrenic patients: relationship to neuroleptic drug treatment, abnormal movements and positive symptoms. *J Neural Trans, 75*, 1–10.

Kraepelin, E.P. (1919) *Dementia praecox and paraphrenia*. Translated by R.M. Barclay. Edinburgh: E. & S. Livingstone.

Kruk, J., Sachdev, P. and Singh, S. (1995) Neuroleptic-induced respiratory dyskinesia. *J Neuropsychiat Clin Neurosci, 7*, 223–9.

Kurz, M., Hummer, M., Oberbauer, H. *et al.* (1995) Extrapyramidal side-effects of clozapine and haloperidol. *Psychopharmacology, 118*, 52–6.

Lamberti, J.S. and Bellnier, T. (1993) Clozapine and tardive dyskinesia. *J Nervous Mental Dis, 181*, 137–8.

Lavin, M.R. and Rifkin, A. (1992) Neuroleptic-induced parkinsonism. In J.M. Kane and J.A. Lieberman (eds), *Adverse effects of psychotropic drugs*. New York: Guilford Press, 175–88.

Levinson, D.F., Simpson, G.M., Singh, H. *et al.* (1990) Fluphenazine dose, clinical response and extrapyramidal symptoms during acute treatment. *Arch Gen Psychiatry, 47*, 761–8.

Liddle, P.F., Barnes, T.R.E., Speller, J.C. *et al.* (1993) Negative symptoms as a risk factor for orofacial dyskinesia. *Br J Psychiatry, 163*, 776–80.

Lieberman, J.A., Saltz, B.L., Johns, C.A. *et al.* (1991) The effects of clozapine on tardive dyskinesia. *Br J Psychiatry, 158*, 503–10.

Lipinski, J.F.Jr., Keck, P.E.Jr. and McElroy, S.L. (1988) Beta-adrenergic antagonists in psychosis: is improvement due to treatment of neuroleptic-induced akathisia. *J Clin Psychopharmacol, 8*, 409–16.

Lipinski, J.F., Mallya, G., Zimmerman, P. *et al.* (1989) Fluoxetine-induced akathisia: Clinical and medical implications. *J Clin Psychiatry, 50*, 339–42.

Loo, H., Poirier-Littre, M-F., Theron, M. *et al.* (1997) Amisulpride versus placebo in the medium-term treatment of the negative symptoms of schizophrenia. *Br J Psychiatry, 170*, 18–22.

McCreadie, R.G., Robertson, L.J. and Wiles, D.H. (1992) The Nithsdale Schizophrenia Surveys. IX: Akathisia, parkinsonism, tardive dyskinesia and plasma neuroleptic levels. *Br J Psychiatry, 161*, 793–9.

Macpherson, R. and Collis, R. (1992) Tardive dyskinesia: patients' lack of awareness of movement disorder. *Br J Psychiatry, 160*, 110–12.

Marder, S.R. and Meibach, R.C. (1994) Risperidone in the treatment of schizophrenia. *Am J Psychiatry, 151*, 825–35.

Marder, S.R., Van Putten, T., Wirshing, W.C. *et al.* (1991) Subjective experiences of extrapyramidal side-effects in schizophrenia. In G. Racagni *et al.* (eds), *Biological psychiatry*, Vol 1. Amsterdam: Elsevier Science Publishers, 590–2.

Marsden, C. D. and Jenner, P. (1980). The pathophysiology of extrapyramidal side-effects of neuroleptic drugs. *Psychol Med*, **10**, 55–72.

Marsden, C.D. and Quinn, N.P. (1990) The dystonias. *Br Med J*, **300**, 139–44.

Marsden, C.D. (1985) Is tardive dyskinesia a unique disorder? In D.E. Casey, T.N. Chase, A.V. Christensen and J. Gerlach (eds), *Dyskinesia – research and treatment*. Berlin: Springer-Verlag, 64–71.

Miller, C.H., Fleishhacker, W.W., Ehrmann, H. *et al.* (1990) Treatment of neuroleptic-induced akathisia with the 5-HT$_2$ antagonist ritanserin. *Psychopharmacol Bull*, **26**, 373–6.

Miller, C.H., Hummer, M., Pycha, R. *et al.* (1992) The effect of ritanserin on treatment-resistant, neuroleptic induced akathisia: case reports. *Prog Neuropsychopharmacol Biol Psychiatry*, **16**, 247–51.

Modestin, J., Krapf, R. and Boker, W. (1981) A fatality during haloperidol treatment: Mechanism of sudden death. *Am J Psychiatry*, **138**, 1616–17.

Moller, H-J. (1996) Extrapyramidal side-effects of neuroleptic medication: Focus on risperidone. In J.M. Kane, H.-J. Moller, F. Awouters (eds), *Serotonin in antipsychotic treatment: mechanisms and clinical practice*. New York: Marcel Dekker, 345–56.

Morgenstern, H. and Glazer, W.M. (1993) Identifying risk factors for tardive dyskinesia among long-term outpatients maintained with neuroleptic medications. *Arch Gen Psychiatry*, **50**, 723–33.

Munetz, M.R. (1986) Akathisia variants and tardive dyskinesia (Letter). *Arch Gen Psychiatry*, **43**, 1015.

Newcomer, J.W., Miller, L.S., Faustman, W.O. *et al.* (1994) Correlations between akathisia and residual psychopathology: A by-product of neuroleptic-induced dysphoria. *Br J Psychiatry*, **164**, 834–8.

Owens, D.G.C., Johnstone, E.C. and Frith, C.D. (1982) Spontaneous involuntary disorders of movement: their prevalence, severity and distribution in chronic schizophrenics with and without treatment with neuroleptics. *Arch Gen Psychiatry*, **39**, 452–61.

Pandurangi, A.K. and Aderibigbe, Y.A. (1995) Tardive dyskinesia in non-western countries: a review. *Eur Arch Psychiatry Clin Neurosci*, **246**, 47–52.

Pantelis, C., Barnes, T.R.E. and Nelson, H.E. (1992) Is the concept of subcortical dementia relevant to schizophrenia? *Br J Psychiatry*, **160**, 442–60.

Paulsen, J.S., Caligiuri, M.P., Palmer, B. *et al.* (1996) Risk factors for orofacial and limbtruncal tardive dyskinesia in older patients: a prospective longitudinal study. *Psychopharmacology*, **123**, 307–14.

Peuskens, J. and Link, C.G.G. (1997) A comparison of quetiapine and chlorpromazine in the treatment of schizophrenia. *Acta Psychiatr Scand*, **96**, 265–73.

Playford, E.D., Passingham, R.E., Marsden, C.D. *et al.* (1992) Abnormal activation of striatum and dorsolateral prefrontal cortex in dystonia. *Neurology*, **42** (Suppl 3), 377.

Puri, B.K., Barnes, T.R.E., Chapman, M.J. *et al.* (1999) Spontaneous dyskinesia in first-episode schizophrenia. *J Neurol Neurosurg Psychiatry*, **66**, 76–8.

Pycock, C.J., Kerwin, R.W. and Carter, C.J. (1980) Effect of lesion of cortical dopamine terminals on subcortical dopamine receptors in rats. *Nature*, **286**, 74–6.

Raja, M. (1995) Tardive dystonia: prevalence, risk factors and comparison with tardive dyskinesia in a population of 200 acute psychiatric inpatients. *Eur Arch Psychiatry Clin Neurosci*, **245**, 145–51.

Rapoport, A., Stein, D., Grinshpoon, A. *et al.* (1994) Akathisia and pseudoakathisia: clinical observations and accelerometric recordings. *J Clin Psychiatry*, **55**, 473–7.

Reynolds, G.P., McCall, J.C. and Mackay, A.V.P. (1989) Post-mortem neurochemical studies of tardive dyskinesia. *Schizophr Res*, **2**, 106.

Reynolds, G.P. and Cutts, A.J. (1992) Dopamine D2 receptor changes in the pallidum: their relationship with antipsychotic drug treatment and dyskinesias in schizophrenia. *Schizophr Res,* **6**, 137.

Reynolds, G.P., Brown, J.E., McCall, J.C. *et al.* (1992) Dopamine receptor abnormalities in the striatum and pallidum in tardive dyskinesia: a post mortem study. *J Neural Transm,* **87**, 225–30.

Rifkin, A., Quitkin, F. and Klein, D.F. (1975) Akinesia: A poorly recognised drug-induced extrapyramidal behavior disorder. *Arch Gen Psychiatry,* **32**, 672–4.

Romo, R. and Schultz, W. (1992) Role of primate basal ganglia and frontal cortex in the internal generation of movements: Neuronal activity in supplementary motor area. *Exp. Brain Res,* **91**, 396–407.

Rupniak, N.M.J., Jenner, P. and Marsden, C.D. (1986) Acute dystonia induced by neuroleptic drugs. *Psychopharmacology,* **88**, 403–19.

Saltz, B.L., Woerner, M., Kane, J.M. *et al.* (1991) Prospective study of tardive dyskinesia in the elderly. *J Am Med Assoc,* **266**, 2402–6.

Sachdev, P. (1995) *Akathisia and restless legs.* Cambridge: Cambridge University Press.

Sandyk, R. (1984) Persistent akathisia associated with early dyskinesia (letter). *Postgrad Med J,* **60**, 916.

Seeman, P. (1985) Brain dopamine receptors in schizophrenia and tardive dyskinesia. In D.E. Casey, T.N. Chase, A.V. Christensen and J. Gerlach (eds), *Dyskinesia – research and treatment (Psychopharmacology,* Suppl 2). Berlin: Springer-Verlag, 2–8.

Shapleske J., McKay A.P. and McKenna P.J. (1996) Successful treatment of tardive dystonia with clozapine and clonazepam. *Br J Psychiatry,* **168**, 516–18.

Shriqui, C.L. and Annable, L. (1995) Tardive dyskinesia. In C.L. Shriqui and H.A. Nasrallah (eds), *Contemporary issues in the treatment of schizophrenia.* Washington, DC: American Psychiatric Press, 585–632.

Silver, H., Geraisy, N. and Schwartz, M. (1995) No differences in the effect of biperiden and amantadine on parkinsonism and tardive dyskinesia-type involuntary movements: a double-blind, cross-over, placebo-controlled study in medicated chronic schizophrenic patients. *J Clin Psychiatry,* **56**, 167–70.

Small, J.G., Hirsch, S.R., Arvanitis, L.A. *et al.* (1997) Quetiapine in patients with schizophrenia. *Arch Gen Psychiatry,* **54**, 549–57.

Song, F. (1997) Risperidone in the treatment of schizophrenia: a meta-analysis of randomized, controlled trials. *J Psychopharmacology,* **11**, 65–71.

Sokoloff, P. and Schwartz, J-C. (1996) Multiple dopamine receptors: their significance for disease states. In R.J. Beninger, T. Palomo and T. Archer (eds), *Dopamine disease states.* Madrid: CYM (Fundacion Cerebro y Mente), 237–50.

Stahl, S.M. (1996) *Essential psychopharmacology.* Cambridge: Cambridge University Press, 249–88.

Struve, F.A. and Wilner, A.E. (1983) Cognitive dysfunction and tardive dyskinesia. *Br J Psychiatry,* **143**, 597–600.

Stein, M.B. and Pohlman, E.R. (1987) Tardive akathisia associated with low-dose haloperidol use. *J Clin Psychopharmacol,* **7**, 202–3.

Swett, C. (1975) Drug-induced dystonia. *Am J Psychiatry,* **132**, 532–4.

Tamminga, C.A., Mack, R.J., Granneman, G.R. *et al.* (1997) Sertindole in the treatment of psychosis in schizophrenia: efficacy and safety. *Int Clin Psychopharmacol,* **12** (Suppl 1), 29–35.

Tamminga, C.A. and Thaker, G.K. (1989) Tardive dyskinesia. *Curr Opin Psychiatry,* **2**, 12–16.

Tassin, J.P., Stinus, L., Simon, H., *et al.* (1978) Relationship between the locomotor hyperactivity induced by A10 lesions and the destruction of the frontocortical dopaminergic innervation in the rat. *Brain Res,* **141**, 267–81.

Thaker, G.K., Tamminga, C.A., Alphs, L.D. *et al.* (1987) Brain gamma-aminobutyric acid abnormality in tardive dyskinesia. Reduction in cerebrospinal fluid GABA levels and therapeutic response to GABA agonist treatment. *Arch Gen Psychiatry,* **44**, 522–9.

Thaker, G.K., Nguyen, J.A., Strauss, M.E. *et al.* (1990) Clonazepam treatment of tardive dyskinesia: a practical GABAmimetic strategy. *Am J Psychiatry,* **147**, 445–51.

Tonda, M.E. and Guthrie, S.K. (1994) Treatment of neuroleptic-induced movement disorders. *Pharmacotherapy,* **14**, 543–60.

Umbricht, D. and Kane, J.M. (1996a) Understanding the relationship between extrapyramidal side-effects and tardive dyskinesia. In J.M. Kane, H.-J. Moller and F. Awouters (eds), *Serotonergic mechanisms in antipsychotic treatment.* New York: Marcel Dekker, 221–51.

Umbricht, D. and Kane, J.M. (1996b) Medical complications of new antipsychotic drugs. *Schizophr Bull,* **22,** 475–83.

Van Putten, T., Marder, S.R. and Mintz, J. (1990) A controlled dose comparison of haloperidol in newly admitted schizophrenic patients. *Arch Gen Psychiatry,* **47**, 754–8.

Van Putten, T. and Marder, S.R. (1987). Behavioural toxicity of antipsychotic drugs. *J Clin Psychiatry,* **48**, (Suppl 9); 13–19.

Waddington, J.L. (1989) Schizophrenia, affective psychoses, and other disorders treated with neuroleptic drugs: the enigma of tardive dyskinesia, its neurobiological determinants and the conflict of paradigms. *Int Rev Neurobiol,* **31**, 297–353.

Waddington, J.L. (1992) Mechanisms of neuroleptic-induced extrapyramidal side-effects. In J.M. Kane and J.A. Lieberman (eds), *Adverse effects of psychotropic drugs.* New York: Guilford Press, 246–65.

Waddington, J.L. and Youssef, H.A. (1996) Cognitive dysfunction in chronic schizophrenia followed prospectively over 10 years and its longitudinal relationship to the emergence of tardive dyskinesia. *Psychol Med,* **26**, 681–8.

Waddington, J.L., O'Callaghan, E., Buckley, P. *et al.* (1995) Tardive dyskinesia in schizophrenia. Relationship to minor physical anomalies, frontal lobe dysfunction and cerebral structure on magnetic resonance imaging. *Br J Pschiatry,* **167**, 41–4.

Waddington, J.L., O'Callaghan, E., Larkin, C. *et al.* (1993) Cognitive dysfunction in schizophrenia: organic vulnerability factor or state marker for TD? *Brain and Cognition,* **23**, 56–70.

Waddington, J.L., Youssef, H.A. and Kinsella, A. (1990) Cognitive dysfunction in schizophrenia followed up over 5 years, and its longitudinal relationship to the emergence of tardive dyskinesia. *Psychol Med,* **20**, 835–42.

Walters, A.S., Hening, W., Chokroverty, S. *et al.* (1989) Restlessness of the arms as the principal manifestation of neuroleptic-induced akathisia. *J Neurol,* **236**, 435.

Weiden, P.J., Dixon, L., Frances, A. *et al.* (1991) Neuroleptic non-compliance in schizophrenia. In C. Tamminga and S.C. Schulz (eds), *Advances in neuropsychiatry and psychopharmacology,* Vol 1. New York: Raven Press, 285–95.

Wilcox, P.G., Bassett, A., Jones, B. *et al.* (1994) Respiratory dysrhythmias in patients with tardive dyskinesia. *Chest,* **105**, 203–7.

Williams, J.H., Wellman, N.A., Geaney, D.P. *et al.* (1997) Intravenous administration of haloperidol to healthy volunteers: lack of subjective effects but clear objective effects. *J Psychopharmacology,* **11**, 247–52.

Winslow, R.S., Stiller,V., Coons, D.J. *et al.* (1986) Prevention of acute dystonic reactions in patients beginning high potency neuroleptics. *Am J Psychiatry,* **143**, 706–10.

Wojcik J.D., Falk, W.E., Fink, J.S. *et al.* (1991) A review of 32 cases of tardive dystonia. *Am J Psychiatry,* **148**, 1055–9.

World Health Organization: Heads of centres collaborating in WHO co-ordinated studies on biological aspects of mental illness. (1990) Prophylactic use of anticholinergics in patients on long-term neuroleptic treatment: a consensus statement. *Br J Psychiatry,* **156**, 412.

Yagi, G. and Itoh, H. (1987) Follow-up study of 11 patients with potentially reversible tardive dyskinesia. *Am J Psychiatry,* **144**, 1496–8.

Yassa, R. and Jeste, D.V. (1992) Gender differences in tardive dyskinesia: a critical review of the literature. *Schizophr Bull,* **18**, 701–15.

Yassa, R. and Lal, S. (1986) Respiratory irregularity and tardive dyskinesia. *Acta Psychiatr Scand,* **73**, 506–10.

Yassa, R., Ghadirian, A.M. and Schwartz, G. (1985) Tardive dyskinesia: developmental factors. *Can J Psychiatry,* **30**, 344–7.

Yassa, R., Iskandar, H. and Nastase, C. (1988) Propranolol in the treatment of tardive akathisia: a report of two cases. *J Clin Psychopharmacology,* **8**, 283–5.

Yassa, R., Nair, N.P.W., Iskandar, H. et al. (1990) Factors in the development of severe forms of tardive dyskinesia. *Am J Psychiatry,* **147**, 1156–63.

Youssef, H.A. and Waddington, J.L. (1987) Morbidity and mortality in tardive dyskinesia: associations in chronic schizophrenia. *Acta Psychiatr Scand,* **75**, 74–7.

Zubenko, G.S., Barriera, P. and Lipinski, J.F. (1984a) Development of tolerance to the therapeutic effect of amantadine on akathisia. *J Clin Psychopharmacology,* **4**, 218–20.

Zubenko, G.S., Lipinski, J.F., Cohen, B.M. et al. (1984b) Comparison of metoprolol and propranolol in the treatment of akathisia. *Psychiatry Res,* **11**, 143–9.

Zubenko, G.S., Cohen, B.M. and Lipinski, J.F. (1987) Antidepressant-induced akathisia. *J Clin Psychopharmacol,* **7**, 254–7.

CHAPTER 11

New strategies with conventional antipsychotics

STEPHEN R. MARDER, WILLIAM C. WIRSHING AND DONNA AMES WIRSHING

Introduction

The introduction of newer antipsychotics, particularly the serotonin–dopamine antagonists, has raised questions about the role of the older conventional drugs for the treatment of schizophrenia. These older agents are highly effective for the treatment of schizophrenia and other illnesses associated with psychosis, but they are limited by their side-effects, particularly extrapyramidal side-effects (EPS). Concerns about their side-effects have resulted in the recommendation by some that these agents should only be considered when newer agents cannot be used. However, a number of treatment strategies have been developed that can minimize EPS while still permitting patients to take advantage of these highly effective agents.

The classification of newer and older drugs is somewhat controversial at this time. This chapter will classify these agents based on their presumed mechanism of action. The older drugs will be designated dopamine receptor antagonists or DAs, since they appear to decrease psychotic symptoms by their antagonism of D2 receptors. These agents are, in turn, classified as low potency (for example, chlorpromazine or thioridazine), mid-potency (for example, molindone or loxapine) and high potency (for example, fluphenazine or haloperidol), depending on the amount of drug required for antipsychotic effects. This chapter will not discuss the serotonin–dopamine antagonists such as clozapine, risperidone, olanzapine and sertindole, which have affinity for both D2 and 5HT2A receptor activity.

Strategies for managing acute schizophrenia

SELECTION OF AN ANTIPSYCHOTIC

Factors that will influence the selection of an antipsychotic include the patient's prior drug history, the patient's preference, and whether the clinician plans to use a long-acting compound. Although all of the DAs are equally effective, a patient will sometimes respond better to one rather than the others. This responsiveness may be related to the patient's tolerance of side-effects. Van Putten and co-workers (1991) studied patients who were assigned to one of three doses of fluphenazine. Using logistic regression Van Putten and co-workers developed dose–response curves for the proportion of individuals who met their criteria for clinical improvement and disabling side-effects. The two curves were very close together indicating that many patients experienced side-effects at doses that were very near to the doses needed for treating psychosis. In most patients, the disabling side-effect was EPS, particularly akathisia. This supports the common clinical observation that poor response to an antipsychotic may be related to an intolerance of that agent's side-effects. Under these conditions, changing to another DA, perhaps a lower potency agent with less potential for causing that side-effect, may be helpful. Alternatively, it may be helpful to treat the patient prophylactically with an antiparkinsonian agent when starting a high potency DA. The same principle would affect individuals who have difficulty tolerating sedation or hypotension associated with a low potency DA. In this case the clinician may select a higher potency drug.

One of the important factors to consider is the patient's preference. That is, if a patient reportedly responded well previously to a particular drug, that drug may be the best choice. Van Putten and coworkers (1984) searched for indicators available early in treatment that would predict how well a patient would respond to a particular antipsychotic. They found that one of the most reliable predictors was the patient's early subjective response to that agent. In other words, patients responded better to a medication that made them feel better. A substantial part of this effect may have resulted from better compliance with medications that did not result in uncomfortable side-effects (Van Putten et al., 1984).

One of the important advantages of the DAs in comparison to SDAs (serotonin-dopamine antagonists) is that DAs are available as short- or long-acting injectable formulations. Therefore, if the clinicians has decided that the maintenance plan will include a depot formulation, the oral form of the depot drug – haloperidol or fluphenazine in the United States and other agents elsewhere – remains a logical choice. Depot drugs are usually a poor choice for acute treatment. The reason is that these drugs take three months or more to reach a stable steady state and are excreted very slowly (Marder et al., 1986). As a result the clinician is not able to titrate clinical response against dose. Moreover, if too high a dose is selected, the patient may not experience relief for weeks or longer. Also, if the clinician has decided to treat a patient with a long-acting depot for maintenance treatment, the gradual transition from oral to depot should begin as early in treatment as possible.

IMPLEMENTING ACUTE TREATMENT

Understanding certain characteristics of antipsychotics can guide an acute treatment strategy. Perhaps the most important principle is that their antipsychotic effects do not emerge immediately, but may require days or weeks. It appears that these agents must first exert effects on target receptors before the drug actually manifests its clinical effects. This observation is supported by findings from both PET scanning and the measurement of plasma homovanillic acid which suggest that clinical improvement is not associated with the immediate effects of the drug on dopamine receptors, but on processes that occur later (Kahn and Davis, 1995).

For clinicians these observations suggest that the goal of the first days of treatment is to administer a drug dose that occupies an adequate proportion of D2 receptors and to keep the patient comfortable until the drug's effect becomes apparent. If a patient does not respond in the first week or two, this does not indicate that the current treatment is inadequate. Since most of the improvement on an antipsychotic occurs during the first 6 weeks, patients should be observed for this interval before changing a drug (Janicak *et al.*, 1993). Also, the strategy of using 'as needed medications' (PRNs) as a guide to finding the optimal dose makes very little sense since the immediate and delayed responses are very different. The calming that is seen soon after an antipsychotic is administered to an excited or agitated patient can be extremely helpful under many conditions. However, the doses needed to induce and maintain this calming can result in patients being treated with doses of the drug that are higher than the doses needed to treat the psychosis. As a result, it is probably better to manage agitation with a benzodiazepine that is targeted at agitation and an antipsychotic to reduce psychotic thought processes.

Another important principle in treating acute psychosis is that patients demonstrate a drug response in a particular dose range. Studies suggest that this range is between 300 and 1000 mg of chlorpromazine or 5 and 20 mg of haloperidol (Baldessarini *et al.*, 1988). Clinicians are often tempted to increase the dose above the usual range when patients are responding slowly to treatment or not responding at all. However, a number of well-designed studies indicate that raising the dose does not lead to a better or a more rapid response (Van Putten *et al.*, 1990; Kinon *et al.*, 1993).

This property of antipsychotics supports the treating of patients with a dose in the therapeutic range for that drug and waiting about 6 weeks for a drug response. If a patient fails to respond after an adequate trial, the clinician should confirm that the patient was receiving an adequate dose (and that the patient was compliant) by monitoring the plasma concentration. If the plasma level is adequate, the clinician is faced with a number of alternatives: (i) wait longer for a response; (ii) change drugs; or (iii) initiate a high dose trial. As mentioned previously, increasing the drug dose is unlikely to be effective. If the patient has improved but has not reached the level of improvement that was hoped for, the clinician should consider waiting since it is common for patients to continue to improve for as long as 6 months after beginning treatment with an antipsychotic. If the decision is made to change drugs, the clinician should decide whether to change to a newer SDA or to another DA. Studies (Kinon *et al.*, 1993) indicate that patients who have failed to respond to one conventional agent are unlikely to respond to others even if the clinician changes to a drug from a different class. There is evidence (Kane *et al.*, 1988; Bondolfi *et al.*, 1995) that changing to a newer SDA may be the most effective intervention.

Measuring plasma concentrations

Dopamine receptor antagonists (DAs) should be ideal drugs for plasma level monitoring since there are wide inter-individual variations in blood levels for patients given the same dose of a DA and there is a relatively narrow dose range in which the drug is effective with minimal side effects (Van Putten *et al.*, 1991). On the other hand, studies (reviewed in Marder *et al.*, 1995) have produced mixed results, with the more recent ones suggesting certain circumstances where monitoring a drug's plasma level may be helpful.

At this time, there is no evidence that routine monitoring should be a part of a treatment strategy. However, when patients have been treated with a DA and the clinical response is questionable, ordering a plasma level determination may provide some useful information if the patient is receiving a drug for which there is adequate information about therapeutic levels. At this time, haloperidol is the best studied drug, but there is reasonable information about therapeutic levels of perphenazine, fluphenazine, and trifluoperazine. A low level (for example less than 5 ng/ml of haloperidol, 1 ng/ml of trifluoperazine, or 1 ng/ml of fluphenazine) suggests that raising the dose may be helpful. A higher level (for example, greater than 15 ng/ml of haloperidol) may indicate that side-effects are interfering with therapeutic response and that lowering the dose may be helpful.

A plasma level determination may also be useful when patients are receiving certain drugs such as heterocyclic antidepressants, fluoxetine, beta-blockers, and cimetidine which may increase plasma levels by competing for enzyme binding sites, or barbiturates and carbamezepine which may decrease plasma levels by enhancing metabolism of the antipsychotic. For example, when carbamazepine is added to haloperidol it may reduce the haloperidol level by as much as 50%. Under these circumstances a plasma level measurement may be helpful in confirming that the addition of these agents has not had a serious effect (Van Putten *et al.*, 1991).

MANAGEMENT OF NEGATIVE AND COGNITIVE SYMPTOMS

Recent studies of psychopathology in schizophrenia indicate that there are three dimensions to psychopathology: psychotic, negative, and disorganized or cognitive symptoms. Psychotic symptoms include hallucinations, ideas of reference, and delusions. These are symptoms that tend to result in hospitalization and to disrupt the lives of patients. Negative symptoms include decreased motivation, emotional blunting, and impoverished speech and thought. These symptoms are associated with the social and vocational impairments in schizophrenia. Disorganized symptoms include disorganized speech and behaviour as well as impairments in attention, memory, and information processing. These symptoms are also associated with the social and vocational impairments in schizophrenia. Given the importance of negative and cognitive symptoms it is important for clinicians to consider their management in developing a treatment strategy.

In managing negative symptoms, it is helpful to classify them as either primary or secondary negative symptoms. Secondary negative symptoms may result from other conditions such as untreated positive symptoms, depression, or extrapyramidal side-effects (EPS). EPS are a common cause of secondary negative symptoms particularly when patients are experiencing akinesia, a side-effect that can be manifest in decreased speech, decreased motivation, and decreased spontaneous gestures. Positive or psychotic symptoms, may be misinterpreted as negative symptoms. For example, a patient who is withdrawn or uncommunicative as a result of suspiciousness may appear to have affective blunting. Also, patients with schizophrenia may also suffer from symptoms of depression. These symptoms may appear as emotional withdrawal or impoverished speech.

The management of secondary negative symptoms begins with the management of the condition that caused these symptoms. For depression this may include the addition of an antidepressant medication; for EPS this may involve the addition of an antiparkinsonian medication, a dose reduction or a change to an antipsychotic, usually an SDA, that is associated with less EPS. If secondary negative symptoms result from inadequately managed positive symptoms, the clinician may consider reevaluating the drug dose or changing to another antipsychotic.

If the causes of secondary negative symptoms have been ruled out, the patient is likely to be suffering from primary negative symptoms that may be difficult to manage. Although novel treatments such as SSRIs (selective serotonin reuptake inhibitors), stimulants, and other agents have been studied, none have proven themselves effective for primary negative symptoms. There is some evidence suggesting that the SDAs are more effective in treating negative symptoms than DAs. However, these agents have not as yet been studied in individuals who have documented primary negative symptoms. Until this issue is decided by adequate controlled studies, it is probably reasonable for clinicians to consider changing to an SDA for patients with substantial negative symptoms.

It may also be helpful to categorize disorganized or cognitive symptoms as primary or secondary. In this case, cognitive symptoms can be secondary to anticholinergic or sedating medications that may impair cognition. These symptoms can frequently be managed by decreasing the use of anticholinergics and managing EPS by decreasing drug dose or changing to a different agent. Similarly, changing to a less sedating drug may be helpful for some patients. Once these symptoms are ruled out, the patient is likely to be suffering from impairments in attention and information processing that are common in schizophrenia. These cognitive impairments can also interfere with the social and vocational rehabilitation of patients, even when their psychotic symptoms have been well controlled. At this stage, there is controversial evidence suggesting that newer SDAs may be more effective than DAs for cognitive symptoms.

Managing side-effects during acute treatment

One of the difficulties in managing acute treatment is that patients will usually experience the side-effects of an antipsychotic well before they experience clinical improvement. For low potency drugs the experience is likely to include sedation, postural hypotension, and anticholinergic effects, whereas high potency drugs are likely to cause EPS. These often disturbing experiences tend to occur at the time that patients are most ill and, as a result, they are suspicious and unco-operative. Under these conditions, unexpected side-effects may further undermine the relationship between the physician and the patient. Warning patients about side-effects and responding quickly when they occur may be helpful. Patients who have difficulty describing their internal experiences may require assistance. Warning patients about the potential side-effects of medication can lead to prompt management and will often improve the trust between patient and clinician.

The most common form of EPS from DAs is akathisia, consisting of a subjective feeling of restlessness. Patients who experience severe akathisia will often pace continuously or move their feet restlessly while they are sitting. Severe akathisia can cause patients to feel anxious or irritable, and some reports suggest that severe akathisia can result in aggressive or suicidal acts. The incidence of akathisia on DAs may be underestimated since it is frequently misinterpreted as psychotic agitation. When Van Putten *et al.* (1991) specifically asked his patients about akathisia, he found that 75% of patients treated with haloperidol experienced some form of restlessness. Braude *et al.* (1983) reported that 25% of their patients experienced akathisia.

Another reason for carefully managing side-effects is that they can affect a patient's attitude toward drug treatment in subsequent episodes. Van Putten (1974) found that 89% of his patients who were reluctant to accept a DA had experienced some form of EPS. In these patients, this was most commonly akathisia.

Since patients may experience akathisia as irritability or agitation, asking them whether they are restless or have difficulty sitting still may be helpful in the early stages of treatment. At this point, a dosage adjustment, a beta-blocker, or an anticholinergic antiparkinson drug may provide considerable relief. Also, patients who have a history of developing severe akathisia that responds poorly to these treatments are likely to do better if they are treated with a newer SDA.

Clinicians may consider prescribing prophylactic antiparkinsonian medications for patients who are likely to experience disturbing EPS. These include patients who have a history of EPS sensitivity or those who are being treated with relatively high doses of high potency drugs. Prophylactic antiparkinsonian medications may also be indicated when high potency drugs are prescribed for young men who tend to have an increased vulnerability for developing dystonias. Again, these patients may also be candidates for newer drugs.

Strategies for maintenance therapy

One of the most useful properties of dopamine receptor antagonists is their ability to prevent relapse in patients who have been stabilized. Although studies differ depending on the population, approximately 70% of stable patients who are changed to a placebo will relapse each year whereas only about 30% of patients on an antipsychotic will relapse (reviewed by Davis, 1975). This very large drug-placebo difference supports the practice of maintaining patients on an antipsychotic even after they have recovered from a psychotic episode. Clinicians are often tempted to discontinue medications in patients who have been well and stable for prolonged periods. Unfortunately, these patients also have high relapse rates when their medications are discontinued (Hogarty *et al.,* 1976).

Relapse rates for first episode patients are somewhat lower than rates for patients who have had multiple episodes. This raises the difficult question as to how long to continue maintenance medications after an initial episode. The question is complicated by the fact that patients who are experiencing their first psychotic episode are usually able to return to the community and thus have the most to lose if a relapse occurs. A reasonable strategy for most first episode patients would probably involve continuing drugs for at least a year following an episode, with consideration of dosage reduction or observation off drugs during the following year (Kissling, 1991).

ROUTE OF ADMINISTRATION FOR MAINTENANCE TREATMENT

Clinicians who are developing a long-term maintenance strategy can administer DAs as either oral or long-acting depot compounds. As mentioned previously, depot drugs are poor choices for acute treatment because clinicians are unable to titrate dose against either side-effects or clinical improvement. However, these agents have two potential advantages over oral therapy. First, depot drugs provide a mechanism of drug delivery that does not require the patient to comply with taking oral medications. This gives these agents an advantage for patients who are vulnerable to being non-compliant or partially compliant. Second, depot drugs are more bioavailable. Since these agents are not vulnerable to variations in gastrointestinal absorption or first-pass hepatic and gut metabolism, drug levels are more reliable (Marder *et al.,* 1989).

Both open label and controlled studies have compared oral and depot drugs. The open-label studies found much larger differences favouring depot treatment. The difference probably results from the populations studied. Open-label studies will usually compare typical clinical populations and include individuals who may be non-compliant. Double-blind studies usually include individuals who are selected because they are co-operative and compliant. Moreover, research staffs will tend to monitor patients more carefully, thereby undermining the advantage of depot drugs in less compliant patients. It is therefore not surprising that double-blind studies are less conclusive. In a review of six studies, Davis *et al.* (1993) found that in five of them the results favoured depot. When the results were weighted for sample size, there was a significant difference favouring depot. In addition, the comparison that lasted the longest (Hogarty *et al.*, 1979) found an advantage for depot.

These advantages of depot therapy suggest that clinicians should consider this route of administration for a substantial proportion of patients in long-term therapy. In places where only a small proportion of patients are treated with depots – such as the United States – there is a tendency to reserve long-acting drugs for patients who have a clear history of non-compliance or unco-operativeness. This may result in an underutilization of these agents since it has been estimated that as many as 60% or more of patients with schizophrenia cannot be relied upon to take their medication as prescribed. It is likely that a high proportion of these patients will have a better outcome if they are treated with a depot.

DOSAGE REDUCTION STRATEGIES

Making decisions about the optimal drug dosage during the maintenance phase of treatment can be particularly difficult because the patient is usually clinically stable. As a result, drug dose cannot be titrated against clinical response. If the dose is too low, this may not be apparent until the patient relapses. If the dose is higher than necessary, the patient may be exposed to unnecessary side-effects. In addition, there are data suggesting that higher doses may expose patients to a greater risk of developing tardive dyskinesia. For these reasons, a number of strategies have been proposed for decreasing the maintenance doses of antipsychotics.

A number of investigators (Pietzcker *et al.*, 1986; Carpenter *et al.*, 1987; Jolley *et al.*, 1989; Herz *et al.*, 1991) have proposed a strategy called targeted or intermittent therapy. Patients who are stable have their drug dose gradually decreased until medications are completely discontinued. They are then followed very closely until there are signs that the individual is beginning to relapse. At the earliest sign of a recurrence, drugs are reinstituted. To make this strategy work, patients and their families are trained to detect the early prodromal signs of impending psychotic breakdown. This makes sense since a number of studies indicate that most schizophrenic patients do not relapse abruptly. For example, Herz and Melville (1980) found that a majority of patients and their families were aware of a relapse more than a week before it occurred. Signs were often apparent weeks before the relapse.

All four studies found that targeted treatment resulted in patients sustaining substantially higher relapse rates than continuous treatment. Schooler (1991) reviewed these studies and found that the one-year relapse rate (using a sample-sized weighted mean) with continuous treatment was 17% compared to 37% with targeted treatment. Two-year rates were 24% for the continuous group and 50% for the targeted group. A review by Davis and co-workers (1993) also found a highly statistically significant difference favouring continuous treatment. Moreover, reported rehospitalization rates were significantly higher with targeted treatment. The results from the study at National Institute of Mental Health Treatment Strategies in Schizophrenia (Schooler *et al.*, 1997) also indicated that relapse and rehospitalization rates were unacceptably high with targeted treatment. Although these results are discouraging, it is conceivable that patients with insight and well-characterized prodromal symptoms may be effectively managed with targeted treatment.

Another strategy proposed treating patients with much lower doses of a DA than are usually prescribed. Studies by three groups (Kane *et al.*, 1983; Marder *et al.*, 1987; Hogarty *et al.*, 1988) indicated that a substantial number (but by no means all) 'maintenance' patients do well on doses of fluphenazine decanoate that are only 20% of the usual doses. These doses were in the range of 5 to 10 mg of fluphenazine decanoate every 14 days. In the Kane study (1983) much lower doses in the range of 1.25 to 2 mg were associated with substantially higher relapse rates. Although the Marder and Hogarty studies reported a greater risk of mild psychotic exacerbations with doses in the 20% range, these episodes were usually rather mild and were seldom associated with a need for rehospitalization. These minor exacerbations were usually easily controlled by a small dosage adjustment. In addition, patients receiving the lower dose had fewer side-effects, and those in the Marder study complained less of anxiety and depression and had a lower drop-out rate. Kane *et al.* (1983)

reported that patients on lower doses also had lower dyskinesia ratings, suggesting that the low dose strategy may reduce vulnerability to tardive dyskinesia. These findings suggested that there are likely to be benefits associated with the use of the lowest effective dose of maintenance neuroleptic.

Marder and co-workers (1994) proposed a strategy that combines characteristics of both low dose and targeted treatment. In this strategy, patients are treated with low doses of fluphenazine decanoate and are monitored for prodromal symptoms. If prodromal symptoms are identified, oral fluphenazine is prescribed until the episode is adequately treated. This strategy was tested in a study by managing patients with 5 to 10 mg of fluphenazine decanoate every 14 days. When patients met study criteria for a prodrome they were randomly assigned to either 5 mg twice a day of oral fluphenazine or placebo. The results indicated that there was no difference between the active supplementation group and the placebo group during the first year. However, in the second year, patients who received active supplementation spent a significantly lower proportion of time in an exacerbated state.

MONITORING OF PRODROMAL SYMPTOMS

The strategy of monitoring patients for prodromal symptoms appeared to be successful in the study by Marder *et al.* (1994) but it also revealed some limitations. Only 45% of patients demonstrated a prodromal episode during the study suggesting that prodromal monitoring would not be useful for all patients. Also, in the placebo group, fewer than half of prodromal episodes were followed by a psychotic exacerbation. This suggests that prodromal episodes are not a completely reliable indicator of relapse risk. Nevertheless, as Herz and Lamberti (1995) have pointed out, characterizing prodromal states as periods of increased vulnerability to relapse is not the same as expecting that the process of relapse is irreversible when patients have entered a prodromal state. Another study by Herz and Lamberti (1995) found that crisis intervention when patients demonstrated prodromal symptoms was effective in reducing the risk of relapse.

These studies suggest that the routine monitoring of prodromal symptoms is a useful activity for many patients in long-term maintenance therapy. The Marder *et al.* study (1994) found that the strategy tended to become more effective over time. This appeared to be a result of the regular prodromal rating occasions during which the patient and a nurse would review and revise the prodromal symptom rating list. These interactions may have led the patient and the clinician to become better at predicting when a patient was on the verge of an exacerbation.

INTEGRATING PHARMACOTHERAPY AND PSYCHOSOCIAL TREATMENTS

The most effective long-term treatments for individuals with chronic schizophrenia will probably involve combinations of pharmacotherapy and psychosocial treatments. The literature on combining pharmacological and psychosocial interventions in schizophrenia indicates that these treatments can have complex interactions. The effectiveness of the combination is likely to be influenced by the timing of each treatment, the intensity of the treatments (dosage for the drug), the adverse effects associated with the form of treatment and the selection of individuals. In addition, psychosocial treatments that have been administered to schizophrenic patients can be very different in content and therapeutic goals. It is therefore important not to overgeneralize the results from one type of psychosocial treatment – for example individual therapy or group psychotherapy – to make assumptions about the interactions of drugs with skills training or family therapy.

A number of models have been proposed for understanding interactions between pharmacological and psychosocial interventions. In one very useful model (Falloon and Liberman, 1983), patients with schizophrenia have a genetically inherited trait that renders them vulnerable to undergoing a schizophrenic breakdown. A number of stressors including overstimulating environments, certain life events, stimulant drugs, loss of social supports, or increased emotionality in the family can move the person toward psychotic decompensation. On the other hand, biological protective factors such as antipsychotic medications or social protective factors such as social supports, well functioning families and coping skills operate to stabilize the individual. This provides the clinician with a number of avenues for intervening. These could include assuring optimal drug treatment (as well as drug compliance), decreasing family interactions that are destructive, or improving the patient's ability to cope with the symptoms and deficits that are associated with schizophrenia.

This model suggests possible advantages of thoughtfully combining pharmacological and psychosocial strategies. Examples are included in Table 11.1

The literature on combining treatments has established a number of important principles (Table 11.2). Psychosocial treatments are most effective when patients have been stabilized on drugs and not when they are acutely ill. In an NIMH collaborative study (Hogarty *et al.*, 1974), patients who received a placebo as opposed to an active drug, had a worse outcome when assigned to a form of individual psychotherapy called Major Role Therapy. The opposite was true when patients

Table 11.1 Possible interactions between pharmacological and psychosocial treatments in schizophrenia

- Patients receiving an effective psychosocial treatment might require a lower dose of antipsychotic medication
- Patients who are receiving adequate medication might tolerate more intrusive and stimulating forms of psychosocial treatment than those who are unmedicated or improperly medicated
- Patients who are receiving psychosocial interventions may be more compliant with prescribed medications
- The effects of combining treatments would be more than additive since each would enhance the effectiveness of the other
- Drugs and psychosocial treatments may affect different outcome domains (for example, drugs may affect psychotic symptoms or relapse rates and psychosocial treatments may affect social and vocational skills)

Table 11.2. Studies on interactions between antipsychotic and psychosocial treatments

Treatment	References	Findings
Social treatment	Hogarty *et al.*, 1974	Improved social adjustment; interaction with drug
Behavioural family treatment criticism	Falloon and Liberman, 1983	Lower relapse, decreased
Family education	Goldstein *et al.*, 1978	Lower relapse, improved functioning
	Hogarty *et al.*, 1991	
Social skills training	Wallace *et al.*, 1985	Lower relapse;
	Hogarty *et al.*, 1991	improved social adjustment

received antipsychotics; that is, drug-treated patients demonstrated positive effects from the psychosocial treatment including a better social outcome and lower relapse rates.

A different interaction was suggested by a study by Falloon and Liberman (1983). These authors found that patients who received a form of family therapy demonstrated better compliance with drug taking than those in a control group. This may explain why patients in family treatment appeared to require lower doses of an antipsychotic. Alternatively, family therapy may have resulted in an overall reduction in the level of stress that patients experienced within the family. The previously described model by Falloon and Liberman (1983) suggested that the lower level of stress would be associated with a decreased requirement for antipsychotic medications.

The role of medication in improving the effectiveness of a psychosocial treatment is illustrated in an important study in which patients received social therapy and either fluphenazine decanoate or fluphenazine hydrochloride (Hogarty *et al.*, 1979). Relapse rates were substantially lower for individuals who received depot fluphenazine and social therapy. This suggested that social treatments work best when patients are guaranteed drug delivery.

Our laboratory has designed a study that is aimed at maximizing the possible interaction between drug and social skills training (Marder *et al.*, 1994, 1996). As noted below the psychosocial method was developed with the specific intention of improving drug compliance and improving the relationship between patients and drug prescribers. For this study we included two drug conditions and two psychosocial conditions. The drug conditions are described in a prior section on Dosage Reduction Strategies. Outpatients with schizophrenia were stabilized on a low dose of fluphenazine decanoate (5 to 10 mg every 14 days) and supplemented with either active oral fluphenazine (5 mg twice daily) or a placebo when they first met criteria for a prodromal period. For the psychosocial conditions, patients were randomly assigned to receive either behavioural skills training (SST) or supportive group therapy (SGT) administered twice weekly for two years. We monitored the rates of psychotic exacerbation as well as scores on the Social Adjustment Scale II (SAS II).

We found significant main effects favouring SST over SGT on two of the six SAS II cluster totals examined (Personal Well-Being, $P=0.010$ and the total SAS II, $P = 0.016$). We also found statistically significant interactions between psychosocial treatment and drug treatment for three items (External Family, $P = 0.011$, Social–Interpersonal, $P = 0.022$, and total SAS II, $P = 0.032$). In each case, these interactions indicated that the advantage of SST over SGT was greatest when combined with active drug supplementation. Although SST appeared to affect social adjustment, it did not appear to affect relapse rates. In contrast, we found that the early intervention strategy with oral medication reduced the risk of relapse during the second year of the study, but did not affect social adjustment.

These findings also support the idea that pharmacological and psychosocial treatments affect different outcome dimensions. Drugs affect relapse risk whereas skills training affects social adjustment. The interaction between social and pharmacological treatments may be explained as follows: a pharmacological treatment that includes intervention when patients demonstrate early signs of relapse will reduce the risk of relapse. If this strategy is combined with skills training, those individuals who are best protected against relapse will derive the most benefit from skills training.

References

Baldessarini, R.J., Cohen, B.M., Teicher, M.H. (1988) Significance of neuroleptic dose and plasma level in the pharmacological treatment of psychoses. *Arch Gen Psychiatry*, **45**, 79–90.

Braude, W.M., Barnes, T.R. and Gore, S.M. (1983) Clinical characteristics of akathisia. A systematic investigation of acute psychiatric inpatient admissions *Brit J Psychiatry*, **143**, 139–50.

Bondolfi, G., Bauman, P., Patris, M. *et al.* (1998) Risperidone versus clozapine in treatment-resistant chronic schizophrenia: a randomized double-blind study. *Am J Psychiatry*, **155**, 499–504.

Carpenter, W.T., Heinrichs, D.W. and Hanlon, T.E. (1987) A comparative trial of pharmacologic strategies in schizophrenia. *Am J Psychiatry* **144**, 1466–70.

Davis, J.M. (1975) Overview: maintenance therapy in psychiatry. I. Schizophrenia. *Am J Psychiatry*, **132**, 1237–45.

Davis, J.M., Janicak, P.G., Singla, A. and Sharma, R.P. (1993) Maintenance antipsychotic medication. In T.R.E. Barnes (ed.) *Antipsychotic drugs and their side effects*. New York: Academic Press, 182–203.

Falloon, I.R. and Liberman, R.P. (1983) Interactions between drug and psychosocial therapy in schizophrenia. *Schizophr Bull*, **9**(4), 543–54.

Goldstein, M.J., Rodnick, E.H., Evans, J.R. *et al.* (1978) Drug and family therapy in the aftercare of acute schizophrenics. *Arch Gen Psychiatry*, **35**,1169–77.

Herz, M.I., Glazer, W.M., Mostert, M.A. *et al.* (1991) Intermittent vs. maintenance medication in schizophrenia: two-year results. *Arch Gen Psychiatry*, **48**, 333–9.

Herz, M.I. and Lamberti, J.S. (1995) Prodromal symptoms and relapse prevention in schizophrenia. *Schizophr Bull*, **21**, 541–51.

Herz, M.I. and Melville, C. (1980) Relapse in schizophrenia. *Am J Psychiatry*, **137**, 801–12.

Hogarty, G.E., Andersen, C.M., Reiss, D.J. *et al.* (1991) Family psychoeducation, social skills training, and maintenance chemotherapy in the aftercare treatment of schizophrenia. Two-year effects of a controlled study on relapse and adjustment. *Arch Gen Psychiatry*, **48**(4), 340–7.

Hogarty, G.E., Goldberg, S.C., Schooler, N.R. and Ulrich, R.F. (1974) Drug and sociotherapy in the aftercare of schizophrenic patients. II. Two-year relapse rates. *Arch Gen Psychiatry*, **31**, 603–8.

Hogarty, G.E., McEvoy, J.P., Munetz, M. *et al.* (1988) Environmental/Personal Indicators in the Course of Schizophrenia Research Group. Dose of fluphenazine, familial expressed emotion, and outcome in schizophrenia: results of a two-year controlled study. *Arch Gen Psychiatry*, **45**, 797–805.

Hogarty, G.E., Schooler, N.R., Ulrich, R.F., Mussare, F., Ferro, P. and Herron, E. (1979) Fluphenazine and social therapy in the aftercare of schizophrenic patients: Relapse analysis of a two-year controlled study of fluphenazine decanoate and fluphenazine hydrochloride. *Arch Gen Psychiatry*, **36**, 1283–94.

Hogarty, G.E., Ulrich, R.F., Mussare, F. and Aristigueta, N. (1976) Drug discontinuation among long-term, successfully maintained schizophrenic outpatients, *Prac J Psychiat/Neurol*, **9**, 494–503.

Janicak, P.G., Davis, J.M., Preskorn, S.H. and Ayd, F.J. (1993) *Principles and practice of psychopharmacology*. Baltimore: Williams and Wilkins, 93–184.

Jolley, A.G., Hirsch, S.R., McRink, A., Manchanda, R. (1989) Trial of brief intermittent neuroleptic prophylaxis for selected schizophrenic outpatients: clinical outcome at one year. *Br Med J*, **298**, 985–90.

Kahn, R.S. and Davis, K.L. (1995) New developments in dopamine and schizophrenia. In F.E. Bloom and D.J. Kupfer (eds), *Psychopharmacology: The Fourth Generation of Progress*, New York: Raven Press, 1193–203.

Kane, J.M., Honigfeld, G., Singer, J., Meltzer, H., and the Clozaril Collaborative Study Group (1988) Clozapine for the treatment-resistant schizophrenic: a double-blind comparison versus chlorpromazine/benztropine. *Arch Gen Psychiatry*, **45**, 789–96.

Kane, J.M., Rifkin, A., Woerner, M. *et al.* (1983). Low dose neuroleptic treatment of outpatient schizophrenics: I. preliminary results for relapse rates. *Arch Gen Psychiatry*, **40**, 893–96.

Kinon, B.J. Kane, J.M. Johns, C. *et al.* (1993) Treatment of neuroleptic-resistant schizoprenic relapse. *Psychopharmacol Bull*, **29**, 309–14.

Kissling, W. (ed.) (1991) *Guidelines for neuroleptic relapse prevention in schizophrenia*. Berlin: Springer-Verlag.

Marder, S.R., Hubbard, J.W., Van Putten, T. and Midha, K.K. (1989) The pharmacokinetics of long-acting injectable neuroleptic drugs: clinical implications. *Psychopharmacology*, **98**, 433–9.

Marder, S.R., Hubbard, J.W., Van Putten, T. *et al.* (1986) Plasma fluphenazine levels in patients receiving two doses of fluphenazine decanoate. *Psychopharmacol Bull*, **22**, 264–6.

Marder, S.R. and Van Putten, T. (1995) Antipsychotic medications. In A.F. Schatzberg and C.B. Nemeroff (eds) *The American Psychiatric Press textbook of psychopharmacology*. Washington, DC: American Psiatric Press, 435–56.

Marder, S.R., Van Putten, T., Mintz, J., Lebell, M., McKenzie, J. and May, P.R.A. (1987) Low and conventional dose maintenance therapy with fluphenazine decanoate: two year outcome. *Arch Gen Psychiatry*, **44** , 518–21.

Marder, S.R. Wirshing, W.C., Mintz, J. *et al.* (1996) Behavioral skills training versus group psychotherapy for outpatients with schizophrenia: two-year outcome. *Am J Psychiatry*, **153**, 1585–92.

Marder, S.R. Wirshing, W.C., Van Putten, T. *et al.* (1994) Fluphenazine versus placebo supplementation for prodromal signs of relapse in schizophrenia. *Arch Gen Psychiatry*, **51**, 280–7.

Pietzcker, A., Gaebel, W., Kopcke, M. *et al.* (1986) A German multicentre study of the neuroleptic long term therapy of schizophrenic patients: preliminary report. *Pharmacopsychiatry,* **19**, 161–6.

Schooler, N.R. (1991) Maintenance medication for schizophrenia: strategies for dose reduction. *Schizophr Bull,* **17**, 311–24.

Schooler, N.R., Keith, S.J., Severe, J.B. *et al.* (1997) Relapse and rehospitalization during maintenance treatment of schizophrenia. The effects of dose reduction and family treatment [*see* comments]. *Arch Gen Psychiatry,* **54**, 453–63.

Van Putten, T. (1974) Why do schizophrenic patients refuse to take their drugs? *Arch Gen Psychiatry,* **31**, 67–72.

Van Putten, T., Marder, S.R. and Mintz, J. (1990) A controlled dose comparison of haloperidol in newly admitted schizophrenic patients. *Arch Gen Psychiatry,* **47**, 754–8.

Van Putten. T., Marder, S.R., Wirshing, W.C., Aravagiri, M. and Chabert, N. (1991) Neuroleptic plasma levels. *Schizophr Bull,* **17**, 197–216.

Van Putten T., May, P.R.A. and Marder, S.R. (1984) Response to antipsychotic medication: the doctor's and the consumer's view. *Am J Psychiatry,* **141**, 16–19.

Wallace, C.J. and Liberman, R.P. (1985) Social skills training for patients with schizophrenia: a controlled clinical trial. *Psychiatry Res,* **15**(3), 239–47.

CHAPTER 12

New antipsychotic drugs: preclinical evaluation and clinical profiles in the treatment of schizophrenia

JOHN L. WADDINGTON

Evolving concepts in the search for new antipsychotics

CURRENT STATUS OF CONVENTIONAL AGENTS

This volume coincides with the 45th anniversary of the identification of the anti-psychotic and other effects of chlorpromazine as the progenitor of what has become the wide range of conventional neuroleptic drugs that have dominated the pharmaco-therapy of schizophrenia over subsequent decades. Recent reviews have documented contemporary perspectives of these agents, but it is chastening to note the extent to which we still fail to understand fully their pharmacological actions and optimal clinical usage (Waddington, 1995; Kane, 1996).

In pharmacological terms, antagonism of brain D2 dopamine (DA) receptors (now more appropriately referred to as 'D2-like;' *see also* Waddington, 1993a) has become recognized as the one action that appears common to all such conventional agents identified to date. However, it is necessary to consider whether this action is

(i) 'sufficient' for antipsychotic efficacy, (ii) 'necessary' for such efficacy in association with adjunctive properties, or (iii) an epiphenomenon that confounds a more primary role for those adjunctive properties: Furthermore, it cannot be excluded that there exist distinct mechanisms that are independently 'sufficient' for antipsychotic efficacy (Waddington, 1995). In clinical terms, evidence continues to emerge that (i) antipsychotic efficacy can be evident in association with few extrapyramidal or other adverse effects at doses of conventional agents, such as haloperidol, that are considerably lower than those often prescribed routinely; (ii) these lower doses appear to be associated with high occupancy of D2 receptors as evaluated *in vivo* by positron emission tomography (PET), and (iii) adequate prevention of relapse may be obtainable at yet lower dosages and levels of D2 receptor occupancy (Stone *et al.*, 1995; Waddington, 1995; Kapur *et al.*, 1996).

APPROACHES TO IDENTIFYING NEW ANTIPSYCHOTICS

While the above findings should engender a more positive approach to the use of such conventional agents, they cannot negate either their sometimes serious adverse effects which can be a major impediment to effective treatment and compliance (Owens, 1996; Barnes and McPhillips, 1996), or the particularly problematic issue of limited- or non-response in a significant proportion of patients (Meltzer, 1995a; Kane, 1996); and though it appears that conventional agents *can*, and thus *should*, be used more effectively than is sometimes appreciated, their evident limitations underpin the continuing search for new agents.

That search has proceeded via numerous routes. In mechanistic terms, compounds of greater selectivity for a single receptor sub-type and compounds having either a 'tailored' combination of actions or a yet broader spectrum of pharmacological activity, in accordance with prevailing theoretical concepts, have all been sought. Evolving insights into the pathobiology of schizophrenia itself has generated new behavioural models for evaluating putative antipsychotics, while advances in molecular neuroscience have generated new neurochemical models for their evaluation. However, beneath most of these new, neuroscience-led approaches lies, at least in part, some influence of serendipitous clinical findings.

New preclinical considerations

CLASSICAL CONCEPTS AND THEIR LIMITATIONS

Recognition of D2 receptor antagonism as a common denominator among conventional antipsychotics of pharmacological diversity resulted initially in the exploration of a large number of selective D2 antagonists, e.g. sulpiride, piquindone, nemonapride, remoxipride, raclopride, none of which has yet constituted a fundamental therapeutic advance. These compounds were evaluated initially, in the main, using animal models that sought to dissociate those aspects of DA-dependent psychomotor behaviour, neurochemistry and electrophysiology that were held to be limbically mediated, and thus to predict antipsychotic activity, from those aspects held to be striatally mediated, and thus to predict extrapyramidal side-effects (EPS) (Ellenbroek, 1993; Kinon and Lieberman, 1996). However, such preclinical approaches carry with them the risk of entering false-positive agents into clinical trials. For example, savoxapine was identified preclinically as a D2 receptor antagonist, having a higher affinity for hippocampal than for striatal receptors and a presumed greater potency to antagonize limbically – as opposed to striatally – mediated behaviour; however, clinical trials revealed moderate antipsychotic efficacy *and* EPS, with subsequent PET studies revealing appreciable occupancy of basal ganglia D2 receptors (*see* Waddington, 1995). Also, such emphasis on anatomical specificity may be incomplete (Lidsky, 1995). Such approaches continue to evolve, both in rodents (Ellenbroek, 1993; Ogren and Archer, 1994; Hoffman and Donovan, 1995; Arnt, 1995) and in non-human primates (Casey, 1996).

NEW FAMILIES OF DOPAMINE RECEPTOR SUB-TYPES

For several years now, hypotheses of antipsychotic drug action have had to take into account new evidence from the application of molecular biology and gene cloning techniques, suggesting that the number of DA receptor sub-types appears considerably larger than envisaged originally within the D1/D2 schema; current theory encompasses at least six DA receptor sequences which, on the basis of their known pharmacological characteristics, are best grouped into two families: D1-like (D1A/1, D1B/5; and D2-like (D2L/S, D3, D4) receptors (*see* Seeman, 1992; Waddington, 1993a, 1995).

For D2, read D2-like receptors

Earlier emphasis on D2 antagonism has required recasting to substitute D2 with D2-like, given the inability of most conventional antipsychotics to distinguish among cloned D2L/S, D3 and D4 receptors; indeed, it has proved difficult to identify new agents having appreciable selectivity for D2L/S over their D3 and D4 counterparts.

There endures a good correlation between the affinities of conventional antipsychotics for the cloned rat or human D2 receptors and their free concentrations in patient plasma (Seeman, 1992), though it has been reported that among diverse antipsychotics, none was able to distinguish materially between either the cloned 'long' and 'short' splice variants of human D2 or of rat D2 receptors in striatal or limbic tissue (Schotte *et al.*, 1996).

Partial D2-like agonists

This approach to antipsychotic therapy is based on the putative action of partial agonists to attenuate ongoing D2-mediated neurotransmission to an extent commensurate with antipsychotic efficacy without inducing the degree of blockade that is thought to underlie EPS; unfortunately, clinical studies to date appear to have involved compounds with so low a partial efficacy that they are antipsychotic but also induce some degree of EPS, or else with so high a partial efficacy as to induce some psychotic exacerbation (Waddington, 1993a). It has been argued that a partial

D2-like efficacy of the order of 50%, as is the case for CI-1007 (Meltzer *et al.*, 1995) may be more optimal; however, clinical data are needed to substantiate this proposition.

D3 receptors

In contrast to the classical distribution of their D2L/S counterparts, the predominantly 'peristriatal' limbic localization of D3 receptors, in juxtaposition with their high affinity for most antipsychotic drugs, has engendered considerable interest as a potential novel therapeutic target. However, no known antipsychotics show any material selectivity for D3 over D2L/S receptors, and the correlation between the free concentrations of such drugs in patient plasma and their affinities for the D3 receptor does not appear to be as strong as that for the cloned D2 receptor (Seeman, 1992). Compounds with >10-fold selectivity for D3 over D2L/S and D4 receptors are now emerging, but there endures some controversy over whether a D3 antagonist or agonist is the optimal antipsychotic candidate.

A conventional perspective, i.e. generalization from the efficacy of D2-like antagonists, would suggest D3 antagonists as the more likely option, yet the pharmacological profile of emergent compounds (e.g. GR 103691, nafadotride, U 99194A), of which some appear to enhance psychomotor behaviour, particularly at lower, more selective doses (Clifford and Waddington, 1998a), is far from straightforward; conversely, there is overlap between the effects of D2-like antagonists and emergent D3 agonists, some of which (e.g. PD 128907) appear to attenuate psychomotor behaviour, particularly at lower, more selective doses (*see* Bristow *et al.*, 1996a). Furthermore, debate continues as to whether the relevant D3 receptors are located presynaptically, to inhibit the synthesis/release of DA, or postsynaptically to directly inhibit behaviour. The urgent need is for the identification and availability of much more selective D3 agonists, antagonists (and inverse agonists) to clarify these fundamental aspects of D3 receptor function and to define their psychopharmacological effects both in a broad range of antipsychotic models and in the clinic.

D1 receptors

Enthusiasm for the antipsychotic potential of selective D4 antagonists derived indirectly from: (i) their *extrastriatal*, corticolimbic localization: (ii) a putative elevation in their density in the *striatum* in schizophrenia; and (iii) some preferential affinity of clozapine, a superior efficacy, low EPS antipsychotic (see p. 232), for D4 over D2L/S and D3 receptors (Seeman, 1992), despite the absence of any selective D4 antagonist with which these issues might be addressed more directly. However, the most recent evidence suggests that the site so identified in the human striatum is *not* the D4 receptor and is *not* elevated in schizophrenia, while the originators of the findings now refer themselves to this site as a 'D4-like' entity whose status is otherwise undefined; furthermore, conventional antipsychotics such as haloperidol, fluphenazine and trifluoperazine are >50-fold selective for D2L/S over D4 receptors, while any putative preference of clozapine for D4 over D2L/S receptors is very modest and of uncertain relevance (Roth *et al.*, 1995).

Recently, the first selective D4 antagonists have become available, and for one of these, L-745 870, both preclinical and clinical findings are now available. This compound appears psychopharmacologically 'silent' by virtue of its inactivity in several models of dopaminergic behaviour or antipsychotic activity (Bristow *et al.*, 1996b; Clifford and Waddington, 1998b), and in both control subjects and patients with schizophrenia; indeed, clinical trials in schizophrenia with L-745 870 were terminated prematurely because of somewhat *higher* overall symptom ratings in treated patients relative to those receiving placebo. It is important to emphasize that further studies with additional selective D4 antagonists are necessary to clarify these issues. Such compounds continue to emerge (e.g. CP-293 019, NGD 94-1, RO 61-6270, U 101387), with the latter exhibiting the provocative effect of attenuating amphetamine sensitization.

D1-like receptors

Given the weight of evidence for some primacy of D2 blockade in the therapeutic action of conventional antipsychotic drugs, considerable surprise was engendered by the activity of the first selective D1 (i.e. D1-like) antagonist SCH 23390 in essentially all conventional models held to predict antipsychotic activity (Waddington and Daly, 1992); this profile appeared to have its basis in D1-like–D2-like interactions which regulate critically the totality of dopaminergic neurotransmission (Waddington *et al.*, 1994). Newer selective D1 antagonists with more appropriate pharmacokinetics have become available subsequently; these have entered clinical trials in schizophrenia, to allow both their therapeutic potential and the predictive power of such models to be evaluated.

Initial open, uncontrolled studies with SCH 39166 in modest numbers of patients have failed to indicate antipsychotic activity (Karlsson *et al.*, 1995; de Beaurepaire *et al.*, 1995; Den Boer *et al.*, 1995); there were few EPS. Among patients given NNC 01-687, some improvement both in positive and in negative symptoms was apparent, with an increased level of functioning, in the absence of EPS (Karle *et al.*, 1995). This apparent lack of material antipsychotic activity, particularly for SCH 39166, challenges the validity of numerous conventional preclinical, usually rodent, models; however, it should be noted that SCH 23390, unlike conventional antipsychotics, appears active in putative non-human primate models both of positive *and* of negative symptoms (Ellenbroek, 1993). Thus, the therapeutic potential of selective D1 antagonists remains open; a third compound (BTS 73 947; Needham *et al.*, 1996a) may provide important additional information on these issues. No antagonist identified to date can distinguish between rodent D1A and D1B receptors, or between D1 and D5 receptors as their human homologues, hence any differential role for these D1-like sub-types in antipsychotic activity has yet to be explored.

NEW BEHAVIOURAL MODELS

Classical behavioural models continue to evolve but focus primarily on the empirical dissociation of DA-mediated phenomena associated putatively with antipsychotic efficacy from those so associated with EPS liability (see p. 216).

However, the past several years have seen the emergence of new models which involve processes that are thought to be dysfunctional in schizophrenia itself, in terms either of specific behavioural/cognitive impairment or of pathophysiology; thus, these models have putative *face* and potential *construct validity* as against *predictive validity* as preclinical models of schizophrenia/antipsychotic drug action (Ellenbroek, 1993).

The challenge remains to develop models that are able to identify not only antipsychotic efficacy and EPS liability but also activity against primary negative (deficit) symptoms, either empirically or homologous/isomorphic with these features of the illness, in the face of their considerably greater insensitivity to pharmacotherapy (Kirkpatrick and Carpenter, 1995).

Prepulse inhibition

The action of a preceding weak stimulus (prepulse) to attenuate the normal startle response to a strong stimulus subsequently delivered is referred to as prepulse inhibition (PPI), and this putative index of sensorimotor gating is deficient in patients with schizophrenia. Homologous/isomorphic phenomena occur in rodents; PPI can be disrupted by DA agonists or by manipulations of brain systems implicated in the pathophysiology of schizophrenia (temporofrontal and corticostriatopallidothalamic network dysfunction; Waddington, 1993b), and apomorphine-induced disruption thereof is reversed by conventional antipsychotics in proportion to both clinical antipsychotic potency and affinity for D2 receptors (Swerdlow *et al.*, 1994a).

However, data on whether D1-like antagonists are active in this model are inconsistent, and whether antipsychotics *enhance* PPI when given alone or whether disruption of PPI due to isolation rearing might constitute a more appropriate model remains unclear (Swerdlow *et al.*, 1994a; Wilkinson *et al.*, 1994; Varty and Higgins, 1995). There is preliminary evidence that the D3 agonist PD 128907 can disrupt PPI (Bristow *et al.*, 1996a) and that among new selective D4 antagonists, NGD 94-1 but not L-745 870 partially reverses the disruptive action of apomorphine; there may be some alteration of PPI in transgenic mice with D4 receptor 'knock-out'.

Latent inhibition

Retarded conditioning to a stimulus that has been presented repeatedly without reinforcement is referred to as latent inhibition (LI) and this putative index of capacity to ignore irrelevant stimuli may be impaired in patients with schizophrenia. Homologous/isomorphic phenomena occur in rodents; LI can be attenuated by DA agonists or by manipulation of brain systems implicated in the pathophysiology of schizophrenia (hippocampal- and perihippocampal-temporofrontal network dysfunction; Waddington, 1993b), and amphetamine-induced attenuation of LI can be reversed by conventional antipsychotic drugs (Dunn *et al.*, 1993; Gray *et al.*, 1995; Weiner *et al.*, 1996).

However, LI is not disrupted by isolation rearing in the manner of PPI (Wilkinson *et al.*, 1994). Furthermore, whether facilitation of LI by antipsychotics when given alone might constitute a more appropriate model remains unclear, and a recent study fails to identify specific LI deficits in schizophrenia (Swerdlow *et al.*, 1996); this would challenge the *face validity* of the model but not necessarily its *predictive validity*.

Neonatal hippocampal lesion

Excitotoxic neonatal lesions of the ventral hippocampus are associated with behavioural abnormalities, including hyperlocomotion, exaggerated locomotor responsivity to amphetamine and disruption of PPI, which emerge only in early adulthood, are attenuated by antipsychotic drugs and appear to involve brain systems implicated in the pathophysiology of schizophrenia (Lipska *et al.*, 1995); in particular, this ontogeny of impairment is congruent with schizophrenia, in which a putative early, neurodevelopmentally determined abnormality of perihippocampal and other (temporofrontal and corticostriatopallidothalamic) brain regions is associated with the emergence of psychosis, only in early adulthood on completion of maturation in fundamental physiological processes (Waddington, 1993b).

Thus, this model is of particular heuristic significance, in that it appears to evidence homology/isomorphism with, and thus *construct validity* for, schizophrenia at several levels, from putative pathophysiology through developmental trajectory to neurocognitive deficit.

NEW NEUROCHEMICAL MODELS

Classical neurochemical models, like their behavioural counterparts, continue to evolve but focus generally on the empirical dissociation of DAergic indices in corticolimbic regions from those in striatal regions that relate putatively to antipsychotic activity versus EPS liability, respectively (p. 148). However, new models have recently emerged which involve novel neuronal processes. As yet, these phenomena bear little specific relationship to schizophrenia itself but may constitute important empirical indices that can be explored with considerable anatomical precision in relation to antipsychotic efficacy versus EPS liability.

Intermediate-early gene expression

Neuronal expression of Fos, the protein product of the intermediate-early gene *c-fos* and a marker for neurons that are metabolically activated, is increased by D2-like antagonists and this effect generalizes in a characteristic way over a wide range of antipsychotic drugs: all elevate *c-fos* in the nucleus accumbens (particularly its shell region) and medial striatum, with variable effects in prefrontal cortex, lateral septum and thalamic regions, while *c-fos* induction in the dorsolateral striatum appears in proportion with EPS liability (Deutch *et al.*, 1992; Robertson *et al.*, 1994).

Interestingly, in the neonatal hippocampal lesion model (see p. 231), the acute but not later phases of action of amphetamine to also increase *c-fos* expression was attenuated in the prefrontal cortex, cingulate cortex, septum and striatum; *c-fos* was barely detectable in the nucleus accumbens under any condition (Lillrank *et al.*, 1996).

These findings suggest some time-dependent involvement of *c-fos* in this important heuristic model, which is probably complex; it may suggest transcription factors and/or their target genes as targets for antipsychotic drugs. Intriguingly, the selective D4 antagonists CP-293 019 and RO 61-6270 may each increase *c-fos* in frontal and cingulate cortices but not in striatum.

NEW CONCEPTS: GLUTAMATERGIC PROCESSES

The action of non-competitive antagonists of NMDA-like glutamate receptors, such as phencyclidine (PCP), to induce psychopathology similar to both the positive and the negative symptoms of schizophrenia is an important element of a more general and rapidly evolving glutamatergic hypothesis of schizophrenia (Heresco-Levy *et al.*, 1996; *see also* Kerwin, this volume).

Susceptibility to the psychotoimimetic effects of such agents may be minimal in childhood but becomes maximal in early adulthood. Strikingly, recent studies indicate that the related compound dizocilpine (MK-801) is neurotoxic to rodents in areas such as the cingulate cortex and other corticolimbic regions in an age-dependent manner; such neurotoxicity appears to become evident only in early adulthood, with antipsychotic drugs able to offer some protection against these effects, reflecting, at least in part, the developmental trajectory of schizophrenia itself (Farber *et al.*, 1995). Furthermore, conventional antipsychotics are able to antagonize PCP and dizocilpine-induced stimulation of behaviour, though not PCP-induced social withdrawal (Corbett *et al.*, 1995).

Clinical considerations

IMPACT OF CLOZAPINE

In 1983, Pierre Deniker, who with Jean Delay had played a landmark role in the introduction of chlorpromazine some 30 years earlier, wrote:

Stille and Hippius in Munich (1970) claimed that they had found in clozapine a potent antipsychotic without any neurological effect; the theory of Delay and Deniker appeared to be under serious attack. In reality it was only a false exception; we ourselves had studied this drug and abandoned it because of the strong neurovegetative side effects . . . Clozapine has by the way been abandoned [p.179].

Neuronal mechanisms

Clozapine is a highly non-selective compound which demonstrates an extensive range of pharmacological actions at multiple levels of neuronal function involving diverse neurotransmitter systems; yet within its complex profile must reside important clues to improved antipsychotic activity. These actions have been extensively reviewed (Waddington, 1995; Wagstaff and Bryson, 1995; Ashby and Wang, 1996; Schotte *et al.*, 1996) and are not easily summarized. However, one might note that clozapine is at best a modest antagonist of both D2-like

(D4>D2L/S >D3) and D1-like (D1/1A > D5/1B) receptors whose 'preferential' affinity for the D4 receptor may have been both overestimated in magnitude and overinterpreted in relation to antipsychotic activity; conversely, it shows considerably higher antagonist affinity for adrenergic ($\alpha1 > \alpha2$), histaminergic (H1 > H3), muscarinic [M1 > M5 > M4 (agonist) > M3 > M2] and serotonergic (5HT2A = 5HT6 > 5-HT2C> 5-HT7 > 5-HT3 > 5-HT1A-F) receptors. In patients with schizophrenia, PET studies indicate clozapine to occupy 36–59% of D1-like and 20–67% of D2-like receptors in the basal ganglia, and 84–94% of cortical 5HT2 receptors (Nordstrom *et al.*, 1995; *see also* Kerwin, this volume). It is important to emphasize that the functional effects of drugs may not be reliably predicted solely on the basis of their receptor binding profiles; in particular, clozapine appears to exert much more prominent and preferential attenuation of D1-like-mediated behaviour than would be predicted from its binding affinities (*see* Waddington and Daly, 1992; Deveney and Waddington, 1996).

In relation to the new models discussed above (see p. 229), there are both positive and negative findings with clozapine regarding restoration of disruption of PPI induced by DA agonists, PCP and dizocilpine, while clozapine appears to share a general action of antipsychotics to restore isolation rearing-induced disruption of PPI (*see* Swerdlow *et al.*, 1994a; Varty and Higgins, 1995). Similarly, there have been variable findings as to any action of clozapine in the LI model, though the most recent studies report it both to facilitate the development of LI and to reverse disruption of LI induced by DA agonists (see Dunn *et al.*, 1993; Moran *et al.*, 1996; Weiner *et al.*, 1996). In particular, clozapine protects more effectively than do conventional antipsychotics against MK-801-induced neurotoxicity (Farber *et al.*, 1996) and can attenuate PCP-induced social isolation, a paradigm in which conventional antipsychotics appear inactive (Corbett *et al.*, 1995; Sams-Dodd, 1996).

Clozapine shares the ability of conventional antipsychotics to elevate *c-fos* in the shell region of the nucleus accumbens; but in addition elevates *c-fos* preferentially in the thalamic paraventricular nucleus and selectively in the prefrontal cortex (Deutch *et al.*, 1992, 1995; Robertson *et al.*, 1994), brain regions that currently attract considerable interest regarding the pathobiology of schizophrenia in the context of corticostriatopallidothalamic network dysfunction (Waddington, 1993b). Furthermore, chronic administration of clozapine, unlike that of haloperidol, elevates the *c-fos*-encoded protein ΔFosB in the lateral septal nucleus and prefrontal cortex (Vahid-Ansari *et al.*, 1996). It must be emphasized that despite considerable efforts (see for example Deutch *et al.*, 1995), the neuronal basis of these regionally selective effects of clozapine on *c-fos* as against conventional antipsychotics remains unclear but may contain fundamental clues for the development of new agents.

Clinical impact

Probably no agent introduced since chlorpromazine has modified so profoundly our view of antipsychotic drug development as has clozapine. The renaissance of this agent has a very practical basis: it is the only antipsychotic known to have efficacy superior to that of conventional agents, including efficacy against negative symptoms in a significant proportion of otherwise refractory patients, in the face of little liability to induce EPS; however, the increased risk for potentially fatal agranulocytosis inherent to clozapine and the necessity for mandatory blood-count-monitoring, together with its liability to induce seizures, sedation, hypotension, hypersalivation and weight gain, means that it is perceived by many as a critical 'reserve' drug for patients who are unresponsive to or intolerant of conventional antipsychotics. Its clinical properties have recently been documented extensively (Pickar, 1995; Waddington, 1995; Wagstaff and Bryson, 1995; Kane, 1996), and have engendered considerable controversy in relation to therapeutic use and pharmacoeconomics (e.g. Carpenter *et al.*, 1995; Meltzer, 1995b). The contributions(s) of its diverse effects to the antipsychotic efficacy and low EPS liability of clozapine is uncertain but likely contributes materially to its profile of adverse effects. On this basis we have argued: 'Thus, the breadth of this range of actions of clozapine can be considered either a rich reservoir for theorizing on or, alternatively, extremely muddy waters in which to fish for' the substrate of its advantageous clinical effects; indeed it cannot be excluded that clozapine's particular clinical profile is in fact related to so broad a range of effects on multiple levels of neuronal function, or to a fortuitous balance between them, such that reproducing one or several of its individual properties in a new molecule may fail to reproduce the complete profile of the progenitor compound (Waddington, 1995).

IMPACT OF RISPERIDONE

In contrast to clozapine, risperidone is a new antipsychotic with a more restricted range of pharmacological actions. Importantly, however, the actions of risperidone are among those evidenced by clozapine also, hence similarities and distinctions between these two drugs have the potential to reveal important information as to the relative roles of their overlapping versus disparate mechanisms in several aspects of antipsychotic activity.

Neuronal mechanisms

It is common to refer to risperidone as a serotonin–dopamine antagonist which thus combines two of the actions of clozapine that may be important for improved antipsychotic efficacy and reduced EPS liability; however, its pharmacology appears more complex. Risperidone is a very high affinity antagonist of 5HT (5HT2A > 5HT7 >> 5HT1A-F/2C/3/6) and a high affinity antagonist of D2-like (D2L/S > D3 = D4) adrenergic (α1/2) and histaminergic [H1] receptors; a metabolite, 9-OH-risperidone, has a similar profile and likely contributes to overall duration of pharmacological activity following administration of the parent compound (Schotte *et al.*, 1996).

There is a long-standing and still evolving literature on serotonergic as well as dopaminergic mechanisms in schizophrenia and antipsychotic drug action (Breier 1995); it should be noted that in patients evaluated by PET, risperidone at 6 mg occupies 75–80% of basal ganglia D2-like receptors, a value *indistinguishable* from conventional antipsychotics, together with 78–88% of cortical 5HT2 receptors, a value considerably *higher* than that for conventional antispychotics but similar to that for clozapine (Farde *et al.*, 1995; *see also* Kerwin, this volume). Theoretically, 5HT2 antagonism may release dopaminergic fields from serotonergic inhibition in the striatum to reduce D2 antagonist-induced EPS and in the frontal cortex to attentuate negative symptoms; however, the putative benefits of combined 5HT2–D2-like blockade may be evident only over a limited dose range and may be lost with doses that induce supramaximal D2 blockade (Kapur and Remington, 1996; Wadenberg, 1996).

The actions of risperidone in classical models relating to antipsychotic potential and EPS liability have been reviewed previously in detail (Megens *et al.*, 1994). In relation to the new models described above, risperidone restores disruption of PPI induced by DA agonists, dizocilpine and isolation rearing (Varty and Higgins, 1995) but, unlike clozapine, fails to reverse PCP-induced social withdrawal (Corbett *et al.*, 1995). Like other antipsychotics, risperidone elevates *c-fos* in the shell region of the nucleus accumbens; however, unlike clozapine, it induces a modest elevation in the dorsolateral striatum but does not result in elevations in the prefrontal cortex, lateral septal nucleus or thalamic paraventricular nucleus (Robertson *et al.*, 1994; Deutch *et al.*, 1995).

This profile would, subject to the validity of these models, suggest that risperidone is at least as effective an antipsychotic as conventional agents while having some advantage with regard to EPS liability, at least at low–moderate doses; however, any advantage in relation to negative symptoms may fall short of that attained with clozapine.

Clinical impact

In terms of engendering debate as to the scope of antipsychotic activity, risperidone is second only to clozapine and has received extensive clinical evaluation using methodologies more advanced than those applied to essentially all previous agents. There is little evidence for any significant superiority over typical antipsychotics in terms of efficacy against positive psychotic symptoms, though a debate endures as to any ability to effect greater reduction in negative symptoms (Umbricht and Kane, 1995); recent meta-analyses have suggested that patients taking an *optimal* dose of risperidone (6 mg) may be 1.43-fold more likely than patients taking typical antipsychotics to experience a 20% reduction in negative symptom scores (i.e. 7 out of 10 risperidone-treated versus 5 out of 10 otherwise-treated patients), with 60% of that change appearing to be secondary to primary changes in EPS, positive symptoms and depressive features (Carmen *et al.*, 1995; Moller *et al.*, 1995). There are as yet no systematic, controlled studies in schizophrenia as to the efficacy of risperidone in long-term maintenance therapy of carefully defined populations of patients who are refractory to conventional antipsychotics; particularly, there are no thorough comparisons with clozapine in such populations.

There is consistent evidence that lower doses of risperidone (4–8 mg) induce no more EPS than does placebo, while higher doses (10–16 mg) induce levels of EPS that approach those induced by 10–20 mg haloperidol; thus, risperidone appears to induce EPS in a dose-dependent manner, with its advantage over conventional antipsychotics restricted to the lower end of the dose range to which optimal therapeutic efficacy is restricted similarly. Risperidone can also induce, usually but not invariably in a dose-dependent manner: dysphoria, sedation, autonomic/cardiovascular effects, prolactin elevation, sexual dysfunction and weight gain (Umbricht and Kane, 1995; Owens, 1996).

It is important to emphasize that the above considerations derive from extensive phase III trials conducted primarily for regulatory purposes; the rarefied atmosphere of the controlled clinical trial in carefully defined patients may differ from 'front-line' usage in more heterogeneous populations. In such naturalistic settings, there is a preliminary report that risperidone can induce EPS at doses lower than has been noted previously, with implications for cost-effectiveness (Carter *et al.*, 1995); furthermore, there is a preliminary report that some patients can experience a loss of effectiveness after some months (Stip *et al.*, 1995). It is equally important to note that such caveats may reflect in part the substantial clinical and pharmacoeconomic attention directed to risperidone; it would be necessary to direct the same degree of attention to more recently introduced agents (see p.238) before comparative judgements can be made.

IMPLICATIONS OF MDL 100907

The proposal (Meltzer, 1995a) that some combination of high affinity 5HT2A antagonism with varying extents of D2-like antagonism confers material advantage on an antipsychotic in terms of EPS liability and, less certainly, efficacy against negative symptoms, has attracted considerable attention; both clozapine and risperidone evidence this combination of actions together with varying affinities for other receptors, and this proposal endures in its influence on antipsychotic drug development. An extreme variant is that 5HT2A antagonism is not *necessary*, in combination with D2-like antagonism, but is *sufficient* even in the absence of D2-like antagonism, for superior antipsychotic activity; however, appropriate agents for evaluating this proposition are only now becoming available.

MDL 100907 is a highly selective 5HT2A antagonist with little or no affinity for D2-like or numerous other receptors, and which demonstrates high occupancy of neocortical 5HT2A but not D2-like or D1-like receptors as evaluated in non-human primates by PET. In classical preclinical models it evidences a profile that would predict antipsychotic efficacy with very low EPS (Kehne *et al.*, 1996) and recently, MDL 100907 has been examined in some of the new preclinical models. It reverses the disruption of PPI induced by 5HT releasers or by 5HT2A/C agonists in a manner independent of D2-like receptor involvement (Padich *et al.*, 1996), as do clozapine and risperidone (Varty and Higgins, 1995), and reverses DA agonist-induced disruption of LI (Moser *et al.*, 1996). Though no permutation of 5HT2, D2-like and α1 antagonism, including 5HT2 antagonism alone, appears able to reproduce the characteristic ability of clozapine (but not of risperidone) to elevate *c-fos* in the prefrontal cortex (Fink-Jensen *et al.*, 1995), the primary agent utilized, ritanserin, is a mixed 5HT2A/C antagonist; thus, generalization to MDL 100907 may be inappropriate.

To date, there are few clinical findings in the public domain concerning any effects of MDL 100907 in patients with schizophrenia. However, this agent is likely to challenge a number of 'perceived wisdoms'. It is the only agent advanced in clinical investigation that has among its properties *no* affinity for D2-like receptors; thus, evidence for antipsychotic activity would necessitate revision of the long-standing presumption of primacy for at least some degree of D2-like antagonism, while evidence to the contrary would question the validity of a number of classical and new preclinical models.

Concept of atypicality in relation to antipsychotic activity

CURRENT STATUS

It is common to refer to clozapine as the progenitor *atypical* antipsychotic and to remoxipride (now withdrawn), risperidone and putative successor compounds as the new atypicals, to distinguish them in advantageous terms from conventional or *typical* agents. However, this terminology is inconsistent and has neither clear theoretical underpinnings nor rigour in application (Gerlach and Casey, 1994; Kinon and Lieberman, 1996; Waddington and O'Callaghan, 1997). Either the concept of atypical antipsychotic activity is so ill defined that it should be abandoned or some attempt should be made to give the concept firmer roots and defining criteria. The approach adopted here seeks to combine the essentials of these two strategies. Given that the epithet *atypical* has over the past decade acquired a 'life of its own', often driven by commercial considerations, its use is likely to continue. Therefore, the designation is retained, but a recasting using clear operational criteria is proposed. Redefining 'atypical' requires consideration of contemporary usage.

One influential perspective of atypicality is antipsychotic action in most patients at doses that do not cause significant acute or subacute EPS or 'an antipsychotic with a clear advantage with regard to EPS. Differences or similarities with regard to overall efficacy, effect on negative symptoms or prolactin stimulation are considered irrelevant for atypical classification' (Meltzer, 1995a). However, this widely accepted definition is satisfied by thioridazine, which is clearly not recognized as atypical in any contemporary sense and whose clinical usage is not advocated on a radical basis; clozapine, remoxipride and risperidone offer clear advantages over thioridazine at several levels, including superior efficacy (clozapine) and reduced liability for several adverse effects *other than/additional to* EPS (remoxipride: less sedation, postural hypotension, anticholinergic effects, sexual dysfunction and weight gain; *see* Waddington and O'Callaghan, 1997).

A NEW PERSPECTIVE

In addition to (i) reduced EPS liability, we (Waddington and O'Callaghan, 1997) have proposed the following advantages for patient well-being, quality of life and compliance, family cohesion and cost of health care in the course of antipsychotic therapy: (iia) superior general efficacy, particularly against negative symptoms/deficit features and (iib) efficacy in otherwise treatment-refractory patients; (iii) lack of subjective dysphoria; (iv) reduced sedation; (v) reduced autonomic/cardiac effects; (vi) lack of prolactin elevation and other endocrine effects; (vii) lack of sexual dysfunction; (viii) lack of weight gain. Other factors such as reduced liability for tardive dyskinesia and very rare but serious idiosyncratic/haematological reactions, and lack of association with unexpected sudden death, are also of great importance, but they are rarely clarified in the course of extensive but short phase III trials, which are often designed primarily in a regulatory context, and usually become evident only on a more widespread usage following regulatory approval.

As a definition of atypicality based essentially on EPS liability both generates evident contradictions (e.g. thioridazine) and encompasses under a unitary heading agents (clozapine, remoxipride, risperidone) having fundamentally distinct clinical properties, we have proposed (Waddington and O'Callaghan, 1997) the following alternative, operationalized definition: (A) reduced EPS liability (i) *and either* (B) superior general efficacy (iia) or efficacy in otherwise refractory patients (iib), *or* (C) two or more of the additional properties (iii)–(viii); criterion A *and* either criterion B or criterion C must each be met. This operationalized definition would exclude thioridazine from the atypical category; furthermore, this definition not only categorizes clozapine, remoxipride and (at lower doses) risperidone as atypical, but also indicates clearly that their atypical profiles are distinct and specifies the nature of these differences.

These criteria are inherently more conservative than those rooted solely in EPS liability, and require further specification: how are characteristics (ii)–(viii) to be interpreted, and should the requirement be for two or three (or more) of characteristics (iii)–(viii)? The above schema is offered heuristically to indicate yet higher aspirations for the treatment of psychotic patients with the encouraging array of new atypical antipsychotics that is currently emerging, by distilling those agents which are likely to be of *yet greater* benefit to patients, beyond a welcome reduction in likelihood of EPS.

New antipsychotics

AGENTS GIVEN REGULATORY APPROVAL OR IN ADVANCED CLINICAL DEVELOPMENT

At this critical juncture, a number of new antipsychotics have traversed the process of regulatory approval or are well advanced in clinical development.

Amisulpride

This substituted benzamide analogue of sulpiride is a selective antagonist of D2-like [D2L/S = D3 >> D4] receptors with little affinity for D1-like or non-dopaminergic receptors; in patients with schizophrenia, PET studies indicate lower doses of amisulpride (50–100 mg) to occupy only 4–26% of basal ganglia D2-like receptors, while higher doses (200–800 mg) occupy 38–76% (Martinot *et al.*, 1996). It has been argued on the basis of preclinical studies using conventional models that lower doses of amisulpride preferentially block presynaptic D2-like inhibitory autoreceptors, to give a relative enhancement of DAergic function, while higher doses reduce certain postsynaptic DA receptor-mediated behaviours, but with little or no induction of catalepsy; however, there is as yet little in the way of data using the new preclinical models described above (Coukell *et al.*, 1996).

Initial clinical studies indicate that indeed lower doses (50–300 mg) reduce negative symptom scores relative to placebo without any effect on positive symptoms and with little or no induction of EPS. Recently, more extensive trials have confirmed that 100 mg amisulpride produces a sustained reduction in negative symptom scores without EPS, relative to placebo, though with a high drop-out rate due to recrudescence of psychosis; conversely, 400–800 mg amisulpride was at least as effective as 16–20 mg haloperidol in reducing total BPRS psychopathology and positive symptom score, and was more effective in reducing negative symptom score with fewer EPS. In terms of adverse events, amisulpride can induce some dose-related EPS, insomnia-agitation, dry mouth, prolactin elevation and other endocrine effects, and weight gain, but few cardiovascular sequelae (Boyer *et al.*, 1995; Coukell *et al.*, 1996).

Olanzapine

This thienobenzodiazepine analogue of clozapine is a broad, high affinity antagonist of 5HT (5-HT2A/C = 5HT6 > 5-HT3) = M1–4 = H1 > D2-like (D2L/S = D3 = D4) > D1-like = α (α1 > α2) receptors (Bymaster *et al.*, 1996; Schotte *et al.*, 1996); in patients with schizophrenia, olanzapine occupies 70–80% of basal ganglia D2-like receptors while occupying a higher percentage of cortical 5HT2 receptors (*see* Kerwin, this volume). In conventional preclinical models, the profile of olanzapine is one that would predict antipsychotic efficacy with reduced EPS liability (Moore *et al.*, 1994); it shares some of the action of clozapine to effect a greater attenuation of D1-like-mediated function that would be predicted from its relative affinities for D2-like versus D1-like receptors (Deveney and Waddington, 1996). In new preclinical models, olanzapine shares the particular action of clozapine to restore disruption of PPI induced by PCP or dizocilpine (Bakshi and Geyer, 1995), to reverse PCP-induced social withdrawal (Corbett *et al.*, 1995) and to protect against dizocilpine-induced neurotoxicity (Farber *et al.*, 1996); it shares the action of clozapine to elevate *c-fos* in the prefrontal cortex as well as in the lateral septal nucleus and nucleus accumbens, but unlike clozapine it slightly elevated *c-fos* in the dorsolateral striatum (Robertson and Fibiger, 1996). This profile predicts that olanzapine should be an effective antipsychotic with at least some of the advantageous properties of clozapine and a low (but not zero) liability to induce EPS.

Extensive clinical trials now indicate that olanzapine (5–20 mg) is superior to placebo in reducing total BPRS psychopathology scores and both positive and negative symptom scores. In comparison with haloperidol (5–20 mg), it appears superior in reducing total BPRS psychopathology scores, at least as effective in reducing positive symptom scores, and superior in reducing negative symptom scores; furthermore, it appears superior in alleviating affective symptom scores and improving quality-of-life estimates. Among patients continued on these drugs in an extension phase following conclusion of the acute trial, survival analysis indicated olanzapine to be superior in protecting against relapse. Overall, olanzapine appears indistinguishable from placebo and materially superior to haloperidol in terms of EPS liability, and in extension studies it appears to have a reduced propensity for inducing tardive dyskinesia; it can induce sedation, dry mouth-constipation and weight gain, with only transient increases in prolactin, few cardiovascular sequelae and no agranulocytosis (Beasley *et al.*, 1996a, 1996b, 1996c; Martin, 1996; Tran *et al.*, 1996).

Quetiapine

This dibenzothiazepine analogue of clozapine is a broad, lower affinity antagonist of H1 > 5HT (5HT2A > 5HT7) = α1/2 > D2-like (D2L/S = D3 > D4)> D1-like = M receptors (Fulton and Goa, 1995; Goldstein and Arvanitis, 1995; Schotte *et al.*, 1996); in patients with schizophrenia, quetiapine shares the action of clozapine to occupy only 44% of basal ganglia D2-like receptors while occupying 72% of cortical 5HT2 receptors (Gefvert *et al.*, 1996; *see also* Kerwin, this volume). In conventional preclinical models, the profile of quetiapine is one that would predict antipsychotic efficacy with reduced EPS liability (Fulton and Goa, 1995; Goldstein and Arvanitis, 1995); it does not share the action of clozapine to effect a greater attenuation of D1-like-mediated function than would be predicted from its relative affinities for D1-like versus D2-like receptors (Deveney and Waddington, 1996). In new preclinical models, quetiapine shares the action of known antipsychotics to restore DA agonist-induced disruption of PPI (Swerdlow *et al.*, 1994b), but whether it shares the action of clozapine to restore PCP-induced disruption of PPI and PCP-induced social withdrawal, and to protect against dizocilpine-induced neurotoxicity is not yet clear. It shares the particular action of clozapine to elevate *c-fos* in the prefrontal cortex as well as in the lateral septal nucleus and nucleus accumbens but not in the dorsolateral striatum (Robertson *et al.*, 1994), and on chronic administration to elevate ΔFosB in the prefrontal cortex and lateral septal nucleus (Vahid-Ansari *et al.*, 1996). This profile predicts that quetiapine should be an effective antipsychotic with perhaps some of the advantageous properties of clozapine and a low (but not zero) liability to induce EPS.

Extensive clinical trials now indicate quetiapine (75–750 mg) to be superior to placebo and indistinguishable from haloperidol (12 mg) in reducing total BPRS psychopathology and both positive and negative symptom scores. Overall, quetiapine appears indistinguishable from placebo and materially superior to haloperidol in terms of EPS liability; it can induce sedation-dizziness, constipation, dyspepsia, headache and weight gain with only transient increases in prolactin, few cardiovascular sequelae and no agranulocytosis (Fulton and Goa, 1995; Goldstein and Arvanitis, 1995; Borison *et al.*, 1996; Hirsch *et al.*, 1996; Hellewell and Hurst, 1996).

Sertindole

This indole derivative is a high affinity antagonist of 5HT (5HT2A/C > 5HT7 > α1 > D2-like (D2L/5 = D3 = D4) (Sanchez *et al.*, 1991; Schotte *et al.*, 1996); in patients with schizophrenia, sertindole shares the action of risperidone in occupying a high percentage both of basal ganglia D2-like receptors and of cortical 5HT2 receptors (Pilowsky *et al.*, 1996b; *see also* Kerwin, this volume). In conventional preclinical models, the profile of sertindole predicts antipsychotic efficacy with reduced EPS liability (Sanchez *et al.*, 1991; Dunn and Fitton, 1996). In new preclinical models, sertindole is active on LI (Weiner *et al.*, 1996), but is otherwise rather less extensively explored.

Extensive clinical trials now indicate sertindole (12–24 mg) to be superior to placebo and indistinguishable from haloperidol (4–16 mg) in reducing total PANSS psychopathology and both positive and negative symptom scores. The negative symptom effects of sertindole were statistically significant relative to placebo while those of haloperidol were not; however, the reductions effected by sertindole and haloperidol did not differ significantly from each other. Among patients continued on sertindole in an extension phase, its benefits persisted. Overall, sertindole appears indistinguishable from placebo and materially superior to haloperidol in terms of EPS liability; it can induce nasal congestion, decreased ejaculatory volume, prolongation of cardiac QT/QT_c intervals and weight gain, with little effect on prolactin levels (Baker *et al.*, 1996; Braus *et al.*, 1996; Dunn and Fitton, 1996; Van Kammen *et al.*, 1996). Recently this agent has been withdrawn from clinical use in many countries.

Ziprasidone

This indolone derivative is a high affinity antagonist of 5HT $(5HT2A = 5HT1D/7 > 5HT1A/2C > D2\text{-like} \quad (D2L/S = D3 > D4) > \alpha(\alpha1 > \alpha2) > H1$ receptors with 5-HT1A agonism which also inhibits the reuptake of NA and 5HT (Seeger *et al.*, 1995; Schotte *et al.*, 1996); in human subjects, ziprasidone occupies 77% of basal ganglia D2-like receptors but 98% of cortical 5HT2 receptors (Bench *et al.*, 1996; Fischman *et al.*, 1996). In conventional preclinical models, the profile of ziprasidone would predict antipsychotic and possibly antidepressant efficacy with reduced EPS liability (Seeger *et al.*, 1995), but little or no information is available on its effects in new preclinical models.

Initial phase II studies indicate ziprasidone (40–160 mg) to be superior to placebo and indistinguishable from haloperidol (15 mg) in reducing total BPRS psychopathology, positive and negative symptom scores. Ziprasidone appears superior to haloperidol in terms of EPS liability; it appears to induce sedation, constipation and headache with little effect on prolactin (Gunn *et al.*, 1995). However, more results of ongoing phase III studies must enter the public domain before its profile can be evaluated in greater detail.

Zotepine

This dibenzothiazepine analogue of clozapine is a high affinity antagonist of 5HT $(5HT2A/C = 5HT6/7) = \alpha1 = H1 > D2\text{-like} \ (D2L/S = D3 = D4) > D1\text{-like} \ (D1A>D1B)$ receptors and inhibits the reuptake of NA (Needham *et al.*, 1996b, 1996c; Schotte *et al.*, 1996); it has yet to be evaluated in human subjects using PET. In conventional preclinical models the profile of zotepine would predict antipsychotic efficacy with reduced EPS liability (Needham *et al.*, 1996b) but little or no information is available on its effects in new preclinical models.

Initial phase II studies indicate zotepine (150–300 mg) to be superior to placebo and chlorpromazine (300–600 mg), indistinguishable from haloperidol (10–20 mg) in reducing total BPRS psychopathology and positive symptom scores, and superior to haloperidol but indistinguishable from chlorpromazine in reducing negative symptom scores. Zotepine appears indistinguishable from placebo and superior to chlorpromazine and haloperidol in terms of EPS liability; it appears to induce insomnia, uricosuria and weight gain, and may elevate prolactin, with few cardiovascular sequelae (Barnas *et al.*, 1992; Cooper *et al.*, 1996; Petit *et al.*, 1996). However, more results from phase III studies are necessary before its profile can be evaluated in greater detail.

MECHANISTIC CONSIDERATIONS

Receptor profile

The agents reviewed above fall into three general categories: (i) selective D2-like antagonists (amisulpride); (ii) 5HT2A > D2-like antagonists which exert very high occupancy of both 5HT2A *and* D2-like receptors but whose α1-blocking activity is often ignored (risperidone, sertindole, ziprasidone and the similar but less widely studied agent iloperidone; Szewczak *et al.*, 1995); (iii) 5HT2A > D2-like antagonists which exert very high occupancy of 5HT2A but variable occupancy of D2-like receptors together with a broad range of additional antagonist actions (clozapine, olanzapine, zotepine); (iv) quetiapine is a particularly high affinity H1 antagonist with considerably lower affinity for 5HT2A > D_2-like and several other receptors, which exerts somewhat lower 5HT2A and modest D2-like occupancy, and is less readily categorized. Clinical evidence for superior efficacy particularly in terms of alleviation of negative symptoms, as distinct from a more generic reduction in liability for EPS, appears perhaps most convincing for drugs of category (iii); however, the differing breadths and depths of information available for individual agents must be recognized and the distinction between primary (deficit) and secondary negative symptoms is receiving attention only recently.

Functional profile

It may be relevant to note that the actions of clozapine, olanzapine and zotepine include D1-like antagonism, which may encompass a disproportionate attenuation of D1-like-mediated function (Deveney and Waddington, 1996; Needham *et al.*, 1996b); curiously, while the selective D1-like antagonist SCH 39166 appears to have no activity against positive psychotic symptoms, it appears to reduce negative symptoms (Den Boer *et al.*, 1995) as may the D1-like antagonist NNC 01-687 (Karle *et al.*, 1995). Each of clozapine, olanzapine and quetiapine (but not risperidone) elevates *c-fos* in the frontal cortex, lateral septal nucleus and nucleus accumbens. As there is as yet no evidence that quetiapine shares the greater efficacy of clozapine while olanzapine may show an intermediate profile, the significance of such *c-fos* elevations is unclear; more systematic examination of effects in thalamic nuclei and clarification of the overall *c-fos* profiles of amisulpride, ziprasidone and zotepine may be informative. Both clozapine and olanzapine restore disruption of PPI induced by PCP or dizocilpine, reverse PCP-induced social withdrawal and protect against dizocilpine-induced neurotoxicity; this would complement some overlap in their clinical profiles, but clarification of the profiles of amisulpride, quetiapine, risperidone, ziprasidone and zotepine is necessary to interpret fully this possible commonality.

EXPERIMENTAL APPROACHES

Numerous additional compounds continue to emerge from preclinical programmes as putative atypical antipsychotics, to compete for limited access to clinical development.

Many of these bear some conceptual overlap with clozapine and/or risperidone, though MDL 100907 represents a greater variation on such themes.

There are several alternative approaches to the pharmacotherapy of schizophrenia, two of which may be worthy of particular mention. Glycine acts at a site on the NMDA receptor complex to potentiate NMDA-mediated neurotransmission and this, in physiological terms, acts in an opposite manner to the isomorphic psychotogen PCP (see p.232). It has been examined for therapeutic activity in schizophrenia with inconsistent results. However, the most recent systematic, double-blind, placebo-controlled trials as an adjunct in conventional antipsychotic-treated patients, including poorly or non-responsive cases, indicate amelioration of negative (but not of positive) symptoms and of some aspects of cognitive impairment without increase in EPS (Javitt *et al.*, 1994; Heresco-Levy *et al.*, 1996); D-cycloserine, a partial agonist at the same site, appears to act similarly (Goff *et al.*, 1995). However, the quinolone analogue L-701 324 is a glycine/NMDA receptor antagonist which has a preclinical profile suggestive of antipsychotic efficacy, including reversal of disruption of PPI induced by isolation rearing (Bristow *et al.*, 1996c); were this profile to be sustained clinically, the synaptic basis of the above actions would have to be reconsidered.

Most recently, the monoamine oxidase-B inhibitor selegiline has been given also as an adjunct in similar patients; it appears to reduce negative (but not positive) symptoms and pre-existing EPS (Bodkin *et al.*, 1996). Selegiline may counteract putative decreases in prefrontal DAergic function in schizophrenia (*see* Weinberger and Lipska, 1995) or might point to other, unrelated actions.

Enduring challenges

DEFICIT FEATURES

Antipsychotic drug development has as its 'holy grail' the identification of agents that are active materially against primary negative symptoms (deficit features) and the cognitive debilities of the illness (Kirkpatrick and Carpenter, 1995; Meltzer, 1995a; Kane, 1996). The extent to which emerging drugs constitute progress in this regard remains to be established. However, evolving insights into the pathobiology of schizophrenia, together with the introduction of new preclinical models with apparent face and even construct validity, will be a further spur to research (*see* Weinberger and Lipska, 1995).

THE NATURE OF ANTIPSYCHOTIC DRUG ACTION

Contrary to the long-standing presumption that antipsychotic drugs effect only symptomatic management in schizophrenia, there is an expanding body of evidence to indicate that the longer psychosis proceeds unchecked before initial treatment, the poorer is both the response to such drugs and the long-term outcome of the disease; thus, an alternative perspective is that psychosis reflects some active, morbid process (disease 'progression') that can be ameliorated by antipsychotic medication (Wyatt, 1991; Loebel *et al.*, 1992; Waddington *et al.*, 1995, 1997; Szymanski *et al.*,

1996). As a corollary, earlier intervention and maintenance with antipsychotics might improve further the long-term outcome of schizophrenia (Wyatt, 1995; Waddington *et al.*, 1997). This should be more practicable using new agents that combine high efficacy with reduced side-effects and thus may improve the generally poor level of compliance with conventional agents that so materially impedes their effective use.

Acknowledgements

The authors' studies are supported by the Stanley Foundation and the Royal College of Surgeons in Ireland.

References

Arnt, J. (1995) Differential effects of classical and newer antipsychotics on the hypermotility induced by two dose levels of D-amphetamine. *Eur J Pharmacol*, **283**, 55–62.

Ashby, C. R. and Wang, R. Y. (1996) Pharmacological actions of the atypical antipsychotic drug clozapine. *Synapse*, **24**, 349–94.

Baker, R. W., Mack, R. J., Morris, D. D. *et al.* (1996) The efficacy and safety of three doses of sertindole versus three doses of haloperidol in schizophrenic patients. *Eur Neuropsychopharmacol*, **6** (Suppl 4), 109.

Bakshi, V. P. and Geyer, M. A. (1995) Antagonism of phencyclidine-induced deficits in prepulse inhibition by the putative atypical antipsychotic olanzapine. *Psychopharmacology*, **122**, 198–201.

Barnas, C., Stuppack, C. H., Miller, C. *et al.* (1992) Zotepine in the treatment of schizophrenic patients with prevailingly negative symptoms. A double-blind trial vs. haloperidol. *Int Clin Psychopharmacol*, **7**, 23–27.

Barnes, T. R. E. and McPhillips, M. A. (1996) Antipsychotic-induced extrapyramidal symptoms: role of anticholinergic drugs in treatment. *CNS Drugs*, **6**, 315–30.

Beasley, C. M., Sanger, T., Satterlee, W. *et al.* (1996a) Olanzapine versus placebo: results of a double-blind, fixed dose olanzapine trial. *Psychopharmacology*, **124**, 159–67.

Beasley, C. M., Tollefson, G., Tran, P. *et al.* (1996b) Olanzapine versus placebo and haloperidol: acute phase results of the North American double-blind olanzapine trial. *Neuropsychopharmacology*, **14**, 111–23.

Beasley, C., Tran, P., Beuzen, J. N. *et al.* (1996c) Olanzapine versus haloperidol: long-term results of the multi-centre international trial. *Eur Neuropsychopharmacol*, **6** (Suppl 3), 59.

Bench, C. J., Lammerstma, A. A., Grasby, P. M. *et al.* (1996) The time-course of binding to striatal dopamine D_2 receptors by the neuroleptic ziprasidone (CP-88 059-01) determined by positron emission tomography. *Psychopharmacology*, **124**, 141–7.

Bodkin, J. A., Cohen, B. M., Salomon, M. S. *et al.* (1996) Treatment of negative symptoms in schizophrenia and schizoaffective disorder by selegiline augmentation of antipsychotic medication: a pilot study examining the role of dopamine. *J Nervous Mental Dis*, **184**, 295–301.

Borison, R. L., Arvanitis, L. A., Miller, B. G. *et al.* (1996) ICI 204 636, an atypical antipsychotic: efficacy and safety in a multicenter, placebo-controlled trial in patients with schizophrenia. *J Clin Psychopharmacology*, **16**, 158–69.

Boyer, P., Lecrubier, Y., Puech, A. J. *et al.* (1995) Treatment of negative symptoms in schizophrenia with amisulpride. *Br J Psychiatry*, **166**, 68–72.

Braus, A., Nobulsi, A., Mack, R. *et al.* (1996) Reduction of hospital days in sertindole-treated patients: one year findings. *Eur Neuropsychopharmacology*, **6** (Suppl 4), 109–10.

Breier, A. (1995) Serotonin, schizophrenia and antipsychotic drug action. *Schizophr Res*, **14**, 187–202.

Bristow, L. J., Cook, G. P., Gay, J. C. *et al.* (1996a) The behavioural and neurochemical profile of the putative dopamine D_3 receptor agonist, (+)-PD 128907, in the rat. *Neuropharmacology*, **35**, 285–294.

Bristow, L. J., Saywell, G. P., Cook, J. J. *et al.* (1996b) Lack of effect of the dopamine D_4 receptor antagonist L-745 870 on amphetamine-induced behaviours in rodents. *Br J Pharmacol*, **119** (Suppl), 210P.

Bristow, L. J., Flatman, K. L., Hutson, P. H. *et al.* (1996c) The atypical neuroleptic profile of the glycine/N-methyl-D-aspartate receptor antagonist, L-701 324, in rodents. *J Pharmacol Exp Therap*, **277**, 578–85.

Bymaster, F. P., Calligaro, D. O., Falcone, J. F. *et al.* (1996) Radioreceptor binding profile of the atypical antipsychotic olanzapine. *Neuropsychopharmacology*, **14**, 87–96.

Carmen, J., Peuskens, J. and Vangeneugden, A. (1995) Risperidone in the treatment of negative symptoms of schizophrenia: a meta-analysis. *Int Clin Psychopharmacol*, **10**, 207–13.

Carpenter, W. T., Conlley, R. R., Buchanan, R. W. *et al.* (1995) Patient response and resource management: another view of clozapine treatment of schizophrenia. *Am J Psychiatry*, **152**, 827–32.

Carter, C. S., Mulsant, B. H., Sweet, R. A. *et al.* (1995) Risperidone use in a teaching hospital during its first year after market approval: economic and clinical implications. *Psychopharmacol Bull*, **3**, 719–25.

Casey, D. E. (1996) Behavioural effects of sertindole, risperidone, clozapine and haloperidol in *Cebus* monkeys. *Psychopharmacology*, **124**, 134–40.

Clifford, J. J. and Waddington, J. L. (1998a) Heterogeneity of behavioural profile between three new putative selective D_3 dopamine receptor antagonists using an ethologically based approach. *Psychopharmacology*, **136**, 284–90.

Clifford, J. J. and Waddington, J. L. (1998b) Topographically based search for an 'ethogram' among a series of D_4 dopamine receptor agonists and antagonists. *Schizophr Res*, **36**, 306.

Cooper, S. J., Raniwalla, J. and Welch, C. (1996) Zotepine in acute exacerbation of schizophrenia: a comparison versus chlorpromazine and placebo. *Eur Neuropsychopharmacol*, **6** (Suppl 3), 148.

Corbett, R., Camacho, F., Woods, A. T. *et al.* (1995) Antipsychotic agents antagonize non-competitive N-methyl-D-aspartate antagonist-induced behaviors. *Psychopharmacology*, **120**, 67–74.

Coukell, A. J., Spencer, C. M. and Benfield, P. (1996) Amisulpride: a review of its pharmacodynamic and pharmacokinetic properties and therapeutic efficacy in the management of schizophrenia. *CNS Drugs*, **6**, 237–56.

de Beaurepaire, R., Labelle, A., Naber, D. *et al.* (1995) An open trial of the D_1 antagonist SCH 39166 in six cases of acute psychotic states. *Psychopharmacology*, **121**, 323–7.

Den Boer, J. A., van Megen, H. J. G. M., Fleischhacker, W. W. *et al.* (1995) Differential effects of the D1-DA receptor antagonist SCH 39166 on positive and negative symptoms of schizophrenia. *Psychopharmacology*, **121**, 317–22.

Deniker, P. J. (1983) Discovery of the clinical use of neuroleptics. In M. J. Parnham and J. Bruinvels (eds), *Discoveries in pharmacology, Vol 1: Psycho- and Neuro-pharmacology*. Amsterdam: Elsevier, 163–80.

Deveney, A. M. and Waddington, J. L. (1996) Comparison of the new atypical antipsychotics olanzapine and ICI 204,636 with clozapine on behavioural responses to the selective 'D₁-like' dopamine receptor agonist A 68930 and selective 'D₂-like' agonist RU 24213. *Psychopharmacology*, **124**, 40–9.

Deutch, A. Y., Lee, M. C. and Iadarola, M. J. (1992) Regionally specific effects of atypical antipsychotic drugs on striatal Fos expression: the nucleus accumbens shell as a locus of antipsychotic action. *Mol Cell Neurosci*, **3**, 332–41.

Deutch, A. Y., Ongur, D. and Duman, R. S. (1995) Antipsychotic drugs induce Fos protein in the thalamic paraventricular nucleus: a novel locus of antipsychotic drug action. *Neuroscience*, **66**, 337–46.

Dunn, L. A., Atwater, G. E. and Kilts, C. D. (1993) Effects of antipsychotic drugs on latent inhibition – sensitivity and specificity of an animal model of clinical drug action. *Psychopharmacology*, **112**, 315–23.

Dunn, C. J. and Fitton, A. (1996) Sertindole. *CNS Drugs*, **5**, 224–30.

Ellenbroek, B. A. (1993) Treatment of schizophrenia: a clinical and preclinical evaluation of neuroleptic drugs. *Pharmacol Ther*, **57**, 1–78.

Farber, N. B., Wozniak, D. F., Price, M. T. *et al.* (1995) Age-specific neurotoxicity in the rat associated with NMDA receptor blockade: potential relevance to schizophrenia? *Biol Psychiatry*, **38**, 788–96.

Farber, N. B., Foster, J., Duhan, N. L. *et al.* (1996) Olanzapine and fluperlapine mimic clozapine in preventing MK-801 neurotoxicity. *Schizophr Res*, **21**, 33–7.

Farde, L., Nyberg, S., Oxenstierna, G. *et al.* (1995) Positron emission tomography studies on D_2 and 5-HT_2 receptor binding in risperidone-treated schizophrenic patients. *J Clin Psychopharmacol*, **15** (Suppl 1), 19S–23S.

Fink-Jensen, A., Ludvigsen, T. S. and Korsgaard, N. (1995) The effect of clozapine on Fos protein immunoreactivity in the rat forebrain is not mimicked by the addition of α_1-adrenergic or 5HT_2 receptor blockade to haloperidol. *Neurosci Lett*, **194**, 77–80.

Fischman, A. J., Bonab, A. A., Babich, J. W. *et al.* (1996) Positron emission tomographic analysis of central 5-hydroxytryptamine$_2$ receptor occupancy in healthy volunteers treated with the novel antipsychotic agent, ziprasidone. *J Pharmacol Exp Ther*, **279**, 939–47.

Fulton, B. and Goa, K. L. (1995) ICI-204 636: An initial appraisal of its pharmacological properties and clinical potential in the treatment of schizophrenia. *CNS Drugs*, **4**, 68–78.

Gefvert, O., Lindstrom, L. H., Langstrom, B. *et al.* (1996) Time course for dopamine and serotonin receptor occupancy in the brain of schizophrenic patients following dosing with 150 mg 'Seroquel' tid. *Schizophr Res*, **18**, 139–40.

Gerlach, J. and Casey, D. E. (1994) Drug treatment of schizophrenia. *Curr Opin Psychiatry*, **7**, 65–70.

Goff, D. C., Guochuan, T., Manoach, D. S. *et al.* (1995) Dose-finding trial of D-cycloserine added to neuroleptics for negative symptoms in schizophrenia. *Am J Psychiatry*, **152**, 1213–15.

Goldstein, J. M. and Arvanitis L. A. (1995) ICI 204 636 (SEROQUEL™): A dibenzothiazepine atypical antipsychotic. Review of preclinical pharmacology and highlights of phase II clinical trials. *CNS Drug Rev*, **1**, 50–70.

Gray, J. A., Joseph, M. H., Hemsley, D. R. *et al.* (1995) The role of mesolimbic dopaminergic and retrohippocampal afferents to the nucleus accumbens in latent inhibition: implication for schizophrenia. *Behav Brain Res*, **71**, 19–31.

Gunn, K. P., Harrigan, E. P. and Heym, J. (1995) The safety and tolerability of ziprasidone treatment. In N. Brunello, G. Racagni, S. Z. Langer *et al.* (eds), *Critical issues in the treatment of schizophrenia*. Basel: Karger, 172–7.

Hellewell, J. S. E. and Hurst, B. C. (1996) A review of the efficacy of 'Seroquel' (quetiapine) in the treatment of the positive and negative symptoms of schizophrenia. *Eur Neuropsychopharmacol*, **6** (Suppl 4), 14–15.

Heresco-Levy, U., Javitt, D. C., Ermilov, M. *et al.* (1996) Double-blind, placebo-controlled, crossover trial of glycine adjuvant therapy for treatment-resistant schizophrenia. *Br J Psychiatry*, **169**, 610–17.

Hirsch, S. R., Link, C. G. G., Goldstein, J. M. *et al.* (1996) ICI 204 636: a new atypical antipsychotic drug. *Br J Psychiatry*, **168** (Suppl 29), 45–56.

Hoffman, D. C. and Donovan, H. (1995) Catalepsy as a rodent model for detecting antipsychotic drugs with extrapyramidal side effect liability. *Psychopharmacology*, **120**, 128–33.

Javitt, D. C., Zylberman, I., Zukin, S. R. *et al.* (1994) Amelioration of negative symptoms in schizophrenia by glycine. *Am J Psychiatry*, **151**, 1234–6.

Kane, J. M. (1996) Drug therapy: schizophrenia. *New Engl J Med*, **334**, 34–41.

Kapur, S. and Remington, G. (1996) Serotonin–dopamine interaction and its relevance to schizophrenia. *Am J Psychiatry*, **153**, 466–76.

Kapur, S., Remington, G., Jones, C. *et al.* (1996) High levels of dopamine D_2 receptor occupancy with low-dose haloperidol treatment: a PET study. *Am J Psychiatry*, **153**, 948–50.

Karle, J., Clemmesen, L. Hansen, L. *et al.* (1995) NNC 01-0687, a selective dopamine D1 receptor antagonist, in the treatment of schizophrenia. *Psychopharmacology*, **121**, 328–9.

Karlsson, P., Smith, L., Farde, L. *et al.* (1995) Lack of apparent antipsychotic effect of the D_1-dopamine receptor antagonist SCH 39166 in acutely ill schizophrenic patients. *Psychopharmacology*, **121**, 309–16.

Kehne, J. H., Baron, B. M., Carr, A. A. *et al.* (1996) Preclinical characterization of the potential of the putative atypical antipsychotic MDL 100 907 as a potent 5-HT_{2A} antagonist with a favourable CNS safety profile. *J Pharmacol Exp Ther*, **277**, 968–81.

Kinon, B. J. and Lieberman, J. A. (1996) Mechanisms of action of atypical antipsychotic drugs: a critical analysis. *Psychopharmacology*, **124**, 2–34.

Kirkpatrick, B. and Carpenter, W. T. (1995) Drug development and the deficit syndrome of schizophrenia. *Biol Psychiatry*, **38**, 277–8.

Lidsky, T. I. (1995) Re-evaluation of the mesolimbic hypothesis of antipsychotic drug action. *Schizophr Bull*, **21**, 67–74.

Lillrank, S. M., Lipska, B. A., Bachus, S. E. *et al.* (1996) Amphetamine-induced *c-fos* mRNA expression is altered in rats with neonatal ventral hippocampal damage. *Synapse*, **23**, 292–301.

Lipska, B. K., Swerdlow, N. R., Geyer, M. A *et al.* (1995) Neonatal excitotoxic hippocampal damage in rats causes post-pubertal changes in prepulse inhibition of startle and its disruption by apomorphine. *Psychopharmacology*, **122**, 35–43.

Loebel, A. D., Lieberman, J. A., Alvir, J. M. J. *et al.* (1992) Duration of psychosis and outcome in first-episode schizophrenia. *Am J Psychiatry*, **149**, 1183–8.

Martin, C. (1996) Impact of olanzapine on quality of life in schizophrenia. *Eur Psychiatry*, **11** (Suppl 4), 252S.

Martinot, J. L., Paillière-Martinot, M. L., Poirier, M. F. *et al.* (1996) In-vivo characteristics of dopamine D_2 receptor occupancy by amisulpride in schizophrenia. *Psychopharmacology*, **124**, 154–8.

Megens, A. A. H. P., Awouters, F. H. L., Schotte, A. *et al.* (1994) Survey on the pharmacodynamics of the new antipsychotic risperidone. *Psychopharmacology*, **114**, 9–23.

Meltzer, H. Y. (1995a) Atypical antipsychotic drug therapy for treatment-resistant schizophrenia. In S. R. Hirsch and D. R. Weinberger (eds), *Schizophrenia*. Oxford: Blackwell Science, 485–502.

Meltzer, H. Y. (1995b) Clozapine: is another view valid? *Am J Psychiatry*, **152**, 821–5.

Meltzer, L. T., Christoffersen, C. L., Corbin, A. E. *et al.* (1995) CI-1007, a dopamine partial agonist and potential antipsychotic agent. II. Neurophysiological and behavioral effects. *J Pharmacol Exp Ther*, **274**, 912–20.

Moller, H. J., Muller, H., Borison, R. L. *et al.* (1995) A path-analytical approach to differentiate between direct and indirect drug effects on negative symptoms in schizophrenic patients: a re-evaluation of the North American risperidone study. *Eur Arch Psychiat Clin Neurosci*, **245**, 45–9.

Moore, N. A., Tupper, D. E. and Hotten, T. M. (1994) Olanzapine. Drugs of the future, **19**, 114–17.

Moran, P. M., Fischer, T. R., Hitchcock, J. M. *et al.* (1996) Effects of clozapine on latent inhibition in the rat. *Behav Pharmacol*, **7**, 42–8.

Moser, P. C., Moran, P. M., Frank, R. A. *et al.* (1996) Reversal of amphetamine-induced behaviours by MDL 100,907, a selective 5-HT$_{2A}$ antagonist. *Behav Brain Res*, **73**, 163–7.

Needham, P. L., Heal, D. J., Sargent, B. J. *et al.* (1996a) BTS 93 947, a novel D1/D5 antagonist with predicted atypical antipsychotic activity. *Eur Neuropsychopharmacology*, **6**(Suppl 3), 105.

Needham, P. L., Atkinson, J., Skill M. J. *et al.* (1996b) Zotepine: preclinical tests predict antipsychotic efficacy and an atypical profile. *Psychopharmacol Bull*, **32**, 123–8.

Needham, P. L., Atkinson, J., Cheetham, S. C. *et al.* (1996c) Binding of zotepine to serotonin (5-HT) receptor subtypes. *Schizophr Res*, **18**, 141–2.

Nordstrom, A. L., Farde, L., Nyberg, S. *et al.* (1995) D$_1$, D$_2$, and 5-HT$_2$ receptor occupancy in relation to clozapine serum concentration: a PET study of schizophrenic patients. *Am J Psychiatry*, **152**, 1444–9.

Ogren, S. O. and Archer, T. (1994) Effects of typical and atypical antipsychotic drugs on two-way active avoidance. Relationship to DA receptor blocking profile. *Psychopharmacology*, **114**, 383–91.

Owens, D. G. C. (1996) Adverse effects of antipsychotic agents: do newer agents offer advantages? *Drugs*, **51**, 895–930.

Padich, R. A., McCloskey, T. C. and Kehne, J. H. (1996) 5-HT modulation of auditory and visual sensorimotor gating: II. Effect of the 5-HT$_{2A}$ antagonist MDL 100,907 on disruption of sound and light prepulse inhibition produced by 5-HT agonists in Wistar rats. *Psychopharmacology*, **124**, 107–16.

Petit, M., Raniwalla, J., Tweed, J. *et al.* (1996) A comparison of an atypical and typical antipsychotic, zotepine versus haloperidol in patients with acute exacerbation of schizophrenia: a parallel-group double-blind trial. *Psychopharmacol Bull*, **32**, 81–7.

Pickar, D. (1995) Prospects for pharmacotherapy of schizophrenia. *Lancet*, **345**, 557–62.

Pilowsky, L. S., Busatto, G. F., Taylor, M. *et al.* (1996a) Dopamine D2 receptor occupancy *in vivo* by the novel antipsychotic olanzapine: a ^{123}I-IBZM single photon emission tomography (SPET) study. *Psychopharmacology*, **124**, 148–53.

Pilowsky, L. S., O'Connell, P., Davies, N. *et al.* (1996b) In-vivo occupancy of striatal D2 receptors by sertindole: a ^{123}I-IBZM SPET study. *J Psychopharmacology*, **10** (Suppl 2), A9.

Robertson, G. S. and Fibiger, H. C. (1996) Effects of olanzapine on regional *c-fos* expression in rat forebrain. *Neuropsychopharmacology*, **14**, 105–10.

Robertson, G. S., Matsumura, H. and Fibiger, H. C. (1994) Induction patterns of Fos-like immunoreactivity in the forebrain as predictors of atypical antipsychotic activity. *J Pharmacol Exp Ther*, **271**, 1058–66.

Roth, B. L., Tandra, S., Burgess, L. H. *et al.* (1995) D$_4$ dopamine receptor binding affinity does not distinguish between typical and atypical antipsychotic drugs. *Psychopharmacology*, **120**, 365–8.

Sams-Dodd, F. (1996) Phencyclidine-induced stereotyped behaviour and social isolation in rats: a possible animal model of schizophrenia. *Behav Pharmacol*, **7**, 3–23.

Sanchez, C., Arnt, J., Dragsted, N. *et al.* (1991) Neurochemical and in-vivo pharmacological profile of sertindole, a limbic-selective neuroleptic compound. *Drug Devel Res*, **22**, 239–50.

Schotte, A., Janssen, P. F. M., Gommeran, W. *et al.* (1996) Risperidone compared with new and reference antipsychotic drugs: in-vitro and in-vivo receptor binding. *Psychopharmacology*, **124**, 57–73.

Seeger, T. F., Seymour, P. A., Schmidt, A. W. *et al.* (1995) Ziprasidone (CP-88, 059): a new antipsychotic with combined dopamine and serotonin receptor antagonist activity. *J Pharmacol Exp Ther*, **275**, 101–13.

Seeman, P. (1992) Dopamine receptor sequences: therapeutic levels of neuroleptics occupy D_2 receptors, clozapine occupies D_4. *Neuropsychopharmacology*, **7**, 261–84.

Stip, E., Tourjman, V., Lew, V. *et al.* (1995) 'Awakenings' effect with risperidone. *Am J Psychiatry*, **152**, 1833.

Stone, C. K., Garver, D. L., Griffith, J. *et al.* (1995) Further evidence of a dose–response threshold for haloperidol in psychosis. *Am J Psychiatry*, **152**, 1210–12.

Swerdlow, N. R., Braff, D. L., Taaid, N. *et al.* (1994a) Assessing the validity of an animal model of deficient sensorimotor gating in schizophrenic patients. *Arch Gen Psychiatry*, **51**, 139–54.

Swerdlow, N. R., Zisook, D. and Taaid, N. (1994b) Seroquel (ICI 204 636) restores prepulse inhibition of acoustic startle in apomorphine-treated rats: similarities to clozapine. *Psychopharmacology*, **114**, 675–8.

Swerdlow, N. R., Braff, D. L., Hartston, H. *et al.* (1996) Latent inhibition in schizophrenia. *Schizophr Res*, **20**, 91–103.

Szewczak, M. R., Corbett, R., Rush, D. K. *et al.* (1995) The pharmacological profile of iloperidone, a novel atypical antipsychotic agent. *J Pharmacol Exp Ther*, **274**, 1404–13.

Szymanski, S. R., Cannon, T. D., Gallacher, F. *et al.* (1996) Course of treatment response in first-episode and chronic schizophrenia. *Am J Psychiatry*, **153**, 519–25.

Tran, C., Beasley, J., Street, R. *et al.* (1996) Olanzapine versus haloperidol: acute results of the multi-centre international trial. *Eur Neuropsychopharmacology*, **6**(Suppl 3), 59.

Umbricht, D. and Kane, J. M. (1995) Risperidone: efficacy and safety. *Schizophr Bull*, **21**, 593–606.

Vahid-Ansari, F., Nakabeppu, Y. and Robertson, G. S. (1996) Contrasting effects of chronic clozapine, Seroquel™ (ICI 204,636) and haloperidol administration on ΔFosB-like immunoreactivity in the rodent forebrain. *Eur J Neurosci*, **8**, 927–36.

Van Kammen, D. P., McEvoy, J. P., Targum, S. D. *et al.* (1996) A randomized, controlled, dose-ranging study trial of sertindole in patients with schizophrenia. *Psychopharmacology*, **124**, 168–75.

Varty, G. B. and Higgins, G. A. (1995) Examination of drug-induced and isolation-induced disruptions of prepulse inhibition as models to screen antipsychotic drugs. *Psychopharmacology*, **122**, 15–26.

Waddington, J. L. (1993a) Pre- and postsynaptic D_1 to D_5 dopamine receptor mechanisms in relation to antipsychotic activity. In T. R. E. Barnes (ed.), *Antipsychotic drugs and their side-effects*. London: Academic Press, 65–85.

Waddington, J. L. (1993b) Schizophrenia: developmental neuroscience and pathobiology. *Lancet*, **341**, 531–6.

Waddington, J. L. (1995) The clinical psychopharmacology of antipsychotic drugs in schizophrenia. In S. R. Hirsch and D. R. Weinberger (eds), *Schizophrenia*. Oxford: Blackwell Science, 341–57.

Waddington, J. L. and Daly, S. A. (1992) The status of 'second generation' selective D_1 dopamine receptor antagonists as putative atypical antipsychotic agents. In H. Y. Meltzer (ed.), *Novel antipsychotic drugs*. New York: Raven Press, 109–15.

Waddington, J. L. and O'Callaghan, E. (1997) What makes an antipsychotic 'atypical': conserving the definition. *CNS Drugs*, **7**, 341–6.

Waddington, J. L., Daly, S. A., McCauley, P. G. *et al.* (1994) Levels of functional interaction between D_1-like and D_2-like dopamine receptor systems. In H. B. Niznik (ed.), *Dopamine receptors and transporters*. New York: Marcel Dekker, 511–37.

Waddington, J. L., Youssef, H. A. and Kinsella, A. (1995) Sequential cross-sectional and 10-year prospective study of severe negative symptoms in relation to duration of initially untreated psychosis in chronic schizophrenia. *Psychol Med*, **25**, 849–57.

Waddington, J. L., Scully, P. J. and Youssef, H. A. (1997) Developmental trajectory and disease progression in schizophrenia. *Schizophr Res*, **23**, 107–18.

Wadenberg, M. L. (1996) Serotonergic mechanisms in neuroleptic-induced catalepsy in the rat. *Neurosci Biobehav Rev*, **20**, 325–39.

Wagstaff, A. J. and Bryson, H. M. (1995) Clozapine: a review of its pharmacological properties and therapeutic use in patients with schizophrenia who are unresponsive to or intolerant of classical antipsychotic agents. *CNS Drugs*, **4**, 370–400.

Weinberger, D. R. and Lipska, B. K. (1995) Cortical maldevelopment, anti-psychotic drugs, and schizophrenia: a search for common ground. *Schizophr Res*, **16**, 87–110.

Weiner, I., Shadach, E., Tarrasch, R., Kidron, R. *et al.* (1996) The latent inhibition model of schizophrenia: further validation using the atypical neuroleptic, clozapine. *Biol Psychiatry*, **40**, 834–43.

Wilkinson, L. S., Killcross, S. S., Humby, T. *et al.* (1994) Social isolation in the rat produces developmentally specific deficits in prepulse inhibition of the acoustic startle response without disrupting latent inhibition. *Neuropsychopharmacology*, **10**, 61–72.

Wyatt, R. J. (1991) Neuroleptics and the natural course of schizophrenia. *Schizophr Bull*, **17**, 325–51.

Wyatt, R. J. (1995) Early intervention for schizophrenia: can the course of the illness be altered? *Biol Psychiatry*, **38**, 1–3.

CHAPTER 13

Treatment of schizophrenia in the community

ROBIN G. MCCREADIE

Introduction

The substance of this chapter will draw heavily on two studies; first, the only study which, as far as I am aware, has compared the management of schizophrenic patients in both a rural and an urban setting in the United Kingdom (McCreadie *et al.*, 1997), namely Nithsdale in south west Scotland and Nunhead and Norwood in south London; and second, a study which has compared in Nithsdale the management of schizophrenic patients in the community both in 1981 and 1996 (Kelly *et al.*, 1998).

In a sense, the title of the chapter is tautological as at any given time the vast majority of schizophrenic patients are in the community; thus, the treatment of schizophrenia in the community is in fact the treatment of schizophrenia. For example, in Nunhead and Norwood during the year 1991–92, there were no patients in long-term psychiatric inpatient care; on the census day, in Nithsdale, 1 April 1996, 83% of patients were living outside hospital. However, that being so, what are perhaps the more important issues in the management of schizophrenic patients in the community? I would suggest the following: living arrangements; occupational activities; medication; support services; and legal aspects.

Living arrangements

A generation ago substantial numbers of schizophrenic patients were in long-stay wards of large psychiatric hospitals. The run down and closure of many of these hospitals has meant that alternative accommodation has had to be found as there is little consistent evidence that the incidence of schizophrenia is falling (Jablensky, 1994). Table 13.1 shows the living arrangements of patients in Nithsdale in 1981 and 1996, excluding long-stay inpatients. Several points stand out. First, in 1981 30% of patients, excluding long-stay inpatients, were living with their parents. By 1996 this had fallen to 13%. Put another way, on the census date in 1996, 87% of patients were *not* living with their parents. The picture of the adult schizophrenic patient living with ageing parents, with all the difficulties and problems that might arise in such a situation, especially if one or other parents shows high expressed emotion (Bebbington and Kuipers, 1994) is now a rarity. It seems that the parents of today are less willing to care for their sick adult offspring than those of a generation ago.

The fall in the number of patients living with parents is matched by the number of those living in supported accommodation. Supported accommodation in Nithsdale, and in many other parts of the United Kingdom, consists of patients living in small groups in houses, often in residential parts of town. In Nithsdale the property is owned by the local Mental Health Association (MHA), a voluntary organization. The MHA workers, some of whom have come from a nursing background but many have not, provide a range of support from daily visits to 24-hour staffed waking cover. For the most part, these are not 'half-way houses'. This is permanent accommodation for chronically ill schizophrenic patients, mainly young and usually male, patients who a generation ago would have been moving towards long-term care in a psychiatric hospital, or creating considerable havoc in the parental home. It is a paradox that, in the community care of schizophrenic patients in the United Kingdom today, many of the most disturbed patients are now being cared for by the least trained staff.

Patients in supported accommodation will be encouraged to do much for themselves but may require help with budgeting, shopping, cooking, cleaning and so on. There will be varying degrees of success. A neglected area is the patient's diet. Work in Nithsdale (McCreadie *et al.*, 1998) has found that the dietary intake of many patients in supported accommodation is poor when compared with matched normal

Table 13.1. Living arrangements of patients in Nithsdale, south-west Scotland, 1981 and 1996(%)

Living arrangement*	1981 ($N = 133$)	1996 ($N = 168$)
Parents	30	13
Spouse/Partner	25	24
Supported accommodation	–	22
Alone	27	29
Other	18	12

*Excludes long-stay in patients.

control subjects. Almost all patients smoke and their diet lacks fibre and antioxidants, especially vitamin E. Their vegetable and fruit intake are poor and their intake of saturated fats is high. Patients in Nithsdale, as elsewhere, die early, especially from coronary heart disease (Mortensen and Juel, 1990). There is little doubt that smoking habits and a poor diet have contributed to their early death.

In Nithsdale in 1996 a small number of patients were still in long-stay psychiatric wards. The run down of psychiatric hospitals in Scotland has been slower than in England and it still retains some long-stay NHS beds. The realization that the problems of schizophrenia will not simply go away if there is no long-stay accommodation has led to a more recent view that bed closures may have gone too far. The problem is especially reflected in the bed occupancy rates of so-called acute admission wards. Not only in inner city London (Marshall, 1997) but in rural areas such as Nithsdale, bed occupancy rates in admission wards can be well over 100%. There is therefore often a delay in admitting severely ill schizophrenic patients, and they may be discharged too soon. Alternatively, admission beds may become 'blocked' if the professionals concerned believe that there is a lack of suitable accommodation, inadequate domiciliary based community support and lack of rehabilitation places (Shepherd *et al.*, 1997).

With regard to accommodation, we cannot ignore the private sector in the United Kingdom. The private sector is now a significant provider of inpatient care, especially for seriously disturbed schizophrenic patients. One problem, however, is the situation of these hospitals. Some are large and remote from the catchment area of the patients they are treating. They are in danger of becoming the successors to the Victorian mental hospitals.

In the Nithsdale survey of April 1996, no known schizophrenic patient was 'roofless'. The rural nature of the area with its well developed medical and social services makes it most unlikely that of the few patients not known to the services, any were homeless. The same, however, cannot be said of inner city areas where the prevalence of schizophrenia is higher in hostels for the homeless than among the general population (Geddes *et al.*, 1994). Lack of permanent accommodation will inevitably be associated with a lack of almost everything else, including medication and good physical health. Assertive outreach in the community must take a special interest in those patients.

Occupational activities

In the Nithsdale, Nunhead and Norwood survey, more than three quarters of the patients were not in gainful employment, and in Nithsdale in April 1996 only 8% were in open employment. Unemployment amongst schizophrenic patients has long been a problem; indeed the high general unemployment in Scotland since the end of World War II has meant that most schizophrenic patients there have long been unemployable. The higher rates in the rest of the United Kingdom in recent years have meant that schizophrenic patients are now at the back of a very long queue in the search for jobs. In short, employment is not, and will not in the foreseeable future, be an option for most schizophrenic patients.

Work is an integral part of most people's lives. Without it many people lack self-worth and a sense of purpose. Schizophrenic patients are no exception. Steps there-fore are taken in different parts of the country to provide work. Because of the inher-ent disabilities of schizophrenia, especially the negative symptoms, sheltered work is usually required. This may take the form of workshops for the sole use of the men-tally ill; however, these are few and far between. Alternatively, sympathetic employ-ers may take on patients, and if the work is deemed 'therapeutic' a small wage can be paid over and above the patient's state benefits. Voluntary organizations such as the National Schizophrenia Fellowship and local Mental Health Associations often can provide part-time sheltered work for schizophrenic patients, for example in craft guilds, cafes and in charity shops. Much of this work can be interesting and of value, but at times there is a sense of 'taking in each other's washing'.

Providing work brings not only general benefits but can have a specific role to play in schizophrenia. It has long been known that an understimulating environment can exacerbate negative symptoms (Wing and Brown, 1970). Attending a workplace can provide more stimulation and perhaps ameliorate some of the more severe negative symptoms. Too busy a workplace, of course, may *over*stimulate the vulnerable patient and an acute relapse may occur (Wing *et al.*, 1964).

If work is not an option, and it will not be for most schizophrenic patients, what other activities could or should be provided? The most obvious are activities of daily living. Many patients through their illness, which may have begun in late adoles-cence or early adulthood have never acquired the necessary skills to cope adequately in everyday life. This is where the 'rehabilitation team' or rather the 'habilitation team' has a role to play. Patients may be helped in their own home, at a day hospital, or may need to be admitted to an inpatient rehabilitation unit. Different members of the team should have different roles. The occupational therapist can help with mun-dane but very important areas such as budgeting, cooking, shopping, housework and personal hygiene. The clinical psychologist (few of whom, however, in the United Kingdom are interested in the care of the severely mentally ill, McCreadie *et al.*, 1993) may attempt to improve social skills or increase assertiveness. Nursing staff often take part in these activities and can also help to organize the patient's leisure time, including holidays. However, it must be recognized that many patients simply do not want to take part in organized activities. Wherever there is a day hospital or day centre, one finds that patients attend, quite often on a regular basis, but do not want to do anything, except perhaps smoke a cigarette or have a cup of tea. They seem to enjoy 'being there' but not 'doing anything'. This, of course, can be extremely irritating to some nursing staff who feel that 'patients need therapy'. Their attendance at the unit, however, can be therapy enough for some patients (Mitchell and Birley, 1983).

Medication

Most schizophrenic patients in the community will need antipsychotic medication, either to treat an acute relapse, which is increasingly managed outside hospital, or as maintenance therapy to postpone the next relapse.

Table 13.2 shows the proportion of patients receiving antipsychotic medication in Nithsdale in 1981 and 1996. In the comparison of Nithsdale with Nunhead and

Table 13.2. Antipsychotic medication in Nithsdale, 1981 and 1996 (%)

Antipsychotic medication	1981 (N = 133)	1996 (N = 168)
None	24*	5*
Oral	30	55
Intramuscular	31	26
Oral and intramuscular	15	14

*$P<0.0001$.

Norwood, 48–65% were receiving oral, 42–60% intramuscular and 12–19% oral and intramuscular antipsychotic medication; 24–30% anti-parkinsonian medication; 0–10% a benzodiazepine; and 0–1% clozapine.

The first point of interest about Table 13.2 is that in 1981 about a quarter of all known schizophrenic patients in Nithsdale were *not* receiving antipsychotic drugs. These patients fell principally into two groups: those in long-stay psychiatric wards, where perhaps patients had few positive symptoms but had marked social disabilities; and patients known to their general practitioner but currently untreated. By 1996 only 5% were not receiving antipsychotic medication. Presumably this was the result of more vigorous outreach to patients in the community and the fewer numbers of long-stay inpatients.

The proportions receiving oral or intramuscular medication were about the same. There is no doubt that if patients can be persuaded to take intramuscular drugs, their compliance is improved. However, patients outside hospital often have different ideas. Intramuscular antipsychotic drugs in the United Kingdom have now been available for about 25 years. Large numbers of patients were started on these drugs with high hopes. Early on, it was realized that drug discontinuation was a problem (Johnson and Freeman, 1973); patient refusal, side-effects and loss of contact were the most common reasons for stopping intramuscular drugs. It is my experience that as more time has passed large numbers of patients resent intramuscular medication, especially the perceived indignity of dropping their trousers or raising their skirt month in, month out, year in, year out, at the request of the community psychiatric nurse or at the 'depot clinic'. Now, with the introduction of the newer antipsychotic drugs such as sulpiride, risperidone, olanzapine and quetiapine, with fewer extrapyramidal side-effects (Casey, 1996) the case for intramuscular drugs is further weakened. It has long been known that extrapyramidal side-effects, especially akathisia, are associated with poor compliance (Van Putten, 1974).

But what is the effect of medication in the community care of patients with schizophrenia? Table 13.3 shows the prevalence of positive schizophrenic symptoms in patients living in Nithsdale in 1981 and 1996. Patients were assessed by the Manchester Scale for Chronic Psychosis; a symptom was said to be present if it was scored at two or more. It can be seen that schizophrenic patients in Nithsdale in 1996 were in fact *worse off* than they were in 1981, with a significant increase in the number showing delusions.

Why might this be so? More patients in fact in 1996 were being prescribed

Table 13.3.   Positive schizophrenic symptoms and side-effects in Nithsdale patients, 1981 and 1996 (%)

Symptom	1981 (N = 118)	1996 (N = 146)
Delusions	23*	40*
Hallucinations	10	19
Incongruity of affect	5	11
Incoherence	9	12
Side-effect	(N = 117)	(N = 144)
Tardiue dyskinesia	21**	44**
Tremor	23†	41

*P=0.005.
**P=0.0001.
†P=0.004.

antipsychotic drugs than in 1981. Also, there was no change in the proportion receiving intramuscular antipsychotic medication. Might it be that the shift to community care itself is important? The patients who were deluded in 1996 were especially found among the young males. These are the patients who 15 years ago might have been 'settling down' in long-stay wards. Now they are in the community exposed to the stresses and strains of everyday life and thus more likely to develop an exacerbation of positive symptoms (Bebbington *et al.*, 1996). Also, the young men are the schizophrenic patients most likely to be abusing alcohol and drugs, known to worsen outcome (Menezes *et al.*, 1996). As they are living outside hospital, many of them taking oral medication, and with by definition less supervision, their compliance is likely to be less. Finally, on a more hopeful note, the suicide rate in schizophrenic patients in Nithsdale is low. Most schizophrenic patients who commit suicide do so in the early stages of their illness; perhaps assertive outreach in Nithsdale is keeping alive more of the severely disturbed young patients.

Table 13.3 also compares the prevalence of extrapyramidal symptoms in 1981 and 1996. The prevalence of tardive dyskinesia as measured by the AIMS scale, with Schooler and Kane criteria, had risen substantially over the 15 years, as had at least one parkinsonian feature, namely tremor, as measured by the TAKE scale. The greater number of patients being treated with antipsychotic drugs no doubt contributed to this finding. Also, intermittent compliance may have contributed to the increased prevalence of TD (Gerlach *et al.*, 1986).

In short, the move to community care with the more vigorous use of antipsychotic drugs has considerable drawbacks.

Support services

Patients living outside hospital need support from a wide variety of sources. Mention has already been made of voluntary organizations such as the local Mental Health

Association and the National Schizophrenia Fellowship. Recent years have seen the development of 'community mental health teams'. Where community mental health teams are established they should be multi-disciplinary and include nurses, psychiatrists, occupational therapists, psychologists and social workers. From time to time additional input will be required from clinical pharmacists, dieticians, clinical secretaries and, as stated above, local community workers. The team, of course, should have a leader but it is still not clear who that leader should be. Often the psychiatrist takes the lead role. The team should cover a defined sector and be responsible for delivering a specialized level of care. The functions of the team should include (Scottish Office Department of Health, 1996): assessment and regular review of all care programme approach and community care order patients (see below); identifying at-risk patients and regularly reviewing those so identified; pro-active psychological and physical treatments; assertive outreach to support those requiring acute intervention and their carers; acute care backup with responsibility for admission and discharge; liaison on a regular basis with primary care services; and involvement with a range of day and residential settings from hospitals to domiciliary care, including intensively staffed homes with NHS staff. *The team should give service priority to people with severe and enduring mental health problems.*

A crucial member of the team is the community psychiatric nurse (CPN). It is probable that CPNs first developed services 'on the back' of intramuscular medication. Patients were outside hospital, someone had to give them their injections; who better than a trained nurse, not attached to a general practice but with psychiatric skills? At the start most CPNs were of considerable seniority, equivalent to ward-based charge nurses. They soon became disenchanted with being seen merely as the 'nurse who gives me my injection' and sought other useful things to do. At this point they went off in two different directions. First, they became interested in people with less severe mental illnesses and sought direct referrals from general practitioners. They saw themselves as being able to offer such things as 'anxiety management', 'counselling' and other techniques for individuals with a wide range of problems such as sexual abuse and recurrent depression. CPNs are still very keen to be involved in this area, although there is now something of a backlash, both from the CPNs themselves and their employers. Their success rate is probably low (Gournay and Brooking, 1994), their expertise is limited and thus their job satisfaction is diminished. They are also expensive: for example, in Nithsdale, it is more expensive for the patient to be seen by a CPN than by a junior psychiatrist.

The second direction some CPNs have taken is to help in very practical ways those suffering from schizophrenia. Education is currently perhaps the most popular. There is no doubt that carers and patients, but especially carers, are thirsty for knowledge about all aspects of schizophrenia and CPNs are well placed to give this information. There is little evidence that 'psychosocial education' alone cuts down on the relapse rate in schizophrenia (Tarrier *et al.*, 1989) but education of groups of patients can improve their social functioning and quality of life (Atkinson *et al.*, 1996).

Some CPNs have been trained in 'family management' techniques. Here, a more intensive effort is made to improve the family atmosphere and resolve family difficulties, in the hope of affecting outcome. Disappointment has been expressed at the low uptake of CPNs on training courses in family management. However, CPNs are not unaware that nowadays few adult patients live permanently with their parents.

For many schizophrenic patients living in the community the CPN is now the first port of call in a storm. In some, if not many, cases the CPN may be seen by the patient as a friend, home help, counsellor, nurse, social worker and psychiatrist. CPNs must first realize their limitations and second develop their own special expertise if they are to survive as a respected group. I have no doubt that they should concentrate their efforts on the care of the severely mentally ill, and the care programme approach (see below) may encourage this.

Legal aspects

It is clear that the move to community care may mean less supervision of the seriously mentally ill. This being so, things are more likely to go wrong and occasionally disastrously so. Thus, there has been a call for more effective management of schizophrenic patients living outside hospital.

However, it must first be stated that the vast majority of schizophrenic patients are law abiding. On the census date in Nithsdale in 1996, no schizophrenic patient was in prison and only one was in a State Hospital. A minority of schizophrenic patients, however, do have a criminal record. In the Nithsdale, Nunhead and Norwood review, 8% of Nithsdale patients had at some time been in prison; the percentage was higher in south London, 17–25%. Put the other way though, 92% of Nithsdale patients and 75–83% of Nunhead and Norwood patients had *never* been in prison.

British Government directives in recent years have led to changes in the management of schizophrenic patients in the community. Probably the most important change has been the development of the 'care programme approach' (CPA) (Social Work Services Group, Scottish Office, 1996). The CPA is a crucial element in the Government's policy for people with mental illness. Its aim is to ensure that properly designed and managed individual packages of care are arranged for people with severe and enduring mental illness who require health and social care in appropriate accommodation in the community. The Government has consistently restated the view that no one should be discharged from hospital care until suitable alternative sources of health, social care and accommodation are available in the community and properly resourced. The objectives of the arrangements for the CPA are to ensure that:

- there is effective collaboration and working within and between agencies and professions;
- service users and, where appropriate, their carers are involved as far as possible in individual care decisions and arrangements;
- CPA targets those people most in need, or most at risk to themselves or others;
- people receive a full multi-agency assessment and regular reviews of their needs;
- people receive a sustainable care plan which ensures their needs are met;
- people receive care and support for as long as they need it; including follow-up of those at risk of being lost to the system;
- people receive a fully co-ordinated and comprehensive range of services and support;
- all aspects of the arrangements are regularly monitored and evaluated to ensure that they are fully effective.

A key worker will be identified and his/her main responsibility is to co-ordinate an individual's care programme in close collaboration with the individual, the carer and the other members of the care team. This means ensuring that all parties are kept up-to-date with information about the individual's progress and other relevant information, and that meetings and reviews take place at appropriate times. The key worker should have authority to trigger the required multi-agency review of the individual's case. The consultant psychiatrist must be kept informed by the key worker of significant developments in relation to the individual's mental illness and treatment needs.

The individual care programme should comprise a care plan drawn up by the key worker following a multi-agency, multi-disciplinary meeting, and the care plan should set out the objectives of care and identify the future nature of contact, how the key worker can be contacted, what services will be provided and the financial implications for agencies, the monitoring arrangements, the review procedures and arrangements for discharge. It is emphasized that the care plan is not the end in itself but a means of 'clarifying expectations'.

This is the theory but the practice in many places is very different. Practice is often not 'needs led' but 'facilities led'. Also, psychiatrists and nurses often find that their clinical practice has not changed, but the paperwork and meetings involved in CPA have increased so much that they have in fact less time for their clinical work. There is a clear need for a rigorous multi-centred assessment of the effectiveness of CPA. It is noteworthy that the Royal College of Psychiatrists Research Unit and the Royal College of Nursing Institute are inviting mental health services to participate in a National Audit of CPA.

There has been a further tightening of the management of schizophrenic patients in the community, namely through a Community Care Order (CCO) in Scotland, a Supervised Discharge in England and Wales. The purpose of the CCO is to ensure that a patient who has immediately previously been liable to detention without special restrictions receives appropriate medical treatment from the health service and social care from local authorities to which he or she is entitled (National Health Service in Scotland, Management Executive, 1996). Guidance on the CCO indicates that 'it would be good practice for the care plans of all patients on leave of absence or subject to a CCO to comply with the requirements of the CPA. Also, in England and Wales, but not in Scotland, all provider units have been required to establish supervision registers (NHS Management Executive, 1994) The aim is to identify those with a severe mental illness who may be at significant risk to themselves or others and ensure that they receive appropriate and effective care in the community. Considerable doubts have been expressed about its effectiveness and many consultant psychiatrists have been slow to accept the register (Vaughan, 1996). The register is seen by many clinicians as a rod with which to beat their backs if things should go wrong.

Even with a CPA and CCO, patients in the community cannot be compelled to take medication outside hospital which, according to many psychiatrists, is a fatal flaw. Again, much research is needed with these new developments to find out whether or not they are worth the considerable work involved.

General conclusions

Community care of the schizophrenic patient is here to stay. It is highly unlikely that the large mental hospitals of the past will be recreated. Most long-stay patients discharged from hospital in fact welcome something approximating to a normal life (Leff *et al.*, 1994). However, the scattered distribution of schizophrenic patients in the catchment area of a psychiatric service means that if adequate care is to be provided, assertive outreach is necessary. In the review of services in Nithsdale, it was found that 42% of patients made use of more than one of three community services, namely CPN services, outpatient services and day-patient services; 15% made use of all three services. In contrast, in Nunhead and Norwood 23% and 27%, respectively, made use of more than one service, and only 2–3% of all three services. The level of functioning in Nithsdale as assessed by the Global Assessment of Functioning in DSMIIIR (American Psychiatric Association, 1987) was significantly higher than in Nunhead and Norwood. *Better access to services means a better level of functioning.*

Acknowledgement

I thank Dawn Hiddleston for secretarial help.

References

American Psychiatric Association (1987) *Diagnostic and Statistical Manual of Mental Disorders*, 3rd edition–revised. Washington, DC: American Psychiatric Association.

Atkinson, J. M., Coia, D. A., Gilmour, W. H. *et al.* (1996) The impact of education groups for people with schizophrenia on social functioning and quality of life. *Br J Psychiatry*, **168**, 199–204.

Bebbington, P. and Kuipers, L. (1994) The predictive utility of expressed emotion in schizophrenia: an aggregate analysis. *Psychol Med*, **24**, 707–18.

Bebbington, P., Wilkins, S., Sham, P. *et al.* (1996) Life events before psychotic episodes: do clinical and social variables affect the relationship? *Social Psychiat Psychiatr Epidemiol*, **31**, 122–8.

Casey, D. E. (1996) Extrapyramidal symptoms and new anti-psychotic drugs. Findings in patients and non-human primate models. *Br J Psychiatry*, **168**, (Suppl 29), 32–9.

Geddes, J., Newton, R., Young, G. *et al.* (1994) Comparison of prevalence of schizophrenia among residents of hostels for homeless people in 1966 and 1992. *Br Med J*, **308**, 816–19.

Gerlach, J., Ahlfors, U. G. and Amthor, K. F. *et al.* (1986) Effect of different neuroleptics in tardive dyskinesia and parkinsonism. A video-controlled multi-centred study with chlorprothixene, perphenazine, haloperidol and haloperidol and biperiden. *Psychopharmacology*, **90**, 423–9.

Gournay, K. and Brooking, J. (1994) Community psychiatric nurses in primary health care. *Br J Psychiatry*, **164**, 231–8.

Jablensky, A. (1994) The epidemiology of schizophrenia. *Cur Opin Psychiatry*, **6**, 43–52.

Johnson, D. A. and Freeman, H. (1973). Drug defaulting by patients on long acting phenothiazines. *Psychol Med*, **3**, 115–19.

Kelly, C., McCreadie, R. G., MacEwan, T. and Carey, S. (1998). Nithsdale Schizophrenia Surveys 17. Fifteen year follow-up. *Br J Psychiatry*, **172**, 513–17.

Leff, J., Thornicroft, G., Coxhead, N. *et al.* (1994) The TAPS Project. 22: A five year follow up of long-stay psychiatric patients discharged to the community. *Br J Psychiatry*, **165** (Suppl 25), 13–17.

McCreadie, R. G., MacDonald, E., Blacklock, C. *et al.* (1998) Dietary intake of schizophrenic patients in Nithsdale, Scotland: case/control study. *Br Med J*, **317**, 784–5.

McCreadie, R. G., Leese, M., Tilak-Singh, D. *et al.* (1997) Nithsdale, Nunhead and Norwood: similarities and differences in prevalance of schizophrenia and utilization of services in rural and urban areas. *Br J Psychiatry*, **170**, 31–6.

McCreadie, R. G., Williamson, D. J. and Robertson, L. J. (1993) Scottish rehablilitation services: eight year follow-up. *Psychiatr Bull*, **17**, 341–3.

Marshall, M. (1997) London's mental health services in crisis. *Br Med J*, **314**, 246.

Menezes, P. R., Johnson, S. Thornicroft, G. *et al.* (1996) Drug and alcohol problems among individuals with severe mental illness in South London. *Br J Psychiatry*, **168**, 612–19.

Mitchell, S. F. and Birley, J. L. (1983) The use of ward support by psychiatric patients in the community. *Br J Psychiatry*, **142**, 9–15.

Mortensen, P. B. and Juel, K. (1990) Mortality and causes of death in schizophrenia patients in Denmark. *Acta Psychiatr Scand*, **81**, 372–7.

National Health Service in Scotland, Management Executive (1996) *The Mental Health (Scotland) Act, 1984, as amended by the Mental Health (Patients in the Community) Act, 1995*. Edinburgh: The Scottish Office.

NHS Management Executive (1994) *Introduction of Supervision Register for Mentally Ill People from 1 April 1994*. HSG (94)5.

Scottish Office Department of Health (1996) *Draft Framework for Mental Health Services in Scotland*. Edinburgh: Scottish Office Department of Health.

Shepherd, G., Beardsmoore, A., Moore, C. *et al.* (1997) Relation between bed use, social deprivation, and overall bed availability in acute adult psychiatric units and alternative residential options: a cross sectional survey, one day census data, and staff interviews. *Br Med J*, **314**, 262–6.

Social Work Services Group, Scottish Office (1996) *Community care: care programme approach for people with severe and enduring mental illness including dementia*. Circular No: SWSG 16/96, DD 38/96. Edinburgh: the Scottish Office.

Tarrier, N., Barrowclough, C., Vaughn, C. *et al.* (1989) Community management of schizophrenia. A two year follow-up of a behavioural intervention with families. *Br J Psychiatry*, **154**, 625–628.

Van Putten, T. (1974) Why do schizophrenic patients refuse to take their drugs? *Arch Gen Psychiatry*, **31**, 67–72.

Vaughan, P J (1996) The supervision register: one year on. *Psychiatr Bull*, **20**, 143–5.

Wing, J. K., Bennett, D. A. and Denham, J. (1964) *The Industrial Rehabilitation of Long-stay Schizophrenic Patients*. Medical Research Council memo No 42. London: HMSO.

Wing, J. K. and Brown, G. W. (1970) *Institutionalisation and Schizophrenia*. Cambridge: Cambridge University Press.

Index

Page numbers in *italic* refer to figures and tables. Those in **bold** indicate main discussion.